Russian History through the Senses

Russian History through the Senses

From 1700 to the Present

EDITED BY
MATTHEW P. ROMANIELLO
AND TRICIA STARKS

Bloomsbury Academic
An imprint of Bloomsbury Publishing Plc

BLOOMSBURY
LONDON · OXFORD · NEW YORK · NEW DELHI · SYDNEY

Bloomsbury Academic
An imprint of Bloomsbury Publishing Plc

50 Bedford Square	1385 Broadway
London	New York
WC1B 3DP	NY 10018
UK	USA

www.bloomsbury.com

BLOOMSBURY and the Diana logo are trademarks of Bloomsbury Publishing Plc

First published 2016

© Matthew P. Romaniello, Tricia Starks and Contributors, 2016

All rights reserved. No part of this publication may be reproduced or transmitted in any form or by any means, electronic or mechanical, including photocopying, recording, or any information storage or retrieval system, without prior permission in writing from the publishers.

No responsibility for loss caused to any individual or organization acting on or refraining from action as a result of the material in this publication can be accepted by Bloomsbury or the authors.

British Library Cataloguing-in-Publication Data
A catalogue record for this book is available from the British Library.

ISBN: HB: 978-1-4742-6313-9
PB: 978-1-4742-6312-2
ePDF: 978-1-4742-6314-6
ePub: 978-1-4742-6315-3

Library of Congress Cataloging-in-Publication Data
Names: Romaniello, Matthew P. | Starks, Tricia, 1969-
Title: Russian history through the senses : from 1700 to the present / edited by Matthew P. Romaniello and Tricia Starks.
Description: London : Bloomsbury Academic, an imprint of Bloomsbury Publishing Plc, 2016. | Includes bibliographical references and index.
Identifiers: LCCN 2015047983 (print) | LCCN 2016000300 (ebook) | ISBN 9781474263122 (paperback) | ISBN 9781474263139 (hardback) | ISBN 9781474263146 (ePDF) | ISBN 9781474263153 (ePub)
Subjects: LCSH: Russia--History--1613-1917. | Soviet Union--History. | Russia (Federation)--History. | Senses and sensation--Social aspects--Russia--History. | Senses and sensation--Social aspects--Soviet Union--History. | Senses and sensation--Social aspects--Russia (Federation)--History. | Russia--Social life and customs--1533-1917. | Soviet Union--Social life and customs. | Russia (Federation)--Social life and customs. | BISAC: HISTORY / Europe / Russia & the Former Soviet Union. | HISTORY / Modern / General. | HISTORY / Social History.
Classification: LCC DK43 .R843 2016 (print) | LCC DK43 (ebook) | DDC 947--dc23 LC record available at http://lccn.loc.gov/2015047983

Cover design: Sharon Mah
Cover image: The Merchant's Wife, Boris Kustodiev. Universal Images Group / Getty Images

Typeset by Fakenham Prepress Solutions, Fakenham, Norfolk NR21 8NN

CONTENTS

List of maps vii
List of illustrations viii
Notes on contributors ix
Acknowledgments xi

1 Introduction: The sensory in Russian and Soviet history 1
  Alexander M. Martin

PART ONE Imperial Russia 21

2 Humoral bodies in cold climates 23
  Matthew P. Romaniello

3 Fermentation, taste, and identity 45
  Alison K. Smith

4 Market pleasures and prostitution in St. Petersburg 67
  Abby Schrader

PART TWO Revolutionary Russia 95

5 The taste, smell, and semiotics of cigarettes 97
  Tricia Starks

6 The sounds, odors, and textures of Russian wartime nursing 117
  Laurie S. Stoff

7   The taste of *kumyshka* and the debate over Udmurt culture   141
    Aaron B. Retish

PART THREE   Soviet Russia   165

8   Engineering tastes: Food and the senses   167
    Anton Masterovoy

9   Deafness and the politics of hearing   193
    Claire Shaw

10 Sensing danger: The Red Army during the Second World War   219
    Steven G. Jug

PART FOUR   Reconstructing Russia   241

11 The sensory experience of martyrdom and Soviet collective memory   243
    Adrienne Harris

12 Stalinism's sights and smells in the films of Aleksei German, Sr.   267
    Tim Harte

Selected bibliography   283
Index   291

LIST OF MAPS

0.1 Map of Russia in Europe, 1825 xii
0.2 Map of Russia in Asia, 1825 xiii
2.1 "A map of the route to Mosco & Pekin," 1763 27
7.1 Map of Viatka Province in 1914 144

LIST OF ILLUSTRATIONS

4.1 *View of Sennaia (Haymarket) Square* by Ferdinand Victor Perrot 1841 71
5.1 Advertisement for Kolobov i Bobrov tabachnaia fabrika 107
5.2 Advertisement for Papirosy "Sigarnyia" 109
7.2 Photograph of women and children brewing *kumyska*," c. 1900 146
8.1 Illustration from *Stakhanovets*, 1936 176
9.1 Photograph of a deaf workers' meeting 1935 199
9.2 Photograph of M. Muzafarov, 1982 208
11.1 Photograph of Zoia Kosmodemianskaia by Sergei Strunnikov 244
11.2 School portrait of Zoia Kosmodemianskaia 246
11.3 *Kill the Fascist-Monster!* by Viktor Deni 1942 247
11.4 Photograph of Matvei Manizer's sculpture of Zoia Kosmodemianskaia 249
11.5 Photograph of Zoia Kosmodemianskaia's execution, 1943 251
12.1 Scene from *My Friend Ivan Lapshin*, 1984 271
12.2 Scene from *My Friend Ivan Lapshin*, 1984 272
12.3 Scene from *Khrustalev, My Car!* 1998 275
12.4 Scene from *Khrustalev, My Car!* 1998 276
12.5 Scene from *Khrustalev, My Car!* 1998 278
12.6 Scene from *Khrustalev, My Car!* 1998 279

NOTES ON CONTRIBUTORS

Adrienne Harris is associate professor of Russian at Baylor University. She publishes on Soviet collective memory of the Second World War, heroism, combatants' memoirs, war poetry, gender, and Czech film.

Tim Harte is an associate professor of Russian at Bryn Mawr College. He is the author of *Fast Forward: The Aesthetic and Ideology of Speed in Russian Avant-Garde Culture, 1910–1930* (2010) and has published a variety of articles on Russian literature and Russian and Soviet cinema.

Steven G. Jug, adjunct lecturer of Russian and Areas Studies at Baylor University, received his PhD from the University of Illinois in 2013. He has published articles on Red Army frontline culture in the *Journal of War and Culture Studies* and *Masculinities: A Journal of Identity and Culture*.

Alexander M. Martin is professor of history at the University of Notre Dame and specializes in the social, intellectual, and cultural history of imperial Russia. His most recent book is *Enlightened Metropolis: Constructing Imperial Moscow, 1762–1855* (2013).

Anton Masterovoy is an independent scholar. He is revising his dissertation, *Eating Soviet: Food and Culture in the USSR, 1917–1991* (2013).

Aaron B. Retish, associate professor of history at Wayne State University, is the author of *Russia's Peasants in Revolution and Civil War* (2008), co-editor of *Russia's Revolution in Regional Perspective* (2015), and co-editor of the journal *Revolutionary Russia*. He is completing a book on local rural courts in the early Soviet era.

Matthew P. Romaniello is an associate professor of history at the University of Hawai'i. He is the author of *The Elusive Empire: Kazan and the Creation of Russia, 1552–1671* (2012), and editor of three volumes, including *Tobacco in Russian History and Culture* (2009) with Tricia Starks.

Abby Schrader, professor of history at Franklin and Marshall College, authored *The Languages of the Lash: Corporal Punishment and Identity in Imperial Russia* (2002). Her "Unruly Felons and Civilizing Wives: Cultivating Marriage in the Siberian Exiles System, 1822–1860" won the 2008 Heldt Prize for best article in Slavic/Eastern European/Eurasian women's studies.

Claire Shaw is lecturer in Russian at the University of Bristol. Her research interests include the formation of Soviet identity and the history of marginal and disabled groups. She is currently completing a monograph on the history of the deaf community in Soviet Russia.

Alison K. Smith, professor of history at the University of Toronto, is the author of *For the Common Good and Their Own Well Being: Social Estate in Imperial Russia* (2014) and of *Recipes for Russia: Food and Nationhood under the Tsars* (2008) and a contributor to russianhistoryblog.org.

Tricia Starks, associate professor of history at the University of Arkansas, is the author of *The Body Soviet: Propaganda, Hygiene, and the Revolutionary State* (2008), and co-editor with Matthew P. Romaniello of *Tobacco in Russian History and Culture* (2009). She currently is completing a history of Russian tobacco use.

Laurie S. Stoff is senior lecturer and Honors Faculty Fellow at Arizona State University's Barrett Honors College and author of *They Fought for the Motherland: Russia's Women Soldiers in World War I and the Revolution* (2006) and *Russia's Sisters of Mercy and the Great War: More than Binding Men's Wounds* (2015).

ACKNOWLEDGMENTS

Aside from the outstanding scholars whose essays appear in this volume, we must thank several individuals and institutions for their support. Wendy Walker of the Association for Slavic, East European, and Eurasian Studies was instrumental in bringing together the panels that initiated this volume at the 2013 Boston conference. Stephen Bittner, Ethan M. Pollock, and Christine Ruane enriched the project with their suggestions and ideas. The Wiswell Endowment Fund for the Promotion of Russian Studies at the University of Hawai'i at Mānoa and the Fulbright College of Arts and Sciences of the University of Arkansas provided some financial assistance in support of the publication of this volume. We extend a special thanks to Geoffery L. Stark of Special Collections at the University of Arkansas Libraries, Fayetteville for help in the acquisition of visuals for the volume.

We would also like to thank Bloomsbury for their support of this project, and our editor, Rhodri Mogford, in particular, for his encouraging responses and valuable suggestions. We also appreciate the thoughtful comments of our two no-longer anonymous reviewers, Frances Bernstein and Paula Michaels, whose insight helped us produce a much stronger and more useful volume.

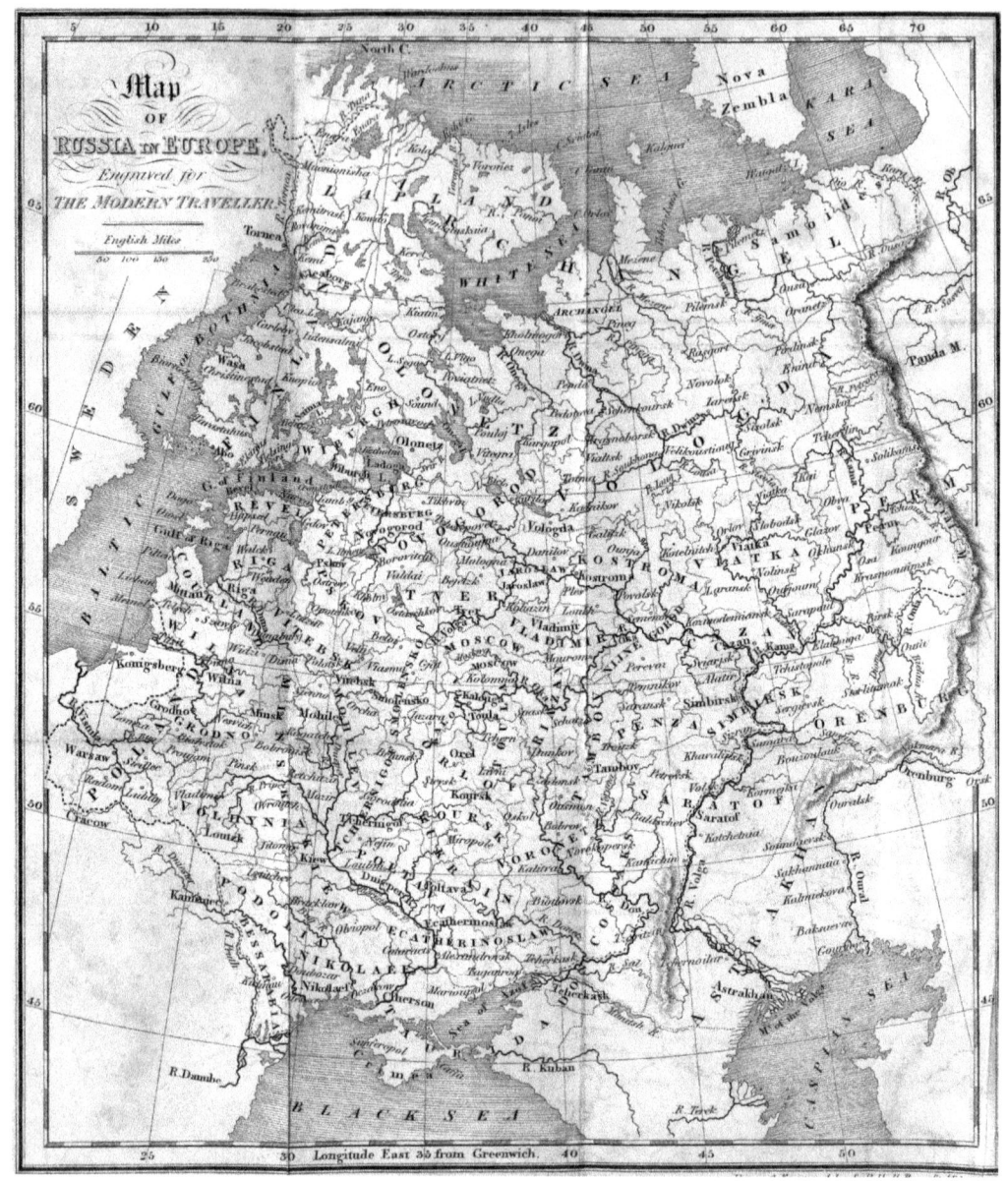

MAP 0.1 *"Map of Russia in Europe,"* The Modern Traveler *10 (1825). Courtesy of the Porter-Pathfinder Library, Special Collections, University of Arkansas Libraries, Fayetteville.*

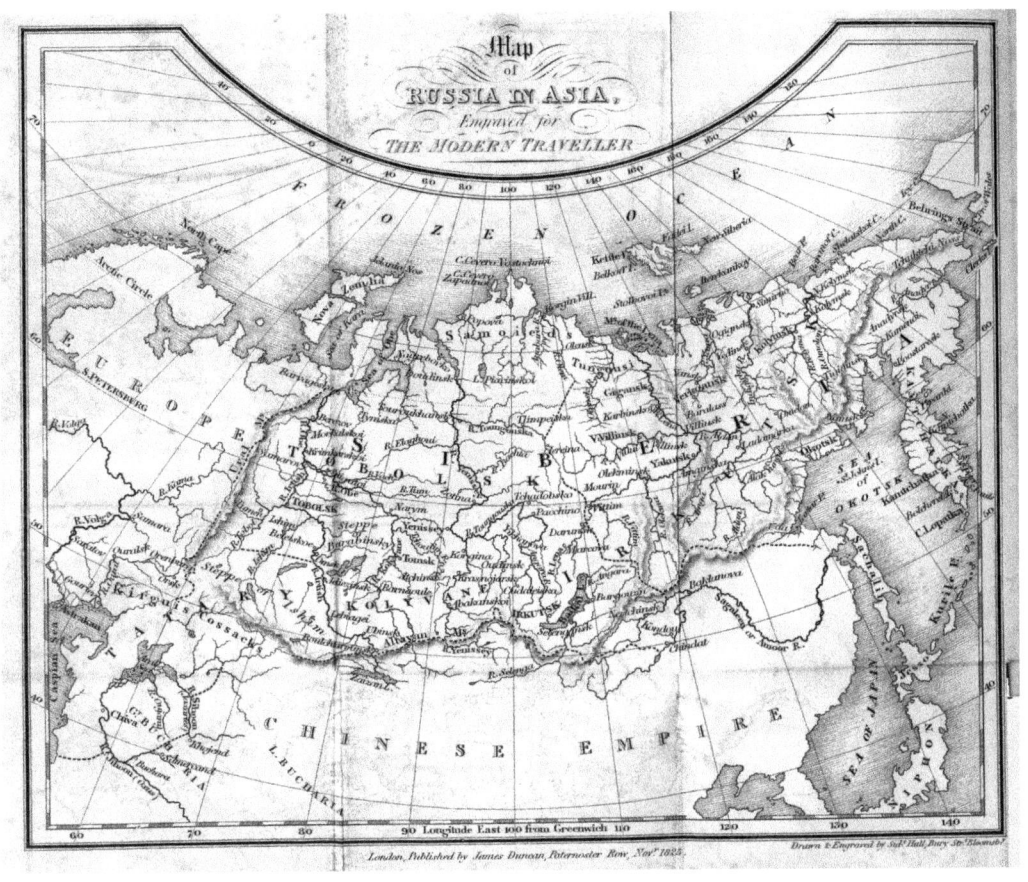

MAP 0.2 *"Map of Russia in Asia,"* The Modern Traveler *10 (1825). Courtesy of the Porter-Pathfinder Library, Special Collections, University of Arkansas Libraries, Fayetteville.*

CHAPTER ONE

Introduction: The sensory in Russian and Soviet history

Alexander M. Martin

Many people interested in the past like historical fiction better than works of scholarship. Of course, fiction writers have the unfair advantage of being able to invent romantic plotlines and probe the intimate thoughts of their characters, but they also manage to give texture to their stories by evoking the primal, almost instinctual ways in which we experience the world around us. What emotions are triggered in us by a religious service, a football game, a battlefield, a favorite movie? What memories stir at the sound of an old pop song, the smell of a freshly mowed lawn, the heat of a summer day, or the sting of an insect bite?

Any depiction of our lives would be incomplete without these fleeting, elusive feelings and perceptions, yet accounting for them confronts the historian with great challenges. My mother spent her childhood during the Second World War in a German city subject to frequent air raids, and that memory left her, and probably many of her generation, with a visceral dislike for the wail of early-warning sirens. Her uncle fought on the Western Front in the First World War and later said that when you approached the frontlines, what struck you from afar was not only the sound but the stench (of sewage, corpses, explosives, and much besides), and one wonders: how did this experience affect him after he returned to civilian life? In both cases—the sound of sirens and the smell of the trenches—a sense impression affected how people experienced and remembered history. Experiences like these are everywhere in history, from the sound of medieval church bells to the coal smoke of Victorian London or the sultry heat of a Southern cotton field. Such things are formative for entire generations, peoples, and social classes, but how do we fit them into the historical record?

In recent decades, historians have increasingly sought solutions to this conundrum. For instance, the French historian Alain Corbin, a pioneer in this field, wrote about why the French upper classes around 1800 developed a distaste for the heavy, musky perfumes that they had traditionally favored. One of the reasons, he found, was that after the upheavals of the French Revolution, these smells had started to remind them uncomfortably of the odor of the poor. As Corbin's study shows, what was thought to smell good or bad could change from one era to the next, and people's sense perceptions evolved in tandem with the larger forces of history.[1]

The senses thus provide an avenue for understanding how people interpret, at a holistic and non-rational level, situations that are difficult or unfamiliar. This brings us to Russia. As the chapters in this volume show, Russian history abounds with cases where people have encountered realities that they found utterly alien. Some of these experiences of alterity, such as deafness or war, occur in all societies, but others are more specific to Russia. The reason is that so many of the people who created our historical sources either came to Russia from abroad, or tried to transform how Russia worked, or felt alienated from the way Russians lived in the present or the past, and in each case, the encounter with Russia affected the senses. Europeans found the Russian winters astonishingly cold. Educated Russians in the nineteenth century constructed their national identity by studying the exotic customs of the common people, including their foods. In the twentieth century, ideas about both the utopian communist future and, once the Soviet Union was gone, the totalitarian past, were associated with a particular smell, taste, feel, look, and sound. Russian history has created experiences that seemed unfamiliar, even bewildering to many people, or at least, to many of those who produced our historical sources. The senses provide an entry point into those perceptions.

In the pages that follow, we will begin with a brief overview of the chapters in this volume. To provide a context, we will then consider the scholarly literatures to which they contribute, and finally, how they are linked together by three larger themes: collective identities, experiments in social engineering, and war.

Overview

The chapters in this collection are divided into four broad categories that reflect the radical discontinuities in Russian history.

In the imperial period of the eighteenth and nineteenth centuries, Russians encountered Europe and faced two new challenges. First, how to define Russia's identity: what made Russia a distinctive nation, and how did that distinctiveness "feel"? Matthew P. Romaniello and Alison K. Smith engage this question by examining weather and food: how did Europeans who froze in the Russian winter interpret that sensation in light of their own theories about climate and the human body, and how did upper-class Russians use the taste of fermented foods to construct a sense of what made something "taste" either Russian or European? Second, like all European and Western societies, Russia faced the challenge that modernity posed to older ways of imagining class, gender, and the place of one's own nation in the larger world. One aspect of this, discussed by Abby Schrader, was consumerism. Shopping traditionally took place in musty, unheated, dimly lit bazaars. Then a competitor arose in the form of elegant arcades, forerunners of today's shopping malls, which transformed the sensory experience of shopping and scrambled the rules governing how the sexes interacted in public places. Tricia Starks examines another sensory experience of modernity, the smoke of cigarettes, and how tobacco—where it came from, how it was blended and marketed, how it smelled—affected Russians' ideas about foreign countries, colonialism, and the class structure of their own society.

The First World War plunged Russia into a crisis that destroyed the monarchy, leading to the Bolshevik Revolution and a calamitous civil war that ended only with the establishment of Soviet rule. Aaron B. Retish's chapter uses a traditional alcoholic drink of the Udmurt people to examine how officials and the educated public dealt with peasants and ethnic minorities throughout the period of war and revolution. Laurie S. Stoff adopts an entirely different perspective: she focuses on middle- and upper-class Russian and European women who volunteered to serve as nurses in the Russian army, and their traumatic encounter with the sights, sounds, and smells of men wounded in battle.

The final two sections of the book are devoted to the Soviet era. The first examines how the senses helped build the new Soviet order, and reveals the mixed results of the regime's attempts to mold a New Soviet Person with specific sensory perceptions. Anton Masterovoy shows how the Soviet state responded to persistent food shortages by engineering new foodstuffs and then trying, without much success, to re-educate people's taste buds accordingly. Steven G. Jug looks at what soldiers during the Second World War saw, smelled, touched, heard, and tasted, and how their experience contradicted the image of the war in the regime's propaganda. Claire Shaw explores the complicated position of the deaf in a Soviet system that wanted to integrate them into mainstream society but was ambivalent about sign language as a legitimate form of communication.

The last section of the book is about the senses and the shaping of Russian memories of the Soviet period. Tim Harte analyzes two movies by the filmmaker Aleksei German, Sr. that capture the oppressiveness of the Stalin era through disturbing evocations of its sights and smells. Adrienne Harris, finally, takes us back to the Second World War through the figure of Zoia Kosmodemianskaia, a young partisan tortured and hanged by the Germans, who for decades persisted in the Russian collective memory through iconic photographs of her mutilated body and the written record of the last words that she spoke.

Historiographical contexts

The chapters in this volume are original pieces of research by the individual authors, but they also form a part of larger intellectual traditions. Let me point out five of these to help provide a framework for understanding the chapters.

One is the work of Walter Benjamin (1892–1940), a German social theorist of the interwar period. Benjamin drew inspiration from Karl Marx's idea of "commodity fetishism." What Marx meant by this is that the actual value of a commodity (that is, a product) comes from the labor of the worker who created it, but capitalism ignores this and instead transforms it into an object of trade by inventing a non-existent commercial value for it, much as a pagan religion might attribute imaginary powers to a wooden fetish or idol. Benjamin took Marx's idea and extended it to the way in which capitalism encourages us to invest consumer goods with our deepest, most unrealizable hopes and dreams. He was writing about nineteenth-century Paris and also had in mind the 1920s and 1930s, but commerce in our own time is no different. Buy our brand of lipstick, the ad whispers to us, and you will look like the photoshopped model on the magazine cover; take your children to our burger joint, and you too will be happy like the smiling family in the TV commercial. Benjamin's point is that capitalism uses consumer goods to encourage utopian fantasies that, by definition, are impossible to fulfill.[2] The fact that Harley-Davidson went to the trouble of trying (unsuccessfully) to trademark the special *vroom* of its motorcycles[3] tells us that our senses, because they are immune to reason, offer especially easy access to our imagination. The same that holds true for advertisers today also applies to historians studying the past, as we see in the chapters by Abby Schrader and Tricia Starks on shopping and cigarette smoke: much can be learned about people by exploring the nexus between their senses and consumerism.

A second source of inspiration for the authors in this book is Benjamin's contemporary, the German-British sociologist Norbert Elias (1897–1990). Elias's book *The Civilizing Process* was first published in 1939, but reached a broad audience only after it was reissued in 1969. It contends that from the Middle Ages to the eighteenth century, as different classes competed for social dominance, refined manners and sensibilities—say, not relieving oneself in public, or eating with forks and napkins, or disgust at certain odors—became a sign of high status. At first, people had to be taught these things, but then they completely internalized them. Our modern attitudes in such matters are therefore not "natural," but neither are they arbitrary; rather, they result from the way our social system has developed.[4] Following Elias's insight, scholars have argued that assertions of dominance often have a sensory component. For instance, people in the past have tried to prove their own group's superiority by claiming that other groups (Africans, Jews,

East Europeans, the poor) smelled bad.[5] Likewise, rulers have used visuality to demonstrate their power by arranging people and things in straight rows: soldiers on parade, neat rows of trees in palace gardens, geometrically aligned avenues in a planned city.[6] The senses can thus be used to demonstrate power. This theme runs through a number of chapters in this volume, including those by Smith, Schrader, Starks, and Retish on the ways in which food, drink, smoking, and shopping helped to establish relations of power.

A third source of ideas is the French philosopher Michel Foucault (1926–84). Foucault's most important idea, for our present purposes, is that the advance of science and technology and of the institutions that support them should not be seen primarily as a triumph of knowledge over ignorance but as a form of power. Foucault makes this argument, for example, in his history of psychiatric hospitals,[7] but one can name many other instances as well. The Nazi doctors who sent disabled people to the gas chambers on eugenic grounds are a grotesque extreme, but in truth, all modern states give immense power to experts—for instance, government child-welfare officials can take away your children if they have (serious) objections to your parenting style. Scholars have taken up Foucault's ideas and asked about the ways in which the cultural authority and legal power of supposed experts have been used to promote a coercive social agenda—and ways in which average people have refused to comply with it.[8] These questions are central to several chapters: Masterovoy's and Retish's on the state's attempts to control what Russians ate and drank, Jug's on its propaganda effort to mold people's perceptions of the Second World War, and Shaw's on its quest to shape how the deaf communicated.

A fourth area of scholarship that lies behind these chapters concerns the development of national identities. We conventionally distinguish between two basic types of nationalism. Romantic nationalism holds that we are one nation if we share a common way of thinking and feeling derived from a folk culture (language, customs, religion, and the like) that we have inherited from our ancestors. According to statist or civic nationalism, on the other hand, what makes us one nation is that we owe allegiance to the same government and have a shared vision of the social system that we want to create. There is no consensus about the moment in time when the English, Germans, Russians, and other European peoples first developed a sense of national identity, but it is in the eighteenth century that intellectuals began aggressively articulating the ideas underlying both forms of modern nationalism.[9] Sensory perceptions played a part in this. The chapters by Romaniello and Smith about climate and folk cuisine contribute to our understanding of romantic nationalist ideas according to which Russians were a distinct people because of their unique ancestral way of life. Retish and Shaw, meanwhile, shed light on statist or civic nationalism by showing how the Russian elites tried to integrate marginalized groups, in this case ethnic minorities and the deaf, into a unified, modern, forward-looking Russian nation.[10]

A fifth and final subfield of scholarship that influences this volume is the study of memory. Two aspects are relevant here. First, how sense perceptions are related to individual memory. In his novel *In Search of Lost Time*, the French writer Marcel Proust (1871–1922) explored how fleeting sensory perceptions, such the taste of a food remembered from childhood, could trigger a sudden flood of personal memories. His depiction of this phenomenon is so famous that scientists speak of a "Proust effect."[11] A contemporary of Proust's, the French sociologist Maurice Halbwachs (1877–1945), proposed the notion that not only do individuals remember the past, but entire groups, such as nations or classes, have a collective "memory" that operates somewhat similarly to the memory of an individual person.[12] These ideas provide a context for the chapter in which Stoff analyzes how Russian nurses articulated their own personal memory of the First World War through recollections of sounds and smells; and also the chapter by Harte, which shows how in the 1980s and 1990s, when most movie-goers presumably had little *personal* memory of the Stalin era, films depicted the feel and smell of that bygone time in hopes of awakening the audience's *collective* memory. The study of memory received a further impulse in the 1980s from the French historian Pierre Nora, who argued that a people's collective memory crystallizes around certain iconic things—places, pictures, speeches—that he called "sites of memory."[13] In American history, examples might include the Alamo, the Ford Model T, the photo of marines raising the flag on Iwo Jima, and the date "9/11." In Russia, the images and final words of Zoia Kosmodemianskaia, which Harris discusses in her chapter, form just such a "site of memory" for the Second World War.

Thematic contexts

The chapters in this book are arranged in chronological order, thus highlighting the distinctive features of each historical period. If we group them according to the questions they address, however, rather than the era they describe, other patterns emerge that are also worth considering. Three of these are group identities, social engineering, and war.

One question addressed in this volume concerns the role of the senses in our collective self-perception. What differentiates the groups (say, social classes) into which our people are divided? What, on the other hand, is it that unites our people as one nation? And, what is our nation's place in the larger system of nations? Sensory perceptions are part of the answer, as anyone knows who has ever found that foreign foods taste strange. Six chapters deal with these questions, but from opposite angles. Smith, Starks, and Masterovoy focus on the role of the senses in creating order and coherence in society by helping in the construction of group identities.

Schrader, Retish, and Shaw, on the other hand, show how sensory experiences could disrupt the coherence of such identities.

In the early nineteenth century, constructing identities in Russia primarily meant defining nationality, and this confronted Russians with a conundrum. The trouble was that the country had no real national identity. Its identity was, basically, only that the tsar was its ruler and Orthodoxy was the dominant (but not exclusive) religion. Nothing compelled the widely dispersed ethnic Slavs to develop a unified Russian culture, and as Russia expanded, they often also mingled with their non-Slavic neighbors. The upper class reflected this diversity, and in addition, as a result of the regime's effort in the eighteenth and nineteenth centuries to make Russia a European country, it absorbed influences from abroad, especially France and Germany. All of this worked against the kind of coherent national identity that both the West and educated Russians themselves thought a civilized European country required. However, attempts to create such an identity produced a Catch-22. Russians—at least, those who embraced romantic nationalism—thought that authentically Russian ways of feeling existed mainly among peasants untouched by foreign influences, yet turning those feelings into a coherent national culture required incorporating them into novels, operas, historical scholarship, and other forms that came out of the traditions of Europe and could be mastered only by Russians steeped in European culture.

Russians never quite overcame the feeling that national authenticity and European education formed a zero-sum game, but as they grappled with this tension, they constructed a sense of nationality that remains powerful to this day and has a significant sensory component. They examined their country's sights, sounds, and tastes; identified a subset as quintessentially "Russian"; and incorporated them into European forms of expression. When done successfully, this allowed Russians to be part of European civilization while continuing to "feel" Russian. For example, artists distilled Russia's diverse natural environments into a unified visual image of a national landscape—generally a flat or undulating plain, often with birch trees, a river, or wooden houses or churches—to be painted according to the rules of Western landscape art.[14] Similarly, ethnographers collected folk melodies that composers then incorporated into operas and symphonies, thus creating European music with a Russian sound.[15]

One area in which this process operated is taste. Russians to this day believe that certain foods are intrinsic to their identity and reflect their national values. For instance, mushrooms, which people gather in the woods, are seen as reflecting a distinctly Russian love of forests and nature. A similar connection between food and national identity also exists in many other countries where people believe they are heirs to shared ancestral customs. The United States departs from this pattern because Americans think of themselves as a people of diverse origin and lean toward civic or statist rather than romantic nationalism; however, a number of American subcultures do use food—jambalaya, soul food, barbeque, gefilte fish—to affirm identities derived from shared ancestry. Foods associated with a particular national culture can create class boundaries, too. In America, on the one hand it is socially prestigious to be a gourmet (appropriately, a French word) who appreciates French cuisine. On the other hand, French food is also a weapon in class and national rivalries, as when effeminate snobs in the 1980s were lampooned as "quiche eaters"[16] or French critics of the Iraq War in the early 2000s were maligned as "cheese-eating surrender monkeys."[17] Food thus has strong associations of class and nationality.

The chapter by Alison Smith ("Fermentation, taste, and identity") explores how Russians came by their modern sense that certain foods taste "Russian." She focuses on one particular taste sensation: that of fermentation. Fermented food can sometimes be good, but rotten food is definitely bad. The trouble, as Smith writes, is that "the boundary between fermented and rotten is based above all on taste," and how the two were differentiated sheds light on the construction of Russian national identity. Some fermented foods (strong cheeses, long-hung meat) came from the West, while others (rye bread, sour cabbage) were folk dishes, and the discussions about their taste formed a microcosm of larger debates about national and class identity. Sophisticated "gastronomes" tried to elevate the national palate by promoting fermented Western foods, while intellectuals debated whether the fermented foods of the common folk were proof of barbarism or on the contrary gave Russians a special hardiness. Before Darwin's theory of evolution and the discovery of disease-causing germs, it was generally believed that human bodies and minds are shaped primarily by their surroundings. By this reasoning, Russia's cold climate—a topic discussed by Matthew Romaniello, whose chapter I will discuss later—and sour foods had the power to make Russians biologically different from other Europeans.[18] The debate about food was thus not only about nationality and class but also Russia's place in the world. This became a dangerous habit of questioning whether common Russians really had any place in the European community of peoples, which reached its destructive climax in the two World Wars.

As Tricia Starks shows in her chapter ("The taste, smell, and semiotics of cigarettes"), tobacco smoke raised some of the same questions as fermented foods. Tobacco, like food, speaks to multiple senses at once. Starks points out that smoking is about both taste and smell. One might add that it is also about visuality, for example when smokers blow smoke rings or use pipes, cigars, or cigarettes as quasi fashion accessories. Smith and Romaniello argue that people believed food and climate to be capable of changing people's bodies; Starks notes that tobacco smoke has such an effect because it clings to the smoker's hair and clothing. Then as now, tobaccos from around the world were blended to produce scents and flavors appealing to different palates, and marketers, implicitly embracing Walter Benjamin's view of products as a trigger for consumers' fantasies, linked tobacco with enticing images of exotic lands and races. Smoking this or that blend allowed Russians both to feel and to demonstrate worldliness, sophistication, and membership in a peer group of gourmets and connoisseurs. Cigarettes, like the foods discussed by Smith, were thus about both nationality and social status. Additionally, unlike those foods, they made Russians feel that they shared Europe's colonialist power over foreign peoples around the globe, and they had a subversive cachet because they suggested that the smoker was a free-spirited individualist not hemmed in by tradition.[19]

The smell of cigarettes was symptomatic of a larger trend that troubled Russia's rulers: the people of the larger cities had so internalized the cultural modernity promoted by the state that they were losing respect for the rules of hierarchy and propriety on which the regime was based. As we learn from Aaron Retish's chapter ("The taste of *kumyshka* and the debate over Udmurt culture"), taste could also suggest the opposite problem: that groups situated at the other end of the sociocultural spectrum remained stubbornly resistant to both the regime and modernity.

Kumyshka was a traditional—and, to educated Russians, foul-tasting—alcoholic drink of the Udmurt ethnicity deep in Russia's remote rural interior. When Udmurts made *kumyshka* and then drank it for ritual purposes, they antagonized Russia's elites on a variety of levels: by cutting into the government's vodka sales; by subverting the Orthodox Church's efforts to control spirituality; and by perpetuating what educated Russians thought was the debilitating primitiveness of Russian rural life. In the chapters by Smith and Retish, educated Russians were looking at the same reality—that peasant food was unsophisticated and resistant to outside influences—but reached opposite value judgments depending on whether their nationalism was of the romantic or of the civic or statist variety. In the former case, described by Smith, peasant foodways were seen as serving the nation by preserving valuable ancestral traditions, whereas in the latter (Retish), they were judged to be backward and just one more obstacle on Russia's road to modernity.

During the First World War and again after the Bolshevik Revolution, the government tried unsuccessfully to suppress *kumyshka* in the name of progress and civilization. This forms part of a larger historical phenomenon: the repeated attempts by those in power to transform both Russia's social system and the thoughts and behaviors of individuals. The country's leaders aimed to be, as Stalin famously put it, "engineers of the human soul."[20] The chapters by Schrader, Masterovoy, and Shaw explore what the senses can tell us about these attempts at social engineering and their ambiguous results.

The chapters we have discussed so far concern real sense perceptions created by specific objects—the taste and smell of fermented foods, tobacco, and *kumyshka*. Abby Schrader's chapter ("Market pleasures and prostitution in St. Petersburg") deals with something more elusive, namely, how people in St. Petersburg responded to changes in the sensory environment that they themselves culturally constructed. In the 1830s and early 1840s, she writes, a disquieting image of St. Petersburg was created by "authors who wrote panoramas, physiologies, travelogues, and feuilletons" about the city. These were new literary genres that combined entertainment, journalism, sociological analysis, and moralizing commentary. They aimed not just for dispassionate description, but to convey how a city "felt," reveal its hidden underside, and render judgment. Vivid evocations of sense perceptions proved a useful literary device for that purpose. Moreover, Russian writers took their cues from British and French authors who were (justifiably) alarmed at the recent deterioration of urban conditions in their own countries. The upshot was that readers were increasingly exposed to depictions of Russian cities as noisy, malodorous places where nights were gloomy and weird characters lurked around every corner.[21]

Were these texts proof of a new urban reality? More likely, the literary technique itself was new. Similarly, coarse language and graphic violence were rare in American movies until the 1960s and 1970s, when they became ubiquitous; this was a result of changes in Hollywood screenwriting conventions, not in real life. Yet as Schrader shows, the change in perceptions was enough to prompt a new experiment in urban design in downtown St. Petersburg: the construction of a covered, enclosed gallery of elegant stores, climate-controlled and illumined by gas light, where the respectable classes could shop in comfort without having to rub elbows with the masses. The appeal was similar to that of shopping malls in Western countries since the Second World War. Named *Passazh* in Russian, after the Parisian "passages" that formed its prototype and that inspired Walter Benjamin's study of consumerism,[22] the new shopping gallery was meant to become a precisely calibrated environment from which the noise, smells, and dirt of the city at large were banished. As a social experiment, Schrader writes, *Passazh* (which survives today as an upscale mall) was ultimately unsuccessful because it led men and women to mingle in an environment dominated entirely by commerce rather than the traditional rules of gender relations. According to the writers of feuilletons and physiologies, women were drawn by the beautiful wares and sometimes prostituted themselves to make money to buy them, which caused disturbing incidents when men failed to distinguish correctly between honorable ladies and prostitutes. Schrader, drawing on Benjamin's analysis of consumer capitalism, argues that both the merchandise and the women who shopped for it were, in effect, goods, commodities put on display to arouse the greedy fantasies of those who saw them.

Schrader's theme is not so much actual sense perceptions as *ideas* about sense perceptions. In fact, when we read about feuilletonists imagining women's fantasies about luscious objects and men's fantasies about women's bodies, the subject becomes *ideas about ideas* about sense perceptions. But no matter. Even in this form, the senses had power, as Schrader concludes, to "destabilize gender relations in the Late Imperial period." Much like the actual taste and smell of real-life cigarettes discussed by Starks, the ideas about fantasies about consumer goods and sex that *Passazh* aroused help us understand the forces that undermined the stability of the tsarist social order.

Social engineering on a much larger scale than *Passazh* was attempted after the Bolshevik Revolution. An overarching goal of the Soviet regime in the 1920s was to promote just the kind of modernity that had disrupted its tsarist predecessor, and sensory perceptions had their place in this program. Abstract painters and constructivist architects sought to create a Soviet visuality that was unmistakably modern. Radio, a new invention, helped create a distinctly Soviet soundscape. Odor, too, could be "Soviet": in 1927, large-scale industrialization was celebrated by a poster that showed factory smokestacks, accompanied by a caption that read, "The smoke of the chimneys is the breath of Soviet Russia."[23]

Eventually, as in the late imperial period, cultural modernity began to undermine the regime. Sensory perceptions were indicative of this process. The regime failed in its attempt to overcome certain forms of backwardness: for instance, despite much propaganda about hygiene, public bathrooms remained so filthy and malodorous throughout the Soviet period that even Westerners sympathetic to the Soviets were appalled. (In the blunt words of one Stalin-era German communist, "The Russians should first learn how to shit before they build industry."[24]) Even where a version of modernity did take hold, it was slow to adapt to the changes occurring from the 1960s on. Western blue jeans and rock 'n' roll, for example, gained huge popularity on the black market because the way they looked, felt, and sounded was more in-keeping with the mood among young urban people than were Soviet apparel and music. In sum, the sensory environment encouraged the perception that the early Soviet regime of the 1920s and 1930s was at the cutting edge of modernity, but that its successor by the 1970s and 1980s was fatally out of touch, leaving its heirs after 1991 to look to their tsarist-era ancestors and to the West for cultural models: hence the ubiquity, in the urban centers of today's Russia, of the sound of church bells and rock music and the aroma of folk cuisine and cappuccino bars.

The evolving fortunes of Soviet attempts to mold the sensory environment are the topics of the chapters by Anton Masterovoy and Claire Shaw. One such effort concerned food. As we see in the chapters by Smith and Retish, the tsarist elites regarded the people's traditional taste favorably if it represented Russian national culture, but unfavorably if it represented backwardness. Masterovoy (in "Engineering tastes: Food and the senses") comes from a different angle: the mismatch between what people liked to eat and what was convenient to produce. A similar mismatch has existed in many countries in the twentieth century as a result of war-related shortages and business's search for profits. In response, industry and scientists have tried to change people's eating habits. One way they have done this is by encouraging society to think of nutrition mainly in terms of calories, vitamins, and minerals—all things that can be measured and manipulated—while downplaying harder-to-control aspects such as taste, smell, texture, and appearance. This is part of a larger modern pattern in which experts devise solutions by reducing complex, multifaceted problems to a single aspect that can be conveniently analyzed and regulated: questions of urban land-use are simplified by designating areas as exclusively either commercial or residential; education is reduced to test scores; multifaceted mental processes, to an IQ number; food, to the intake of particular nutrients. The other approach has been, on the contrary, to create processed foods that appeal to the taste of consumers. Efforts to modify eating habits in these ways have had mixed results, as we see in the United States and other Western countries, where many people ignore government nutrition guidelines and where some industrial foods are widely embraced but others are not.

Masterovoy's chapter, through systematic comparison of Soviet food science with both Western democracies and fascist regimes, is able to identify what was uniquely Soviet and what was not. In many countries, there were attempts to popularize new foods that were more nutritious than tasty. What was distinctively Soviet, however, is how ideology and propaganda drove the regime to alternate between two approaches. While Western nutritionists, anticipating popular resistance to their inventions, "downplayed the unattractive features of replacement foods," their Soviet counterparts at certain times did the opposite: giddy with revolutionary enthusiasm, they actively drew attention to "the disgusting nature" of new food sources (for instance, a sea bird that smelled of pond scum) to make the hoped-for triumph of Soviet science that much more impressive. At other times, on the contrary, to validate the regime's dubious claims about rising living standards, they advocated for a diet of meat and old-fashioned luxuries. The outcome of these two conflicting approaches, according to Masterovoy, has been that modern Russians distrust processed foods and equate the good life with meat, dumplings, and other traditional fare.

This helps explain something that any Western visitor to Russia notices, namely, the old-fashioned quality of Russian eating habits. One could extend the argument to other areas of sensory perception. Few in Russia seem to favor the gender-neutral style of female dress that one often sees in the West; instead, the unappealing drabness of Soviet modernity helped preserve a more traditional, gendered sensibility about women's appearance. Music tells the same story: for all the regime's revolutionary ambitions, its greatest musical achievement turned out to be the preservation of such tsarist inheritances as classical ballet. If today's Russia is often culturally conservative, it is in no small part an ironic legacy of the Soviets.

Claire Shaw's chapter ("Deafness and the politics of hearing") makes similar points, and these also resonate with the chapters by Smith and Retish. First, peasants, ethnic minorities, and the deaf were all groups that were socially isolated and considered backward by the elites. Integrating the deaf by teaching them oral speech, like teaching the masses to appreciate industrial foods, promised to help transform their consciousness and make them into New Soviet People—one of the regime's paramount goals. Second, these efforts produced mixed results. One cause lay in the regime's own fluctuating priorities: for instance, after the bold experiments of the 1920s, the turmoil of the 1930s saw a return to older ways both in culinary preference and in the acceptance of sign language. Another cause was the way in which the transformative promise of technology (processed foods, hearing aids) remained present in propaganda and ideology but was never fulfilled in everyday reality. People's experience of taste and sound therefore took a distinctly Soviet path to modernity because the effort to create New Soviet People continued even as older cultural traditions persisted.

Beyond the themes of collective identity and social engineering, a third problem addressed by the chapters in this volume is the Russian experience of war. In the calamitous decades from 1914 to 1945, the Russian Empire and the Soviet Union experienced warfare of extraordinary scale and destructiveness. A powerful way to understand how these events affected Russians is through the senses.

Laurie Stoff and Steven Jug deal with the effect of the two World Wars on the full range of sensory perceptions. One might imagine that war meant something different for nurses than for frontline soldiers, but Stoff argues that to the contrary, "the experiences of women serving as medical personnel in Russia often closely mirrored those of men on the battlefields and in the trenches." Yet reading the two chapters side by side, one is struck by the difference in the tone of the sources. The nurses in Stoff's chapter on the First World War ("The sounds, odors, and textures of Russian wartime nursing") are shocked by man's cruelty to man, whereas the Second World War soldiers quoted by Jug (in "Sensing danger: The Red Army during the Second World War") are full of zest to kill the enemy. Stoff quotes a nurse who is shocked to see a dead German and tries to convince herself that he is still alive, while in Jug's chapter, a soldier recalls how good it felt "watching the enemy die".

How to account for such differences? Soviet soldiers in the Second World War saw evidence of German atrocities that had no counterpart in the First World War, but in Jug's chapter, the soldiers seem motivated mostly by a desire to avenge fallen comrades, an urge universal to all wars. Another possibility is that, contrary to Stoff's thesis, soldiers and nurses, or men and women, did in fact experience war differently. A third, and perhaps the best, explanation is that the distinct culture of each period influenced what and how people wrote. Going into the First World War, Russian culture still retained its nineteenth-century cosmopolitanism, the ethos of the intelligentsia encouraged devotion to suffering humanity, and women in particular were expected to be loving and compassionate.[25] By the outbreak of the Second World War, by contrast, the Soviet population had been subjected to years of Stalinist rhetoric about the need to exterminate enemies of the Soviet regime. Perhaps this discrepancy in the wider cultural atmosphere is why Russians wrote differently about the two wars. This leaves us, however, with a difficult question: Did the two groups in reality experience similar feelings, and write differently only because the conventions of their time were different, or had they internalized those conventions to the point that their actual feelings were different? This is a fundamental problem confronting anyone who studies the history of the senses, and a hard one to resolve.

The role of cultural traditions in shaping Russian understandings of war, present only obliquely in the chapters by Stoff and Jug, is addressed explicitly in Adrienne Harris's chapter on the martyred partisan Zoia Kosmodemianskaia ("The sensory experience of martyrdom and Soviet collective memory"). Harris does not focus on the tragic story of Zoia herself, but rather on how her persona was subsequently constructed with materials from both the prerevolutionary and the Soviet tradition and became, to use Pierre Nora's term, a "site of memory" that helped structure Russians' understanding of the Second World War. She stresses the impact of the widely reprinted photographs of Zoia's dead body, with its mutilated and partially naked breast and seemingly serene face. Harris links this image with traditional representations of Orthodox saints; one might add that it also aligns with nineteenth-century Russian and European paintings that represented defiled but chaste maidens as eroticized martyrs for patriotic causes.[26] The other source of Zoia's posthumous propaganda value lay in her reported final words, which summoned the people to fight to the death and be loyal to Stalin.

Food for thought about war and Russian culture is also provided by Tim Harte's chapter on the films of Aleksei German ("Stalinism's sights and smells in the films of Aleksei German, Sr."), which convey the evil of Stalinism with images that evoke stench and feelings of claustrophobia. By the early twentieth century, fresh air and open spaces were associated with youth and freedom and progress. Going back at least to Jean-Jacques Rousseau in the eighteenth century, educated Western people imagined nature as a tonic against the congestion, filth, artificiality, and restrictive rules of urban life. "Nature" versus "civilization" meant truth versus falsehood, freedom versus confinement, but also opposing sense perceptions. This helps explain why, in August 1914, many Russians and other Europeans, especially educated young men and (in the case of Stoff's nurses) women, greeted the war as a release from dull routines in the enclosed, musty, or smelly spaces of schools, offices, nurseries, and kitchens.[27] When Stalin launched his social revolution, he evoked a similar response. Look at the photographs of 1914 and of the totalitarian regimes of Stalin and Hitler: what you see are optimistic, fresh-faced young people, marching off into the warm sunshine as though on a nature hike. The idea of war or revolution triggered thoughts of fresh air and freedom in the great outdoors, so it stands to reason that the disappointment of these hopes evoked the opposite sensations of stench and confinement. This is a central theme of Stoff's chapter on First World War nurses, and also of Harte's analysis of German's movies, in which the characters wander in narrow spaces and repulsive odors emanate from the dying Stalin. (By contrast, the Second World War propaganda discussed by Jug ignores smells, and the photographs of Zoia Kosmodemianskaia's frozen corpse suggest that in death she is somehow odorless.) German's use of sensory perceptions is metaphorical, but it also speaks at a visceral level to the very real connection people make between abstract ideas and physical sensations. If Stalin's body stinks, he tells us, and his people are trapped in a maze with no exit, then Stalinism's promise of liberation was a lie all along.

A final chapter that one can connect with the theme of war, although on its face this may seem surprising, is Matthew Romaniello's chapter about foreigners' impression of the Russian winter ("Humoral bodies in cold climates"). The largest groups of Westerners to "visit" the Russian heartland in modern times were the armies of Napoleon and Hitler, and their war memories had a lasting effect on Western perceptions of Russia. The cold was central to the narratives of both invading armies, narratives that in turn became entrenched in Western thinking: the generals claimed that their side had lost because "General Winter" fought on the side of the Russians, and for the soldiers, memories of the cold encapsulated both the miseries of the war and what they thought was the general barbarism of the country.[28] The Nazi brutality described by Jug and Harris had many causes, but one was the despair of German soldiers confronted with the Russian winter.

Unless one is an invading soldier with inadequate gear, however, there is no intrinsic reason why Russia's cold should be viewed in purely negative terms. In Russian paintings, winter can be a season of beauty and joy.[29] Russians to this day distinguish two types of winter weather in their country: a cold, crisp, sunny, snowy "Russian" winter that invigorates body and soul, and a slushy, muddy, overcast, depressing "European" one with temperatures hovering around freezing. In past centuries, the cold allowed for swift travel by sled on frozen rivers. As Romaniello points out, it prevented meat from spoiling, and it suppressed diseases such as plague and malaria that were endemic in warmer climates. Before the twentieth century, when streets in all countries were drenched in filth and sewage, Russian streets smelled less bad when they froze in the winter. (The spring thaw was a different matter!)[30] Compared, say, with the damp, gray winters of England, which until the nineteenth century were thought to drive people to suicide,[31] a snowy day in Russia can be quite magnificent.

Romaniello's chapter shows that the negative attitude toward the Russian winter had historical roots and was culturally constructed. Europeans during the Age of Exploration, in trying to make sense of unfamiliar lands and peoples, drew on medical theories according to which people's physical and mental faculties were a function of their natural environment. Excessive heat exacerbated the passions, while too much cold produced sluggishness of mind and body.[32] In this view, people accustomed to the supposedly ideal climate of Western Europe risked their health when exposed to the Russian cold, and while Russians compensated by taking steam baths, this had the effect of altering their basic physical makeup. Veterans of both Napoleon's and Hitler's Russian campaigns thought that the Russian winter was deadly to Westerners and that Russians could tolerate it only because they were "different" in some fundamental and barbaric way. Romaniello's chapter helps us see the origin of such thinking, especially in the case of Great Britain. Given Europe's climatic diversity, it would also be interesting to know how Russia appeared to people accustomed to weather either warmer or colder than in Great Britain. Did the physical experience of their native climate cause them to experience Russia differently, in other words, did Italians freeze more than Swedes? Or was the cultural construct of the awful Russian winter so powerful that, overriding actual personal experience, it made all Westerners freeze equally?

* * *

The history of the senses opens a window onto many aspects of Russian life, from the construction of identities to social engineering and the experience of war. It engages with historiographies on themes ranging from "commodity fetishism" and the "civilizing process" to the power of scientific experts and collective memory. Above and beyond what it adds to these diverse fields of scholarly endeavor, the history of the senses endows the study of the past with a visceral sense of immediacy. How did the past in Russia look, sound, smell, taste, and feel? Read this book and find out.

Notes

1   Alain Corbin, *The Foul and the Fragrant: Odor and the French Social Imagination*, trans. Miriam Kochan, Roy Porter, and Christopher Prendergast (Cambridge, MA: Harvard University Press, 1986).
2   Max Pensky, "Method and Time: Benjamin's Dialectical Images," in David S. Ferris, ed., *The Cambridge Companion to Walter Benjamin* (Cambridge: Cambridge University Press, 2004), 184.
3   John O'Dell, "Harley-Davidson Quits Trying to Hog Sound," *Los Angeles Times*, June 21, 2000. Available from http://articles.latimes.com/2000/jun/21/business/fi-43145 (accessed September 10, 2015).
4   Norbert Elias, *The Civilizing Process: Sociogenetic and Psychogenetic Investigations*, trans. Edmund Jephcott (Oxford: Blackwell, 2000).
5   Anita Levy, *Other Women: The Writing of Class, Race, and Gender,*

1832–1898 (Princeton, NJ: Princeton University Press, 1991), 51; Vejas Gabriel Liulevicius, *The German Myth of the East: 1800 to the Present* (Oxford: Oxford University Press, 2009), 115; Corbin, *The Foul and the Fragrant*, Chapter 9 ("The Stench of the Poor").

6 This linkage between visuality and power is a theme in James Scott, *Seeing Like a State: How Certain Schemes to Improve the Human Condition Have Failed* (New Haven, CT: Yale University Press, 1999), e.g., 18, 58, 117, 133.

7 Michel Foucault, *Madness and Civilization: A History of Insanity in the Age of Reason*, trans. Richard Howard (New York: Vintage Books, 1988).

8 Scott, *Seeing Like a State*, 130; Christopher Hamlin, *Public Health and Social Justice in the Age of Chadwick: Britain, 1800–1854* (Cambridge: Cambridge University Press, 1998), 12–3; Ann Laura Stoler, *Carnal Knowledge and Imperial Power: Race and the Intimate in Colonial Rule* (Berkeley: University of California Press, 2002), 206–7.

9 On this topic, see, for example: Benedict Anderson, *Imagined Communities: Reflections on the Origin and Spread of Nationalism* (London and New York: Verso, 1983); E. J. Hobsbawm, *Nations and Nationalism Since 1780: Programme, Myth, Reality* (Cambridge: Cambridge University Press, 1990).

10 For a recent discussion of nineteenth-century Russian nationalism, see Olga Maiorova, *From the Shadow of Empire: Defining the Russian Nation through Cultural Mythology, 1855–1870* (Madison: University of Wisconsin Press, 2010).

11 Cretien van Campen, *The Proust Effect: The Senses as Doorways to Lost Memories*, trans. Julian Ross (Oxford: Oxford University Press, 2014).

12 On the development of the notion of historical memory, see Jeffrey K. Olick and Joyce Robbins, "Social Memory Studies: From 'Collective Memory' to the Historical Sociology of Mnemonic Practices," *Annual Review of Sociology* 24 (1998): 105–40.

13 On Nora, see Steven Englund, "Review Article: The Ghost of Nation Past," *Journal of Modern History* 64 (2) (1992): 299–320.

14 On this topic, see Christopher Ely, *This Meager Nature: Landscape and National Identity in Imperial Russia* (DeKalb: Northern Illinois University Press, 2002).

15 On the influence of folk tradition on Russian art music, see for example: Richard Stites, *Serfdom, Society, and the Arts: The Pleasure and the Power* (New Haven, CT: Yale University Press, 2005), 54–6, 84–6.

16 The term was popularized by a satirical book by Bruce Feirstein, *Real Men Don't Eat Quiche: A Guide to All That Is Truly Masculine* (New York: Pocket Books, 1982).

17 The phrase was first used, with no political intent, in a 1995 episode of the satirical animated series *The Simpsons* (https://en.wikipedia.org/wiki/%27Round_Springfield [accessed September 10, 2015]). For an example of its subsequent use in anti-French polemics on the eve of the Iraq War, see Jonah Goldberg, "Frogs in Our Midst," *National Review* (July 16, 2002), http://www.nationalreview.com/article/205247/frogs-our-midst-jonah-goldberg (accessed September 10, 2015).

18 On early modern ideas about the connection between climate, food, and the body, see Rebecca Earle, *The Body of the Conquistador: Food, Race and the Colonial Experience in Spanish America, 1492–1700* (Cambridge: Cambridge University Press, 2012).

19 On the connection of tobacco with consumerism and social class, see also the chapters by Konstantine Klioutchkine and Sally West in Matthew P. Romaniello and Tricia Starks, eds., *Tobacco in Russian History and Culture: The Seventeenth Century to the Present* (New York: Routledge, 2009).

20 Quoted in Cynthia Ann Ruder, *Making History for Stalin: The Story of the Belomor Canal* (Gainesville: University of Florida Press, 1998), 44.

21 On this literature, see Alexander M. Martin, *Enlightened Metropolis: Constructing Imperial Moscow, 1762–1855* (Oxford: Oxford University Press, 2013), 278–84.

22 Walter Benjamin, *The Arcades Project*, trans. Howard Eiland and Kevin McLaughlin (Cambridge, MA: Belknap, 1999).

23 The original Russian texts reads "Dym trub—dykhan'e sovetskoi Rossii."

24 Quoted in Bert Hoppe, "Iron Revolutionaries and Salon Socialists: Bolsheviks and German Communists in the 1920s and 1930s," in *Fascination and Enmity: Russia and Germany as Entangled Histories, 1914–1945*, ed. Michael David-Fox, Peter Holquist, and Alexander M. Martin (Pittsburgh, PA: University of Pittsburgh Press, 2012), 59.

25 Barbara Alpern Engel, *Women in Russia, 1700–2000* (Cambridge: Cambridge University Press, 2004), 85, 114–15, 130.

26 A few examples include: two paintings by Eugène Delacroix glorifying liberal revolutions, *Greece on the Ruins of Missolonghi* (1826) and *Liberty Leading the People* (1830); Konstantin Makovskii's *Turkish Atrocities in Bulgaria* (1877); and two paintings of the Vendée conflict during the French Revolution: Joseph Aubert, *Mass Drowning of Rebels by Republicans at Nantes in 1793* (1882) and François Flameng, *Massacre of Republicans by Royalists at Machecoul in 1793* (1884).

27 On the romantic modernist rebellion against the conventions of bourgeois culture, and on the connection between this rebellion and enthusiasm for the outbreak of the First World War, see Modris Eksteins, *Rites of Spring: The Great War and the Birth of the Modern Age* (Boston and New York: Houghton Mifflin, 1989).

28 The impact of the Russian winter on the Napoleonic army is a central theme in General Philippe Paul de Ségur, *Defeat: Napoleon's Russian Campaign*, trans. J. David Townsend (New York: New York Review of Books, 2008). The expression "General Winter" appears in nineteenth-century French accounts of the Napoleonic invasion, e.g., Alfred Assolant, *1812: Campagne de Russie* (Paris: Armand I. E. Chevalier, 1866), 198; for evidence of its use in Nazi Germany, see Horst Bischoff, *Ich war ein Geburtstagsgeschenk des Führers: Geschichte einer Jugend in der Hitlerzeit—Eine autobiografische Erzählung* (Oschersleben: Ziethen, 2005), 48.

29 See, for example, *Capturing the Snow Fortress* (1891) by Vasilii Surikov,

or two paintings from 1919 by Boris Kustodiev, *Shrovetide* and *Winter: Shrovetide Festivities*.
30 Martin, *Enlightened Metropolis*, 47.
31 Ian Hacking, *The Taming of Chance* (Cambridge: Cambridge University Press, 1990), 67.
32 On this climate theory of peoples and cultures, see for example Roberto M. Dainotto, *Europe (In Theory)* (Durham, NC: Duke University Press, 2007), 56–64.

PART ONE
Imperial Russia

CHAPTER TWO

Humoral bodies in cold climates

Matthew P. Romaniello

In 1781, Elizabeth Dimsdale, the wife of one of Catherine the Great's physicians, noted, "It is almost difficult for an Inhabitant of our temperate Climate, to have any Idea of a cold so great: it may perhaps give some Idea of it to say that when a person walks out in the severe Weather, the cold makes the Eyes water, and that water freezing, hangs in little Icicles on the Eye lashes." While the "Common Peasants" had the protection of their beards over the "Glands of the Throat," others, including the author, had to make due with inadequate clothing.[1] Dimsdale was not alone in her anxiety about the damaging effects of cold on the body. Later that decade, Dr. Matthew Guthrie, a Scottish doctor in Russian service, wrote to *Medical Commentaries* in Edinburgh with some concern that while several physicians "of late years pointed out the influence of hot climates on the human body, and its diseases; but few seem to have investigated the effects of cold." Based on his career in Russia, he suggested that the country provided ample grounds for study, with "the severity of the climate, and the dirty unwholesome mode of living of the common people of this empire, want of proper ventilation, &c." It was well known that Russians were "marked ... as victims to the scurvy and other putrid diseases." Scurvy was known to be a "cold" disease, linked to climate and poor diet, which needed to be treated with fresh vegetables that were difficult to procure in the long Russian winter. Guthrie further discussed the difficulties of using common medicines such as mercury and opium in the Russian climate, as the cold temperatures affected their power.[2] He urged his fellow doctors to take the matter seriously.

The cold was a great concern for the entire West European community living in Russia. Other travelers, diplomats, and merchants would echo the comments of Guthrie and Dimsdale throughout the eighteenth century. It was not just a consequence of feeling colder than at home, but a fear created by the knowledge that the environment could fundamentally alter the body's humors. Humoral theory allowed for frequent variation in individual bodies, even within the same region and climate, but each body was a specific combination of humors (in other words, one's "temperature, constitution, inclination, denomination, temperament, or complexion"), such that, as historian Mark S. Dawson remarked, "one could not hope to alter permanently the complexion with which one was born."[3] While much of Europe was temperate and its peoples were generally sanguine as a result, its northern reaches were cold and filled with phlegmatics. In the sixteenth or seventeenth century, the idea that living in a particular climate could transform your body was accepted widely. By the eighteenth, the idea of bodily transformation may have been viewed with suspicion, but there was no doubt that climate ultimately affected one's personal humoral balance, positively or negatively impacting health.[4] While historians have discussed the medical community's debate about the consequences of hot, colonial climates on the European constitution, the challenges of surviving a cold climate have not received as much attention.[5]

Foreigners arriving from milder climates in the eighteenth century risked their health and well-being in Russia's extreme cold, and the observations of this community provide insight into the Russian conception of both touch and skin, the study of which scholars have called "hapticity." Historian Mark M. Smith argued that hapticity "was a conduit for 'feeling' the plight of others," as understanding tactility provides a mechanism for interpreting both printed material and circulating ideas.[6] Hapticity pushes the field of touch beyond the study of pain and pleasure, which guided earlier investigations into the analysis of historical bodies.[7] Analyzing the body's reaction to foreign climates situates touch at the center of this growing field of study. In an article on colonial bodies in the New World, literary scholar Scott Manning Stevens concludes that observations of the body "exposed to the extremes of heat or cold does not call on us to visualize the body, so much as it requires us to imagine how the body would *feel* in such situations." Touch, in other words, "governs all human interactions with our environment."[8] This article complements these earlier studies of the Atlantic world by adding the Western experience in Russia in the eighteenth century, viewed through a lens of humoral theory, which was fundamental to the medical understanding of the world in the early modern era.

Humoral theory influenced attitudes toward health and the body, thereby affecting the resulting descriptions of pain and illness as well as those of the people of the Russian Empire. West Europeans such as Matthew Guthrie imported a humoral framework for understanding illness into Russia, and projected those ideas onto those they treated, as well as using its conclusions to explain their own health in an unfamiliar climate. While this humoral framework might not have been shared by Russians in the early modern era, Western medical training spread throughout the empire in the eighteenth century from St. Petersburg's medical school and the scientific explorations of the Russian Academy of Sciences.[9] Contextualizing foreign reactions to the ill effects of cold on the body might not uncover a universal experience of health, but it creates a window into some of the bodily sensations that Western visitors experienced in Russia.[10] For these visitors, feeling cold in Russia was not just an issue of low temperatures, but a persistent challenge to the health and well-being of a foreigner in an unfamiliar climate.

Cold bodies

Matthew Guthrie's letter to *Medical Commentaries* was a small addition to a larger eighteenth-century debate regarding the effects of climate on the body. While doctors were active in these discussions, the issue was no less important for any other traveler. It is not surprising that diplomatic correspondence and merchant memoirs are frequently filled with observations on health, both the authors' own and that of the community at large.[11] This information could be vital for physicians as these travelers were frequently the first to record colonial epidemics or experiences with new illnesses, but even the quotidian health issues that potentially affected travel, commercial exchanges, or diplomatic negotiations would be important information for an increasingly mobile society. Historian Mark Harrison suggested that it was necessary to include this information into the discussion of medical debates to challenge the preexisting hierarchies of scientific knowledge and its prejudiced reliance upon "authorities."[12] This is an important caveat, as popular notions of the humoral body would last in personal narratives after the medical community had moved beyond the humors. While a doctor writing in the early nineteenth century would find humoral ideas at odds with newer chemical or miasmatic theories, an educated diplomat might still rely on this "older" assessment to describe his health.[13]

Observations about the climate were not limited to the diplomatic corps in the eighteenth century, nor were concerns about health only about personal illnesses. Many travelers wrote memoirs and letters describing the population of the Russian Empire, and these records confirm the popularity of the belief that climate affected the humors. The physical body, national characteristics, the environment, climate, and lifestyles were all linked into a continuum of health and illness. Samuel Collins, a seventeenth-century English physician in the Russian court, argued that Russians could not escape the effects of venereal diseases, for example, because in "such a cold Countrey as this, she [venereal disease] earths like a Badger so deep, that there's no driving of her out without a Pickaxe or Firebrand."[14] The cold affected the very nature of the people, as Charles Whitworth, Britain's envoy extraordinary at the turn of the century, wrote:

> The Laplanders and Samoiedes are dispersed all along the large woods on the White and Ice seas; their stature is low, their figure very disagreeable,

their apprehension and understanding scarce above that of brutes, and their religion, if any at all, little understood by those who frequent them. Their food is generally raw fish, or whatever they kill or find dead.[15]

The persistent cold had left these Samoyeds in a lesser state of development. For a visitor from Britain such as Collins, Russia was a "humoral" empire spreading from the Baltic Sea to the Pacific Ocean.

These views were hardly limited to British visitors. Eberhard Isbrand Ides, a Dane in Russian service, reflected these attitudes as well. In his account of Peter the Great's first embassy to China in the 1690s, he portrayed several groups of Siberians in a humoral framework. The Ostiaks, for example, compounded the difficulties of a cold climate by living on a diet of river fish, leaving them phlegmatic, and notably feminine. He described them as "all of a middle Stature, most of them Yellowish or Red haired; and their Faces and Noses disagreeably broad; they are weak and unable to labour hard, not at all enclined to Warrs, and utterly uncapable of Military Exercises."[16]

Throughout the eighteenth century, travelers consistently recorded the prevalence of scurvy in Russia. A cold and moist climate produced the disease, making the empire one of its most likely environs. Georg Wilhelm Steller, the German botanist on the Second Kamchatka Expedition (1733–43), for example, described scurvy as a recurring epidemic in Kamchatka, because of "the constant wetness and thick ground fog," but noted that the disease "actually bothers only the new arrivals on Kamchatka," as the locals had developed a diet designed to prevent the disease.[17] The naturalist on the expedition, Johann Georg Gmelin, recorded the struggles of the disease's victims on the expedition. He wrote that "the symptoms of scurvy were pains residing in places where we had injuries or abscesses, fatigue accompanied by extraordinary slumber, swelling of the feet on which appeared here and there blue spots, a violent sneezing which caused an incredible pain in the kidneys, sore teeth, foul breath, swelling throughout the body accompanied by an unquenchable thirst, a dry cough, and a kind of constipation, the effects of which lasted two or three weeks, and the most powerful purgatives were without effect."[18] The cure he outlines was one that would have been familiar to many, avoiding excessive cold, taking in as much fresh air as possible to "drive out the harmful vapors," and hard work. In fact, more than four hours of sleep a day was to be avoided.[19] As even the Russians on the expedition suffered from this "cold" disease, a fear rose that no one could be fully adapted to the extreme temperatures of Siberia, endangering the health of everyone in the empire.

When the Russian Academy of Sciences set out to categorize the peoples of the empire during the reign of Catherine the Great, the health and well-being of the crown's subjects, and their humoral temperament, were a great concern. Johann Gottlieb Georgi's multivolume *Russia: Or A Compleat Historical Account of All of the Nations which Compose that Empire* (1780–3) described each group in accordance with a continuum of health:

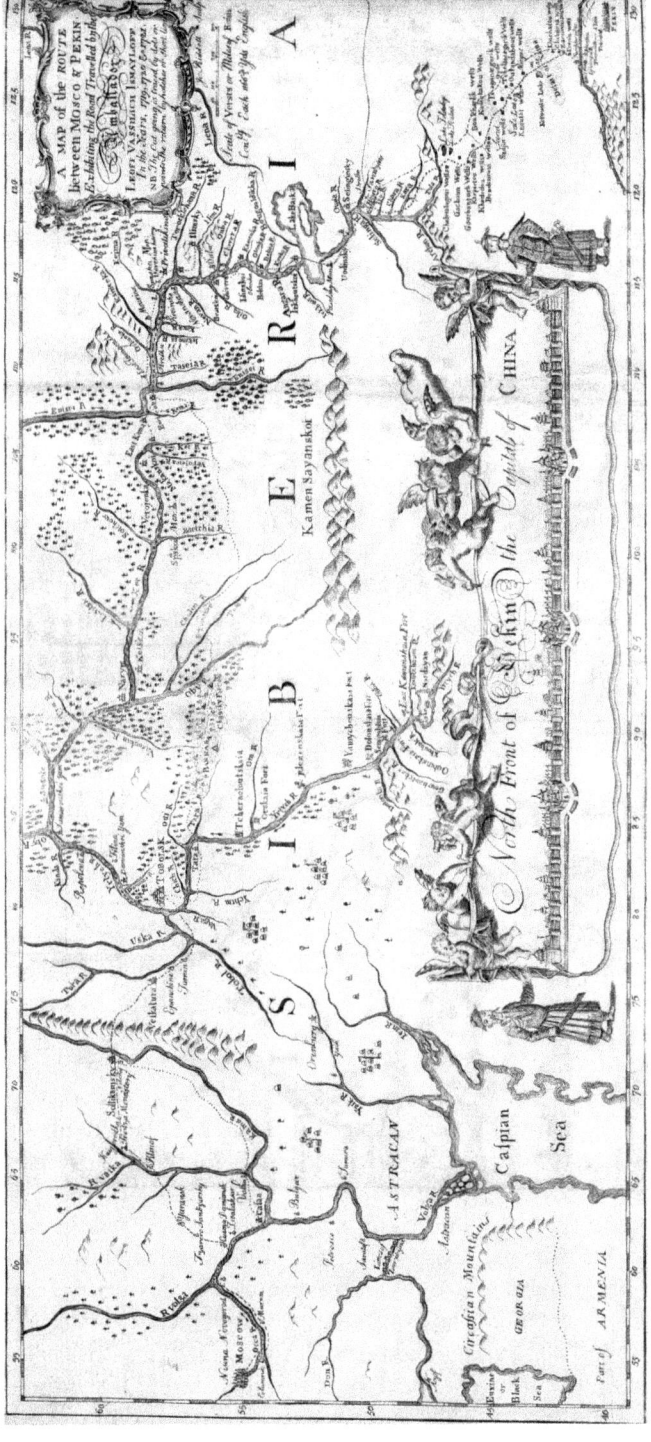

FIGURE 2.1 "A map of the route to Mosco & Pekin," from John Bell, Travels from St. Petersburg in Russia to divers parts of Asia (1763). Courtesy Archives and Manuscript Department, University of Hawaiʻi at Mānoa.

a physical description of the typical man and woman; an examination of their lifestyles and occupations; clothing and customs (with a particular focus on marriage and childbirth); health and illness; and food, climate, and temperament. With few exceptions, the people of the empire were generally classified as phlegmatic or melancholic, the "cold" constitutions. A cold constitution was a challenge for the future of any state, as its subjects would be sexually frigid, if not infertile. The Estonians, for example, were "of a phlegmatic and melancholic disposition. Except life itself, and the pleasures of love, every thing in the world is indifferent to them." Primarily, he concluded, the phlegmatic nature made them "idle, filthy, and addicted to drunkenness."[20]

Few in the empire fared better. The Ostiaks of the Ob River valley "have a flattish face of a pale yellow colour, a thin beard, a dull understanding, and a phlegmatic temperament; consequently, they are timorous, superstitious, and lazy, dirty, and disgusting; but tractable, mild, and good-hearted people." Ostiak girls were "far from being ugly," but "Ostiak women after the birth of their first child become wrinkled and ugly."[21] The "Barabintzes," a Turkic group living on the Baraba steppe south of Ufa, were "almost all of them of a phlegmatic habit, with a pale complexion, to which natural dullness may be added to their poverty and want of instruction." This was the result of "the air of Baraba during the summer [which] is continually charged with vapour." The poor climate of Baraba was such that they were "cold even in their amours, and rarely drink to intoxication."[22] Georgi presented ample evidence that the cold climate, and frequent damp conditions, had produced people of a weak temperament.

It was only along the southern edges of the empire that nature produced more active men and women. The "warm climate" of the Caucasus featured people who engaged in commerce, and those in agriculture produced crops for the market.[23] The Kalmyks were "a mixture of sanguine and phlegmatic, the melancholy is seldom uppermost. They have a good understanding, and a quick comprehension, ... [are] sprightly, hospitable, ready to do kind offices, active and voluptuous."[24] As a result of their healthy temperament, they knew "but little of sickness."[25] The Bukharans enjoyed a "fine climate," and were "cheerful and gay," though this was also the result of their preference for swallowing small cakes made of a mixture of flour, milk, and "hemp flowers." The warm climate also enabled men to be "tolerably at ease [with] two wives,"[26] a notable difference from a group like the Barabintzes, whose phlegmatic traits left them uninterested in sex.

Georgi's general typology of the empire divided it into two distinct types: phlegmatic and melancholic people living throughout most of the state, with a few choleric and sanguine groups in the south. The divide was less clear in the far east. The Tungus, for example, were of a "very sanguine constitution, frank, and always appear to be what they really are. ... They feel no disquietude about the morrow, but chearfully divide the last morsel with the first comer, and the gaiety of the conversation is never diminished by the indigence of the host."²⁷ Their sanguine temperament was not without its flaws, of course, as they could fly into a "rage" over "the merest trifles."²⁸ Despite their hot qualities, the Tungus were located the furthest north of any group identified as sanguine, though living along the coast of the Pacific did produce a different environment than in western or central Siberia. The Buriats were another unusual group; the only one to be classified as both "the sanguine and the phlegmatic."²⁹ This could reflect their position between the Russian Empire and China, producing a mixed quality not seen in the empire at large. Another possibility is that since Georgi did not travel to the far eastern regions of the empire before writing his text, his reliance on earlier texts to classify this group could have created a dissonance from his otherwise distinct separation of humors and climates within the empire.

Nor was Georgi alone in casting a humoral eye over the subjects of the Russian crown. Another was Peter Simon Pallas, a German botanist with Western medical training, who became a professor at the Academy in 1768, and would remain in Russia until the nineteenth century. Following a scientific expedition to Siberia, he published his own multivolume description of the empire, situating its plants and animals within a context of its peoples and their environment.³⁰ Pallas and Georgi traveled together on his first expedition, facilitating a shared view of the effect of the humors on the body. At the southern edge of the empire, for example, Pallas was a great admirer of the Kalmyks, whom he described "as affable, hospitable and honest; they like to render service; they are always cheerful and gay, which distinguishes them from the Kirghiz [of Siberia], who are phlegmatic." However, as nomads, the Kalmyks did have some weaknesses, particularly "uncleanliness, which arose from their lack of education."³¹ Pallas later provided ample evidence of the Kirghizes' phlegmatic nature, as he observed that they commonly suffered from colds, asthma, heart palpitations, and venereal disease, all linked to coldness. He also mentioned that there was no evidence that the Kirghiz suffered from fevers, though this was a common problem among the "warmer" Kalmyks.³²

A humoral assessment of the Russian Empire was not limited to those Westerners working for the Academy of Sciences, as these attitudes were reflected among most visitors to the country. The British diplomat William Richardson, for example, described the Russians in 1768 as "tall, robust, and well-proportioned; their teeth are remarkably good; their hair is in general black, and their complexions ruddy. I have scarcely seen any red-haired persons among them; and those who are fair, are not so good-looking as those who are dark-complexioned."³³ Hair color and complexion are both physical manifestations of the humors. Red hair signified sanguinity hence its rare appearance among the Russians; a "dark complexion" revealed a melancholy temperament. In other words, Richardson described the Russians as phlegmatic and melancholic, as did the later Germanic scholars. Matthew Guthrie might have been the first doctor to request an investigation of the effects of cold on the body, but throughout the century there was ample evidence that Russia's cold climate had permanently affected the development of all of the people within its borders. If Russia's extreme climate was dangerous for its own population, as seen in the prevalence of scurvy, it could only be that much more deadly for a foreigner ill-suited to its temperature.

Experiencing cold

West Europeans suffered from ill health in Russia before the eighteenth century, but the focus shifted to a concern about the consequences of Russia's climate upon the body by the reign of Peter the Great (1682–1725). Britain's diplomatic corps, who maintained a permanent office in Russia after 1700, believed the cold was the primary reason for their persistently poor health. Charles Whitworth, the British envoy to Moscow from 1705 to 1710, was the first to connect the cold to his health, but he would hardly be the last. In 1708, he wrote to the Duke of Marlborough, then one of the foreign secretaries, that he had "for many Months desired leave to return home," because "in this cold Climate I have but an indifferent state of health."[34] Both Whitworth and Charles Goodfellow, the British consul in residence at the same time, purchased crates of fresh lemons and oranges throughout their stay in Russia at significant expense.[35] While it might have been a simple desire for a luxury food, citrus fruits were known to offset the humoral imbalance of a head cold in this period, and it is reasonable to conclude that these men sought whatever remedies were available for surviving life in Russia.

The relocation of the Russian court to the new capital of St. Petersburg only added new difficulties alongside the unbearable climate. In 1715, George Mackenzie, the new British resident, reported to the foreign secretary the devastating effects of St. Petersburg on newly-arrived British sailors. These sailors had been drinking river water, which was "at best known to be unwholesome, it being of a black mossy colour," that sadly had caused the sailors to catch "this distemper, which it ordinarily occasioned of a bloody Flux, and the others are brought down so to the day of squellets, that would move any to compassion."[36]

The inauspicious arrival in St. Petersburg only began a century of discontent in Russia's capital. The cold remained the British bane, producing persistent requests for dismissal by Britain's diplomatic corps. Some of its merchants seemed more adaptable. John Bell, for example, a Scottish doctor turned Russian merchant who spent considerable time in Russia from 1715 until the 1740s, successfully used some of the local cures for the cold in his travels around the country. When suffering from his "face, fingers and toes frozen," he "applied the common cure, that is, rubbing the numbed parts with snow, which [he] found perfectly effectual."[37]

Bell's friend, the consul Claudius Rondeau, would not be as fortunate when he fell ill, "by a great cold, which we often get in this hard climate" in September 1739.[38] Rondeau died within a week of writing that letter, becoming the second consul in succession to die in office.[39] His illness was quite painful, according to an account provided by his nephew. It began with "a Diarrhea that lasted thirteen Days, and then suddenly turned to a nervous feavour and defluxion upon his Breast with a continual delirium until his Death."[40] Undoubtedly the nephew's graphic depiction would have made an impression upon the foreign secretary, if not future diplomats, which might have inspired the significant increase in complaints about Russia's cold climate that followed. It is worth noting, however, that Rondeau had been a very long resident of St. Petersburg, serving the crown for more than a decade in Russia following a long career in diplomatic service across Europe. Though his symptoms may at first appear similar to those of the newly-arrived sailors from more than a decade earlier, his body would likely have been adapted to local conditions before his abrupt death.

Rondeau was the second consecutive envoy to die in office. As a result, it was not surprising that later diplomats reported on the state of their health, regularly citing the cold climate as the cause of ill health. Few would make more consistent use of this narrative than Edward Finch, the ambassador in the early 1740s. Complaints of his poor health quickly became a recurring motif in Finch's letters. For example, on September 17, 1740, he wrote to Lord Harrington, the foreign secretary, that he was "not having been in a Condition to stir out of my Room by the Continuation of my Cold, & a feaverish Indisposition, accompany with a great Oppression upon my Breast, shortness of Breath, a Lassitude all over my Body, & a great lowness of spirits, all which have greatly increased my old Pain in my Side."[41] The following week, Finch let his own blood, "with a very good effect, having found [his] head greatly relieved," though it would only prove a temporary solution.[42] In December, he once again suffered "a Cold accompanied with a feaverish Disorder, violent Headach, & a very sever return of my old pain in my side [which] have confined me to my bed."[43] By the following March, Finch concluded that there was no doubt that Russia itself was the cause of his ongoing illness. St. Petersburg was "much severer Cold than we felt in England," which occasioned "so violent a return of my old Pain in my Side that I was not in a Condition to draw a Dispatch."[44]

As the cold led to persistent illness, which prevented him from serving the king, Finch proposed his only reasonable solution: his departure from Russia. If he could have continued to serve the king, he was willing to set aside his own "private Happiness & Satisfaction," but he suggested that was no longer possible. He requested the foreign secretary allow him leave to return home, "& to take Aix la Chappelle & the Spas in my Way, that I may use the Baths of the first, & drink the Waters of the Past, as the only means which according to the unanimous Opinion of my Physician here & those who have been consulted in England, can possibly remove that pain in my Side." It was a desperate request, as the pain "at least become too violent not to make Me very uneasy with the Prospect of growing every day more miserable, & of a total Incapacity of doing the King's business." He suggested permission be granted immediately, "early enough for Me not to lose the Season of Aix and the Spaw; since a Summer Journey will be infinitely more commodious."[45] His request was successful, if not on his timetable. In late June, he received permission to leave when he concluded a treaty negotiation, as the foreign secretary sympathized with the "ill Health" he labored under "in that Climate."[46] In the fall, Finch departed with plans for stopping in Aix la Chapelle, Bath, and Bristol, writing that he did not expect "a long life" but only a healthier one.[47]

Finch's departure from Russia did not end the objections to the climate. His successor in St. Petersburg, Sir Cyril Wiche, wrote similar complaints throughout his short stay in the post. In July 1743, for example, he protested to the current foreign secretary, John Carteret, that his "Constitution is very much weakened since I have been in this Country, Upon my arrival last summer at Moscow I fell sick, and was above three Months before I recovered." Sadly, the return to Petersburg only made the situation worse, as he "was taken with a violent Fever and Jaundice, which had like to have killed me." However, he remained "very willing to sacrifice in His Majesty's Service," which did set him apart from his predecessor, at least for a short while.[48] By the fall, however, Wiche felt he could no longer bear the climate, as "the Air does not at all agree with my Constitution," and he hoped "at a proper Time" the foreign secretary would "employ him in a more temperate Climate."[49]

Wiche was replaced in office by Lord Tyrawley the following spring. Tyrawley only lasted three months before he requested his recall from St. Petersburg because of its climate. Following the court to Moscow in the summer of 1744, he was "extremely out of order, occasioned by a violent cold," caught by spending three nights at "Balls, Masquerades, Operas, &c." The entertainments unfortunately had been "so excessively hot" followed by being "so exteme chill'd going home" that it had "almost destroyed" Tyrawly. He opined that such a result should have been expected, as he had "never been one day well" since arriving, as the climate did not agree with his constitution at his "advanced stage of life after spending the largest part of it in the soft Climates of Spain and Portugal."[50] Either Tyrawly was more convincing than his predecessors, or his title justified quicker action, for he was recalled soon thereafter, when the foreign secretary agreed that it was necessary to act "upon account of the Increase of Indispositions occasioned by the coldness of that Climate."[51]

By the end of the decade, the Foreign Office should not have been surprised that the protests resumed, this time from the new envoy, John Carmichael, the Earl of Hyndford. He was in court for nearly a year before requesting the right to leave for the spas in Germany. He hoped to be relieved of his office early enough to reach his destination before the season was over to avoid "the great Detriment to my health."⁵² The long delay in receiving permission caused a minor crisis for Hyndford, who not only missed the spa season but also was prevented by his illness from attendance at court. When questioned by the Russian minister, Aleksei Petrovich Bestuzhev, why he desired such a rapid departure from the court, Hyndford could not help but reveal that it was "on account of his Health," revealing that his hands were "full of Scurvy Spots," making it a necessity to take fresh air and the mineral waters of the German spas.⁵³

Following Hyndford, there was no doubt that ill health continued to plague the British diplomatic corps, even if few would turn as often to the climate as the primary cause. One of the last to do so was Sir Charles Hanbury Williams, who suffered from various ailments while in St. Petersburg, where "his Phisicians" informed him that he "cannot support this Climate."⁵⁴ When he was released from office, his departure was derailed outside of Petersburg by "a violent Fever," which was only mitigated by "bleeding and other Medecines," forcing him to forgo a land journey out of the country for a quicker trip by ship across the Baltic.⁵⁵ However, Hanbury Williams' successor, Robert Keith, marked a new era, in which Russia's cold was not identified as the cause of the Britons' poor health. Keith even served in Petersburg for nearly four years, longer than several of his predecessors. He did have to request permission to leave office as his service in Russia was longer than the two or three years he expected, but his request was inspired by his realization that he had not been "of any use to his Majesty's service." He did admit, that "The Consideration of Health is likewise of some Weight," because "two attacks of a Fever" the previous winter made him "dread the approach of that Season."⁵⁶

Keith was followed into office by James Harris, the Earl of Malmesbury. Harris resided in Petersburg for a few years with his new wife and his sister, Katherine Gertrude Harris. Katherine kept a journal of her daily activities throughout her life in Russia, recording varied experiences in the city. While shopping and dining may have been the most common subjects, health and illness were not ignored. On March 22, 1778, for example, her sister-in-law Harriet "was confined with a cold," which was treated the following day with a bloodletting.⁵⁷ In the following August, Harriet was "beginning to be ill," suffering "in much pain the whole day & night & was not deliver'd till a quarter after six … of a boy."⁵⁸ Her matter-of-fact style applied to her own condition as well, reporting in July that while her brother and his wife dined with Count Panin, she stayed at home and "took a vomit."⁵⁹ Katherine's lack of complaint about the cold climate was shared in fact with her brother, who requested and received the right to depart from office without complaints of his health or that of his family.⁶⁰

The Harris family, however, appear to be a unique group among the foreigners in Russia. Most foreigners, particularly the diplomats, had ample evidence of the difficulties created by adjusting to an unfamiliar climate. The requests for duty in warmer climates or a recuperative season at a European spa were requests for humoral balance as much as more congenial posts. The diplomats clearly believed that a cold climate was as dangerous for the humors as a hot climate, even if the Foreign Office may have remained more suspicious.

Treating cold

By the end of the eighteenth century, multiple observers had classified the Russian Empire as a humoral space. Its people were primarily phlegmatic and choleric, "cold" characteristics, reflecting the overall climate. West Europeans, adapted to warmer climates, faced danger in Russia as their experience of living in a cold place rendered them vulnerable to numerous illnesses. In other words, Russia "felt" unhealthy to its foreign residents. While British diplomats requested more temperate posts, residents of Russia had developed their own treatments to mitigate the effects of a cold climate. The most common "cure" was the Russian preference for regular trips to the bania (a Russian bathhouse) to experience the extreme heat. Over the course of the eighteenth century, foreign interest in the bania rose as fears of the cold climate increased, but most foreigners discovered that just like the Russians' native environment, the bania was a treatment best suited to locals.

One of the earliest mentions of the bania was made by Peter Henry Bruce in his memoir of serving in Peter the Great's army in the 1710s. Though his memoir was published later in the century, his comments could serve as a model for all Western reminiscences about the bania:

> [Russians] bathe frequently: people of quality have their own private ones, and bathe twice a week at least; but the public bathing-places are all built near the sides of the rivers. Their stoves are close places with furnaces, which they heat exceedingly, and for the better raising of vapour, frequently throw cold water on the stove: there are benches all round, at some distance, one above another, differing in the degrees of heat, so that every one chooses the temperature that best suits him: upon one of those benches they lay themselves down at full length, quite naked, and having sweated as long as they think proper, they are well washed with warm water, and well rubbed with handfuls of herbs; after which they take a dram of aqua vitae, and go their ways.[61]

According to Bruce, the bath was a necessity, chief among "the universal remedies of the Muscovites, whether for cleanliness of health." As a result, "from their infancy" all Russians were "accustomed to the extremes of heat and cold." Proof of this observation was easy to provide, as men and women who found the heat too intolerable would run out naked and plunge into the nearby river, or, in the winter, roll around in the snow. This had an undoubted positive result. Russians were "stout and hardy, and in general long-lived"; they were "little subject to any distemper" and most of them were "without diseases."[62] While the effectiveness of the baths in terms of enabling Russian well-being was not in doubt, Bruce did raise questions about the morality of the bathhouse, a recurring theme throughout the century:

> These public baths are so carelessly built, that it is an easy matter to see the people in the next room through the aperture of the boards which divide them, which, to the women who frequent them, is of no great consequence, as they are not nicely delicate in being seen naked; both sexes going out and coming in at the same door naked, when they want to cool themselves.[63]

Bruce's judgment on the inappropriate nature of the bania was shared by many of the other foreigners in Russia. During the period of Bruce's service in Russia, a noblewoman committed suicide in a St. Petersburg bania by throwing herself on the coals, which was recorded as a tragedy by the current British envoy, James Jeffreys, because "she pass'd for one of the beautiful ladyes of Russia."[64] Foreign descriptions and images frequently presented the bania as a sexualized arena, or at least one known as an epicenter for scandal.[65]

Despite the suggestion that West Europeans had best avoid such a notorious place, the bania was presented as a necessity for a Russian's health. Alexander Gordon, a Scot in Russian service, believed that before the recent arrival of Western physicians, all the Russians had to support their health was the use of "cold and hot" baths. Hot baths could cure "all their distempers," while cold baths "they only use for achs and rheumatic pains." However, this cold cure was only used directly after sitting in a hot bath. Gordon added that "physicians approved" of these cures, and that this led to Russians living "to a great age, many of them above a hundred years; though temperance is by no means characteristic of the nation."[66]

Bruce and Gordon were among the first Westerners to connect the bania and Russian health, but it became a popular topic among most visitors to the country. Not all of these assessments were positive. L'Abbé Chappe d'Auteroche traveled to Russia in 1761, and wrote a highly critical account of the country, suggesting at one point that as the Russians lacked physicians and surgeons, they could only rely on the bania for "any remedy."[67] The French consul Marbault was a long-term resident in St. Petersburg in the 1750s and 1760s. In his later account of Russia, he suggested that "there was no country where women were more fertile than in Russia" but the harsh environment prevented them from fulfilling their natal destinies. For Marbault, Russia's "excessive cold," combined with poor food quality, damaged both mothers and children, which the bania could not fix.[68]

Few foreigners, however, were as critical. Marbault's countryman, Pierre Nicolas Chantreau, believed Russians' capacity to adjust to extreme temperature changes was an asset. He wrote that their ability "to pass suddenly from excessive heat, extreme cold, when they bathe" produced "the strength of the Russian temperament." For Chantreau, the bania was "the sovereign cure… for all kinds of diseases."[69] An English contemporary of Chantreau, John Richard, also believed Russians' ability to adapt to the extreme temperature changes of the bania was a benefit for them, though he was unique in his assessment that the bania was a result of "tenets of the Greek Church."[70]

Certainly by the end of the century there was a sentiment among the foreigners that Russians had adapted to extreme temperatures from the bania's heat to the climate's cold, and that as a result, there was no doubt that there was an intrinsic difference between Russians and Westerners, emerging from their tolerance of temperature. This observation became a commonplace in references to the Russian constitution. When Samuel Bentham, in his role as director of Siberian mines, toured the countryside, he assumed that his brother would understand that he and his servants were incapable of sleeping in similar conditions, due not to status but to temperature. At several points his servants left him to seek their own accommodations, reminding his brother, "You must understand that Russian peasants are used to sleep in a degree of heat which would be very disagreeable to those who were not accustomed to it."[71]

Bentham reflected a point at which it became accepted knowledge that Russians' were physically different than other Europeans. Medical treatments, therefore, had to adjust to both the environment and the bodies of their Russian patients. John Parkinson, for example, was an English doctor in Catherine the Great's court. His published remarks on Russia argued that the country's cold climate, coupled with a poor diet produced by a short growing season, created a tendency toward scurvy, the classic "cold" disease, among the entire population.[72] Russia's environment challenged accepted medical practices, particularly in treating venereal disease, because mercury failed to produce "the desired effect from the coldness of the climate." Mercury only became effective if the patient was "put into a warm bath."[73] Using heat to offset the cold was a key to this sort of specific treatment, but also their general well-being, as the Russians relied upon the heat of the bania to create an internal balance.[74]

With so much emphasis placed on the integral role of extreme heat for Russian health, it is remarkable that more foreigners did not experiment with the application of heat as the easiest solution for the cold weather. Katherine Harris was once again an exception, having no hesitation on visiting the bania for herself as an essential part of Russian entertainments in the capital. In March 1779, after dining with friends, Katherine went to the bath at Madame Talisin's, and stayed in the heat for twenty minutes. She "did not find the heat so excessive" as she expected, even moving "to the tops & did not perspire for some time, even when the water was thrown on the hot stones which excused a steam that I took at first for perspiration." She did finally perspire, but only after taking a cup of tea after leaving the bath.[75]

While Katherine's reportage fits consistently with her entire assessment of life in Russia, free from humoral fears of cold weather, she remains alone in this position. Far more typical of the foreign community was the Guthrie family. Matthew Guthrie was the Scottish doctor whose comments on a cold climate began this article. His wife, Maria, also recorded her extensive experiences in Russia, which were later published as a travel narrative. She included a thorough depiction of the bania, but not from her own experiences, but rather those of "a Gentleman who went through the whole on purpose narrowly to inspect the inside of the building." She was clear that the bania was dangerous, as she needed to avoid "filling her lungs with the hot aqueous vapour that you are required to respire in the Russian bath … and which is terribly suffocating to a stranger not accustomed to its use like the natives, who, from habit, seem to breathe in water with as much ease as fish."[76] With such an attitude toward the bania, it is not surprising that foreigners failed to pursue the bania's heat as a viable solution to offsetting Russia's dangerous cold.

Conclusion

Over the course of the eighteenth century, a belief in the descriptive power of the humors persisted among Western visitors to Russia, but the connection between the climate and its effect on the body's humors diminished. As the cultural framework for explaining the cold changed, so too did the foreign explanation of the way that the Russian Empire felt upon entering its borders. Feeling cold was no longer the primary explanation for poor health. William Tooke, for example, was a British resident of St. Petersburg in the 1790s, and the translator for Georgi's work into English. When he published his own assessment of the empire, he drew upon Georgi's narrative framework for constructing his own typology of imperial subjects. Unlike Georgi or Pallas, or doctors like Guthrie, he was more critical of the connection between the climate and the humors. Tooke addressed the cold's effect on health at the beginning of his first volume: "Whether the cold be the occasion of certain epidemical diseases, must be left undecided. It may perhaps have been observed in some districts, but never authentically."[77] Furthermore, "one sure proof that in general the climate is not prejudicial to health is the great number of persons that in all these parts attain to a very advanced old age."[78]

While Tooke was dismissive of the probability that the temperature had an effect on the body, he retained a fully articulated belief in the effects of the humors on the body. In the second volume, he began his description of the peoples of the empire by mentioning that "the bodily state of the people is dependent on a thousand things; nature of the soil, climate, weather; way of life, dress, food; manners and usages, even political constitution and religion have a decisive influence on the strength, the durability, the health, in short, the whole physical character of mankind."[79] The Russians were "mostly of a sanguine choleric temperament, and vice versa, with a greater or less mixture of the phlegmatic, seldom of the phlegmatic, still seldomer merely melancholic or phlegmatic; in gait and action they are brisk, lively, and agile."[80] His impressions of the Russians overall were positive, perhaps leading him to be one of the first ever to suggest the Russians were sanguine, as throughout the previous century they clearly had been phlegmatic. Tooke would continue to praise the Russians, who "are endowed with a vitality, of which an instance has scarcely ever yet been found in any other country."[81] The cold was only mentioned in context of the confusion created by "the early maturity of girls," which, could "only to be accounted for, in so cold a climate, by the frequent use of hot bath."[82]

Tooke's work at the beginning of the nineteenth century marks the beginning of an era that would be more critical of the influence of the humors on the body.[83] Throughout the eighteenth century, humoral theory was alive and well among West European diplomats and doctors, creating a rhetorical construct through which they perceived issues of health and illness. The bodies of Russian imperial subjects were innately adapted to their environment, and the bodies of foreign visitors were not, leading inevitably toward illness as the foreigners struggled with Russia's extreme temperatures. While exceptional figures such as Katherine Harris rejected the humoral explanations of changes to her body, she was hardly typical of most visitors from the West. For them, a season in Russia's cold was a danger to their health and well-being, and only a departure from the country could lead to their recovery.

Humoral descriptions of the environment provided foreigners in Russia with one tool for understanding the influence of the climate upon their body. Men such as Matthew Guthrie or Edward Finch felt Russia upon their skin, and expressed these sensations by utilizing familiar ideas and concepts that could translate their experiences across the Baltic Sea to Western Europe. Russia's cold climate, therefore, was not only a physical reality but also a cultural construct employed in correspondence, diaries, and scientific expeditions. This observation was not limited to the sensory experience of the climate as it was clearly paralleled in struggles to define Russia's national tastes as discussed in Alison Smith's work or a the smell of its cities as in Alexander Martin's.[84] Feeling cold in eighteenth-century Russia was one problem; making those feelings convincing to someone who had never experienced that sensation was another.

Notes

1. A. G. Cross, ed., *An English Lady at the Court of Catherine the Great: The Journal of Baroness Elizabeth Dimsdale, 1781* (Cambridge: Crest Publications, 1989), 78.
2. Matthew Guthrie, "A Letter from Dr Matthew Gurthrie Physician at St. Petersburgh to Dr Duncan, on the Effects of a cold Climate on the Land Scurvy, &c.," in *Medical Commentaries for the Year 1787*, vol. II (Edinburgh: C. Elliot, T. Kay and Co., 1788), 328–38.
3. Mark S. Dawson, "Humouring Racial Encounters in the Anglo-Atlantic, c. 1580–1720," in *Old Worlds, New Worlds: European Cultural Encounters, c. 1000–c. 1750*, ed. Lisa Bailey, Lindsay Digglemann, and Kim M. Phillips (Turnhout, Belgium: Brepols, 2009), 139–61, here 146–7.
4. Karen Ordahl Kupperman argued that the link between climate and disease had "become axiomatic" by the eighteenth century. See her "Fear of Hot Climates in the Anglo-American Colonial Experience," *The William and Mary Quarterly*, Third Series 41 (2) (1984): 213–40. In addition, see Joyce E. Chaplin, "Natural Philosophy and an Early Racial Idiom in North America: Comparing English and Indian Bodies," *The William and Mary Quarterly*, Third Series 54 (1997): 229–52; Mark Harrison, *Climates and Constitutions: Health, Race, Environment and British Imperialism in India, 1600–1850* (New York: Oxford University Press, 1999), esp. Chapter 1; Rebecca Earle, *The Body of the Conquistador: Food, Race and the Colonial Experience in Spanish America, 1492–1700* (Cambridge: Cambridge University Press, 2012), esp. 26–30.
5. This debate reached a peak in the middle of the century. See Mark Harrison, *Medicine in an Age of Commerce and Empire: Britain and its Tropical Colonies, 1660–1830* (New York: Oxford University Press, 2010), Chapter 3.
6. Mark M. Smith, "Getting in Touch with Slavery and Freedom," *The Journal of American History* 95 (2) (2008): 381–91, here 382–3.
7. Esther Cohen, "Towards a History of European Physical Sensibility: Pain in the Later Middle Ages," *Science in Context* 8 (1995): 47–74; Robert Jütte, "The Social Construction of Illness in the Early Modern Period," in *The Social Construction of Illness: Illness and Medical Knowledge in Past and Present*, ed. Jens Lachmund and Gunnar Stollberg (Stuttgart: Franz Steiner Verlag, 1991), 23–38.
8. Scott Manning Stevens, "New World Contacts and the Trope of the 'Naked Savage'," in *Sensible Flesh: On Touch in Early Modern Culture*, ed. Elizabeth D. Harvey (Philadelphia: University of Pennsylvania Press, 2003), 125–40, here 135.
9. For a discussion of this transition, see Mirko Grmek, "The History of Medical Education in Russia," in *The History of Medical Education*, ed. C. D. O'Malley (Berkeley: University of California Press, 1970), 303–27.
10. For an introduction to the history of the senses and medicine, see W. F. Bynum and Roy Porter, eds., *Medicine and the Five Senses* (Cambridge:

Cambridge, 1993), and Elizabeth D. Harvey, "Introduction: The 'Sense of All Senses'," in *Sensible Flesh: On Touch in Early Modern Culture*, ed. Elizabeth D. Harvey (Philadelphia: University of Pennsylvania Press, 2003), 1–21.

11 There are numerous biographical and prosopographical works on Western travelers to Russia. Among these are Roger P. Barlett, *Human Capital: The Settlement of Foreigners in Russia 1762–1804* (Cambridge: Cambridge University Press, 1979); Anthony Cross, *By the Banks of the Neva: Chapters from the Lives and Careers of the British in Eighteenth-Century Russia* (Cambridge: Cambridge University Press, 1997); Rebecca Wills, *The Jacobites in Russia, 1715–1750* (East Linton, Scotland: Tuckwell, 2002).

12 Harrison, *Medicine in an Age of Commerce*, 11. Kapil Raj similarly argued for expanding the examination of knowledge networks in his *Relocating Modern Science: Circulation and the Construction of Knowledge in South Asia and Europe, 1650–1900* (Basingstoke: Palgrave, 2007). For an example of this methodology in practice, see Katherine Arner, "Making Global Commerce into Health Diplomacy: Consuls and Commercial Agents in the Age of Atlantic Revolution," *The Journal of World History* 24 (4) (2013): 771–96.

13 For the newer theories, see chapters on miasmata and germ theory in W. F. Bynum and Roy Porter, eds., *Companion Encyclopedia of the History of Medicine*, vol. 1 (London: Routledge, 1993), 292–334.

14 Samuel Collins, *The Present State of Russia* (London: John Winter, 1671), 65.

15 Charles Whitworth, *An Account of Russia as it was in the year 1710* (Strawberry Hill, 1758), 6–7.

16 E. Ysbrant Ides, *Three Years Travels from Moscow over-land to China* (London, 1705), 20.

17 Georg Wilhelm Steller, *Steller's History of Kamchatka: Collected Information Concerning the History of Kamchatka, Its Peoples, Their Manners, Names, Lifestyle, and Various Customary Practices*, ed. Marvin W. Falk, trans. Margritt Engel and Karen Willmore (Fairbanks: University of Alaska Press, 2003), 47.

18 Johann George Gmelin, *Voyage en Sibérie*, 2 vols (Paris: Desaint, 1767), I, 364.

19 Ibid., I, 365–7.

20 Johann Gottlieb Georgi, *Russia: Or, A Compleat Historical Account of All the Nations which Compose that Empire*, trans. William Tooke, 4 vols (London: 1780–3), I: 54.

21 Ibid., I: 178.

22 Ibid., II: 228.

23 Ibid., II: 115.

24 Ibid., IV: 22.

25 Ibid., IV: 39.

26 Ibid., II: 144–5.

27 Ibid., III: 78

28 Ibid., III: 80.
29 Ibid., IV: 132.
30 The original German edition was *Reise durch verschiedene Provinzen des Russischen Reichs*, published in three volumes between 1771–6. The following quotations are taken from the French translation, Peter Simon Pallas, *Voyages de M. P. S. Pallas, en différentes provinces de l'empire de Russie, et dans l'Asie septentrionale*, trans. Gauthier de la Peyronie, 5 vols. (Paris: Maradan, 1788–93), which included the text of his second expedition following the first.
31 Pallas, *Voyages*, I: 499.
32 Ibid., I: 629.
33 William Richardson, *Anecdotes of the Russian Empire in a Series of Letters* (London: W. Straha and T. Cadell, 1783), 201.
34 The British Library (BL), Additional Manuscripts 61149, Blenheim Papers, vol. XLIX, "Whitworth to the Duke of Marlborough," March 10/21, 1708, 54v.
35 BL, Additional Manuscripts 37,354, Whitworth Papers, vol. VIII, f. 317r, Memo from Goodfellow, July 8, 1705; BL, Add. MS. 37,355, Whitworth Papers, Vol. VIII, ff. 306–7, Memo to Whitworth, 1706; BL, Add. MS. 37,356, Whitworth Papers, Vol. IX, ff. 16r., Memo to Whitworth.
36 The National Archives, Kew, Great Britain (TNA), SP 91/8, "Mackenzie to Foreign Secretary," January 24, 1715, ff. 140–1; here 140v.
37 John Bell, *Travels from St. Petersburg in Russia to Diverse Parts of Asia*, 2 vols (Glasgow: John Bell and Robert and Andrew Foulis, 1763), I: 23–4.
38 TNA, SP 91/23, Rondeau to Lord Harrington, September 29, 1739, ff. 295–6, here 296v.
39 John Bell wrote the official notice to the foreign secretary of Rondeau's death. TNA, SP 91/23, John Bell to Harrington, October 6, 1739, f. 309.
40 TNA, SP 91/23, Philip Lernoult to Harrington, October 6, 1739, f. 313.
41 TNA, SP 91/25, Finch to Harrington, September 17, 1740, ff. 94–8, here f. 94r.
42 TNA, SP 91/25, Finch to Harrington, September 27, 1740, f. 120r.
43 TNA, SP 91/25, Finch to Harrington, December 20, 1740, ff. 229–36, here f. 229r.
44 TNA, SP 91/27, Finch to Harrington, March 28, 1741, ff. 140–5, here f. 140r.
45 TNA, SP 91/27, Finch to Harrington, April 8, 1741, ff. 166–7, here 166r–v.
46 TNA, SP 91/28, Harrington to Finch, June 29, 1741, ff. 38–41, here 41r.
47 TNA, SP 91/28, Finch to Mr. Weston, July 15, 1741, f. 116r. For British interest in the spas, see Amanda E. Herbert, "Gender and the Spa: Space, Sociability and Self at the British Health Spas, 1640–1714," *The Journal of Social History* 43 (2009): 361–83.
48 TNA, SP SP 91/35, Wiche to Carteret, July 2, 743, ff. 49–53, here 51r–v.

49 TNA, SP 91/35, Wiche to Carteret, October 8, 1743, ff. 148–52, here 148v.
50 TNA, SP 91/36, Tyrawley to Edward Weston, July 26, 1744, ff. 254–5; here 254r.
51 BL, Trawley Papers, Correspondence of Lord Trawley when Ambassador in Russia, 1742–1745, vol. II, Addition Manuscripts 23,361, Carteret to Tyrawly, September 18, 1744, f. 56.
52 TNA, SP 91/49, Hyndford to Newcastle, February 1749, ff. 150–7; here 153r.
53 TNA SP 91/50, Hyndford to Newcastle, June 5, 1749, ff. 9–17, here 13v.
54 TNA, SP 91/65, Hanbury-Williams to Holderness, January 20, 1757, f. 37.
55 TNA, SP 91/65, George Rineking to Holdernesse, September 6, 1757.
56 BL, Hardwick Papers, vol. CXLV, "Diplomatic Letter-Book of R. Keith, March 3, 1758– August 19, 1762," Add. MS. 35493, Keith to Holdernesse, May 2/13 1760, f. 127.
57 TNA, PRO 30/43/11, Lowry Cole Papers, 30v–31r.
58 TNA, PRO 30/43/11, 51r.
59 TNA, PRO 30/43/11, 49v.
60 The time Harris suggested his time in office might be coming to an end, he left the decision entirely to the Foreign Secretary without argument. TNA, FO 65/2, Harris to Viscount Stormont, March 1781, 13/24, 99–102.
61 Peter Henry Bruce, *Memoirs of Peter Henry Bruce, Esq., A Military Officer, in the Services of Prussia, Russia, and Great Britain* (Dublin: J. and R. Byrn, 1783), 121–2.
62 Ibid., 122–3.
63 Ibid., 122.
64 TNA, SP 91/9, "James Jeffreys to Lord Stanhope," ff. 74–5, February 6, 1719.
65 For a discussion of the foreign depiction of the immoral bathhouse, see A. G. Cross, "The Russian *Banya* in the Descriptions of Foreign Travellers and in the Depictions of Foreign and Russian Artists," *Oxford Slavonic Papers*, New Series 24 (1991): 34–59. Judith Vowles, "Marriage à la russe," in *Sexuality and the Body in Russian Culture*, ed. Jane T. Costlow, Stephanie Sandler, and Judith Vowles (Stanford, CA: Stanford University Press, 1993), 53–72.
66 Alexander Gordon, *The History of Peter the Great, Emperor of Russia*, 2 vols (Aberdeen: F. Douglass and W. Murray, 1755), I: 7.
67 L'Abbé Chappe d'Auteroche, *A Journey into Siberia* (London, 1770), 353. For a discussion of the Russian reaction to this text, see Marcus C. Levitt, "An Antidote to Nervous Juice: Catherine the Great's Debate with Chappe d'Auteroche over Russian Culture," *Eighteenth-Century Studies* 32 (1) (1998), 49–63.
68 Marbault, *Essai sur le commerce de Russia, avec l'histoire de ses découvertes* (Amsterdam, 1777), 28–9.
69 Pierre Nicolas Chantreau, *Voyage philosophique politique et literaire, fait en*

Russie pendant les années 1788 et 1789, 2 vols (Paris: Briand, 1794), vol. 1, 296, 299.

70 John Richard, *A Tour from London to Petersburg, from thence to Moscow, and Return to London by way of Courland, Poland, Germany, and Holland* (London: T. Evans, 1778), 61.

71 BL, Bentham Papers, vol. XVIII, Miscellaneous Papers, Add MS. 33,554, "Diary," f. 7, entry for Dec. 2d, 1781.

72 John Parkinson, *A Tour of Russia, Siberia and the Crimea, 1792–1794*, ed. William Collier (London: Frank Cass, 1971), 68.

73 Ibid., 133.

74 Chantreau, *Voyage philosophique*, 296–9.

75 TNA, PRO 30/43/11, 73r.

76 Maria Guthrie, *A Tour, Performed in the Years 1795–6, Through the Taurida, or Crimea*, ed. Matthew Guthrie (London: T. Cadell, 1802), 201.

77 William Tooke, *View of the Russian Empire during the Reign of Catharine the Second and to the Close of the Eighteenth Century*, 3 vols. (London: T. H. Longman and O. Rees, 1799), I: 21.

78 Ibid.

79 Ibid., II: 1.

80 Ibid., II: 14.

81 Ibid., II: 4.

82 Ibid., II: 3.

83 For discussion of the complex transition away from humors, see Barbara Duden, "Medicine and the History of the Body," in *The Social Construction of Illness: Illness and Medical Knowledge in Past and Present*, ed. Jens Lachmund and Gunnar Stollberg (Stuttgart: Franz Steiner Verlag, 1991), 39–51.

84 See Smith, this volume; Alexander M. Martin, "Sewage and the City: Filth, Smell, and Representations of Urban Life in Moscow, 1770–1880," *The Russian Review* 67 (2) (2008): 243–74.

CHAPTER THREE

Fermentation, taste, and identity

Alison K. Smith

In the early nineteenth century, medical writers in Russia began to think carefully about the relationship of taste to purity and danger, particularly when it came to water. Their concern owed something to a new fad for water cures, something to a more general focus on the healthiness of water, something to interests in sobriety, and something to anxiety about the spread of disease.[1] In their discussions, many such authors found themselves thinking about pure water in terms of negatives, in particular its lack of taste. As one put it, "clean water is completely colorless and transparent, like the most pure crystal; it is completely tasteless, and, when used, it refreshes one's insides and quenches thirst without any stimulation of taste or smell."[2] This idea, that water was above all to be clear, pure, odorless, and tasteless, was the norm for both foreign scholars and Russian ones. Water ought to "have neither taste nor odor."[3] Its purity was above all defined by absence.

Concern for water purity developed alongside new understandings of the processes of fermentation and putrefaction.[4] At the turn of the century, Frenchman Nicolas Appert began to conduct experiments on a new method of preserving food for long periods; the method became the basis of modern canning. Appert's technique was based not in an understanding that particular microbes caused rot—that awaited his countryman Louis Pasteur—but on recognition that rot was a process that could be halted or at least retarded by heat.[5] The process he described also made a particular connection between two alternative forms of transformation: halting rot meant halting fermentation. Appert based his method on the theory that heat destroyed "the fermentation principle" which could go beyond proper fermentation and lead to unwanted results.[6] Several decades later, Pasteur's experiments on fermentation—and in particular on what happened when fermentation went bad—linked processes that led to fermentation on the one hand, and putrefaction on the other, to specific microbial agents that caused the changes.[7]

In these developments, both putrefaction and fermentation were conceived of as opposed to purity. While certain foods could be easily identified as either fermented or rotten, the exact moment when something moved from the former to the latter turned out to be difficult to identify—and yet central to defining what was edible and what was not. Mary Douglas's work on the distinction between purity and danger (in her work defined as the danger of contamination and dirt) focuses above all on the ways that such distinctions created social order in an anxiety-prone world, giving meaning to "disparate elements" and "disparate experience."[8] When purity is opposed not to dirt but to rot, however, the existence of a concept of fermentation complicates this basic distinction. The boundary between these two transformations of raw ingredients is a division that creates order but one particularly difficult to draw in large part because of the problem of taste.

Even biologically it is not necessarily obvious where fermentation ends and putrefaction begins. In one modern handbook of food studies, Alan Davidson's description of fermentation links it specifically to the same processes as putrefaction. For him, fermentation is "a word used loosely to describe desirable changes brought about by living micro-organisms (yeasts, moulds, and bacteria) in food and drink ... When micro-organisms or enzymes cause undesirable changes, for example making food go bad, what happens is called spoilage rather than fermentation."[9] The issue then becomes defining that line between "desirable changes" and the "bad." Studies of the "ecosystem" of fermentation can point to specific processes that produce "acceptable" results, and those that produce "bad" or dangerous ones.[10] That understanding suggests that the line between (proper) fermentation and (undesirable) putrefaction is defined above all biologically—but biology alone turns out to be unable to explain why a single food can be seen by some as properly fermented and by others as undesirably rotten.

Instead, the boundary between fermented and rotten is based above all on taste. The absence of taste can be a marker of purity, as in the many references to ideal, clean water with its taste of nothing. But the presence of taste does not automatically make even something like water necessarily dangerous. Rotted foods might obviously taste somehow bad; the related taste of fermentation was, and continues to be, harder to define. Although it can overlap with them, "fermented" is not exactly one of the four classical tastes identified by scientists: salty, sour, bitter, and sweet.[11] Nor does it quite match the so-called "fifth taste," umami, conceptualized in the early twentieth century as something akin to savoriness, and confirmed as a physiological phenomenon in the early twenty-first century.[12] The chemical act of fermentation, however, activates several of these tastes. Some fermented foods come to be described as bitter or sour, even acidic, above all. And others are, as some modern food writers put it, "umami bombs," carrying with them the glutamates that satisfy this basic taste. Fermented foods have "complex edgy flavors," as one modern fermentation specialist writes, and their very complexity can lead to differing interpretations of those tastes, from pleasant to unpleasant.[13] The taste of fermentation, as opposed to putrefaction, might then be conceptualized as existing at the intersection between unpalatably sour or even bitter, and somehow satisfying. And, in extreme cases, the level of fermentation can cross over the line to purely unpleasant—at least for palates unaccustomed to it.

As a result, as Claude Lévi-Strauss notes, "only observation can tell us what each [specific society] means by 'raw,' 'cooked' and 'rotted,' and we can suppose that it will not be the same for all."[14] Lévi-Strauss illustrated this idea with an anecdote of American GIs burning French cheese factories during the Second World War because they believed that only corpses could create such an odor—an anecdote that suggests that the boundary between what is fermented and what is rotten is culturally constructed as much as it is biologically constructed.[15] It also points to the fact that judgments about smells are as much a part of this process as judgments about tastes, a fact that Yuri Lotman has also made about changes in Russian cuisine in the nineteenth century.[16]

This means that fermented foods can play critical roles in defining a culinary idea of "our" and "other." They serve as excellent markers of particular cultures in part because they can be interpreted as being either within the world of cuisine or beyond it in the realm of the non-edible.[17] The act of recognizing the food as a food serves as a marker of belonging to a particular culture.

In early nineteenth-century Russia, drawing the line between "desirable" and "bad" transformations, and thus of good and bad tastes, played out in two major ways, both of which reflected current cultural issues. First, some Russian writers (like some foreign ones) saw a particular taste for what is essentially controlled rot—long-hung meat, particularly game, and strong cheeses—as part of the world of (foreign, Western) gastronomy. Only educated, gastronomic palates, they believed, could truly appreciate these particular foods; as a result, for them, the line between "desirable" and "bad" indicated a particular social distinction between those with an educated (and thus elite) palate, and those without.[18] Second, and perhaps more importantly, Russians and foreigners alike interpreted a taste for the fermented in national terms. A set of fermented foods—sour rye bread, kvas, and sour cabbage—appeared in many writings as off-putting to foreign palates, and also as being markers of an essential Russian taste. They were, in other words, central to both foreign and Russian conceptions of Russian cuisine.

These issues came to the fore at this particular moment in part because of a conjunction of sources. For one, travelers from Western states, though they had been coming to Russia for centuries, were now not only writing up accounts of their travels but also were being read and responded to by Russians themselves. As a result, their judgments of Russian tastes and habits became part of an internal discourse defining Russianness. In addition, the role of food and cooking in the definition of Russianness gained new prevalence in these decades. There was a clear rise in agricultural journals in the aftermath of a series of crop failures in the early 1830s, and writings on food and cooking followed suit. The few foreign translations of the late eighteenth century were largely superseded by domestically produced cooking advice by the early 1840s, although even those texts borrowed liberally from foreign works. Even so, virtually all shared an interest in constructing and defining Russian cuisine.[19]

Furthermore, early nineteenth-century cookbook authors were joined in their fascination with questions of taste by many writers on health and hygiene. For them, taste was above all a method of defining purity—although here, too, it was far from simple. Mineral waters, quite the new fad for healing in the early nineteenth century, were an exception to the general rule that healthy water ought to be without taste. They were instead primarily defined by their taste, which marked them as somehow outside the norm, and even at times as somewhat off-putting, and yet still healthy. Accounts of mineral waters, both approving and not, focused on these tastes. One Russian commentator complaining about the current fad described them as nothing more than water with a taste.[20] Those who approved also tended to focus on taste. A spring near St. Petersburg was described as having an "astringent" taste, and of providing local peasants with cures for assorted illnesses.[21] Even an account that sought to bring together all current knowledge about mineral waters, and to treat them scientifically, came quickly to the subject of their varied tastes: "every mineral water ... has its own taste or odor (most often sulfurous)."[22]

When it came to water, the problem was that taste was unreliable as a judge of quality, because although taste, and even somewhat unpleasant taste, could be linked with something healthy, it could also indicate something dangerous. In this period before the rise of germ theory, one of the primary ways to recognize unhealthy water was by its taste: bad water had "an unpleasant taste."[23] Descriptions of good water as being without taste often went hand in hand with similarly vague descriptions of the bad taste of bad water.[24] The bad taste of water could even extend past the water itself and spoil the taste of the fish living within it. An account of the different qualities of water available in Kazan' noted that the quality was reflected in fish: in the Volga, where fresh water flowed, the fish were big and tasty, while in the heavily polluted Kazan' they were small and did "not have an excellent taste."[25]

Foods, too, were subject to changes in taste when they were transformed from pure to rotten. Despite this, the presence of some negative taste in things rotten was not necessarily the most common way of recognizing the spoiled. In part, this may reflect the fact that it was difficult to describe bad tastes. A basic description—foods that were spoiled had an "unpleasant taste"—was most common, and furthermore linked to unpleasant outcomes. Bread with the particular "unpleasant taste" of spoilage could lead to "heaviness in the stomach, heartburn, vomiting, pain in the abdomen."[26] Instead, particularly for some spoiled foods, the descriptions of taste are usually less stomach-churning than those of appearance or even smell.[27] In one example, Dr. A. Nikitin described spoiled sausage as having, when cut "a most nasty, sour-sweet, nausea inducing smell," as having "a yellowish or yellowish-green color and mushy texture," but having simply an "unpleasant taste."[28] Even here, though, descriptions largely focused on a basic "unpleasantness"—one description of vegetables gone bad simply noted that they "took on an unpleasant appearance."[29] That appearance was perhaps enough of a warning that taste never played a role.

More generally, the transformation from pure to rotten or from pure to fermented was marked by a transformation in taste—and a transformation in taste that carried meaning in multiple ways. First, the line between pure and spoiled served in part to define gastronomic tastes in the early nineteenth century. A description of the best way to prepare game in the journal *Ekonom* put this clearly:

> Fresh game is not good; it is tough and has a somewhat strange odor, like rawness. A gastronome can never stand to eat fresh game, but lets it lie until it has dried out a bit. Russians who are not used to French cooking do not love game that has rested long, and which has already gotten a sharp odor, just like they do not love the best delicacy in the world, Limburger cheese. But a true gastronome demands game with a bit of gaminess, that is, that has been hung. In order to make peace between the gastronome and those who cannot stand the least bit of gamy odor, we have come to recommend a method that is the average of gastronomic and simple cookery. As a general rule, never eat fresh game. Just let it lie a day in the larder.[30]

A number of issues were embedded within this one quotation. First, its author drew a distinction between Russian and French tastes, the latter of which were additionally conflated with gastronomic pleasures. Second, those gastronomic tastes were considered foreign but also acquirable: a Russian could become used to French taste. Third, the two gastronomic tastes here identified were remarkable most of all for their very strong odor and flavor caused by transgressing (for some palates) the line between pleasure and rot.

The last idea that for the gastronome, meat (and in the example above, Limburger cheese), was transformed for the better by a certain degree of controlled rot was central to certain French "gastronomic" culinary norms. The culinary benefit of partially rotted pheasant, in particular, was touted by Jean-Anthelme Brillat-Savarin in his *Physiology of Taste*. He claimed that though pheasant was the best of all game fowl when properly prepared, one "eaten within a week of its death is not as grand as a partridge or a chicken, for its whole merit lies in its aroma."[31] Later, he went on to describe how a pheasant was brought to its maximum potential: "cooked at the right time, its flesh is tender, sublime, and tasty, for it partakes of both poultry and venison. This desirable stage is reached just as the pheasant begins to decompose; only then does its fragrance develop, combining with an oil which, to be formed, requires a period of fermentation, like the oil of coffee, which is only obtained by roasting."[32]

Agreeing with the author of the *Ekonom* article, above, many other contemporary writers suggested that Russians did not generally have a taste for these kinds of strong, "gastronomic" tastes. In the mid-eighteenth century, at least, one author believed that Russians had not really developed a "taste for cheese."[33] Here the author differentiated between the mild fresh cheeses common to the country, and the strong flavors of aged cheeses imported from Western Europe. Others suggested that one reason for Russian failure to recognize the appeal of aged meat was a peculiarity of Russian foodways. The country's cold weather meant that meat markets in winter usually involved vast amounts of frozen animals—many travelers were taken aback by the sight of frozen carcass after frozen carcass in these markets. But that very fact also, according to one visitor, made Russia's meat "more tasteless than in England."[34] Its quality might be good, but the very ability to use cold against spoilage altered its taste, eliminating the hint of rot that flavored meat elsewhere.

At the same time, however, some of these tastes had clearly been acquired by the early nineteenth century, at least among Russia's elite. Stronger cheeses might have been rare in the mid-eighteenth century, but were common on the tables of the elite by the early nineteenth. One traveler claimed that "a housewife speaks of her supply of Parmesan like in Germany one would speak of the supply of onions or of parsley," and that "the cheeses of England, of Holland, of Switzerland, are the ordinary dessert."[35] That may have been an exaggeration, but in 1833 alone, Russia imported 470,000 rubles worth of cheese, and journals regularly printed articles purporting to give the secrets behind the incredibly popular Parmesan, Dutch, and Swiss cheeses.[36] The Russian medical writer Akim Charukovskii even lamented that Russians were spoiling their digestion by acquiring tastes for cured cheeses (even if he agreed that only the very most gastronomic few could appreciate Limburger).[37]

In addition, Russian culinary writers fairly consistently sought to educate their audience about these properly gastronomic preparations. They informed their readers that beef, for example, ought to be let rest for a day or more in order to tenderize the meat, particularly before roasting.[38] An early nineteenth-century translation of a French text used a footnote to explain the concept to readers.[39] Later, a Russian author noted that "true, real" steak required time spent between slaughter and preparation—and that it should not be frozen. Only by aging beef for four days in summer, for longer in winter, would it have the proper flavor.[40] Fowl and game birds also came in for special attention by culinary authors. One article stated that among the most basic rules of cooking was to never cook fowl on the day it was killed.[41] Certain foods, and particularly game, should be aged even longer. One article on the proper cooking of pheasant claimed that they should be hung in a cold larder for six weeks before eating.[42] Here the gastronomic extremes of even Brillat-Savarin's instructions were made into general advice for average (elite) Russians. The gastronomic—and foreign—both could be, and had been, incorporated as part as the process of becoming European.

Acquired gastronomic appreciation for the rotted was interpreted as a taste for "strong" flavors above all. At the same time a different interpretation, which described fermented flavors as sour or acid, went along with a different means of distinction: taste appropriate to a particular nation. According to a mid-nineteenth-century journalist:

> Russian nature somehow is in general inclined towards everything sour, and if the proverb "what is healthy to a Russian is death to a German" is true, then of course all the more should it be applied to sour foods. Cabbage soup from sauerkraut, beet soup, kvas, rye bread, kisel—all of this is so sour that Western Europeans grimace, while being a delicacy for the Russian stomach.[43]

This Russian writer was quite accurate in his description of Western European responses to "Russian taste." The idea that Russians had a particular "taste for sours," satisfied only by foods that were "atrociously acrid" was a common one.[44] In these cases, however, the word "sour" indicated not the use of vinegar or other acid but rather the result of fermentation. In these foods, the line between fermentation and rot created a kind of national distinction, just as Matthew Romaniello shows in his chapter that only Russians could tolerate a certain weather, so too was their diet theirs alone. For Russians, certain foods were well within the boundary distinguishing the desirable from the bad; for foreigners, those same foods were at best close to the boundary, and at worst far beyond it.

Three foods appeared over and over again in the accounts of travelers as particularly Russian: (sour) rye bread, kvas, and sour (fermented) cabbage. Linking the three foods goes back at least as far as the travels of Macarius in the seventeenth century. In that account, Holy Week was marked in part by a trinity of foods presented to the Emperor: "a large black loaf of rye-bread, of the kind they use in the monastery, carried in the hands of four or five men, and looking like a large mill-stone; ... secondly a barrel of quass, extracted from rye-water, which they are accustomed to drink, enclosed in another empty barrel; and a barrel of pickled cabbage."[45] Each of these foods (or drinks) served as a way to identify those who belonged to the nation, and those excluded from it by their palate. In addition, they served as places for Russians to interact with concepts of taste and of health in ways that complicated this simple national association.

Rye, particularly as rye bread, was central to the conception of Russian foodways. Rye was "the most important and most necessary" of grains and bread "for the whole national society."[46] Rye stood for Russia, and separated it from Western Europe. When St. Petersburg's grain merchants tried to promote the export of rye by donating some to Ireland during its famine, they also realized they would have to send bakers along with it to introduce the grain to a new population.[47] Rye bread even gave certain Russian consumers unique strength:

> In all of Russia, and therefore also in the Russian army, they usually eat rye bread ... the capability of our soldier, unique in the world, to bear, with remarkable strength, all the disadvantages of war, of hunger, of cold, in my opinion, largely depends on a solid foundation of the nutritional juices produced by proper consumption of rye bread—and thus, that which so surprises foreigners about our forces, and what they consider for themselves completely impossible, for a Russian is a natural consequence of his way of life and diet.[48]

Russian bread was marked as "Russian" not only because it was baked of rye flour but also because it was soured (or fermented) in the process of baking.[49] The resulting sourness of Russian rye bread became a focus of the descriptions of many foreigners. J. G. Kohl wrote that "it is incredible how bad the bread is, considering the goodness of the corn; it is all, more or less sour, and why this is so, is not easy to discover."[50] Charles Henningsen agreed, claiming both that Russian bread was "less than by any other mode or preparation, nutritive, economical and palatable," and that "not one Englishman in ten can ever, even in the course of years and with the best will in the world, become accustomed to the effect either on the palate or the bowels of the soft, sour, billet, national bread."[51] Others were more measured in their appraisal, simply commenting on the unusual sourness of the bread, or even, like William Coxe, writing at the end of the eighteenth century, claiming that one could become "reconciled" to it, and then find it "no unpleasant morsel."[52] Faint praise, perhaps, but still Coxe recognized that national tastes could be acquired.

Kohl may have wondered why Russian rye bread was so sour, but Russian medical writers believed—with some just cause—that rye flour benefited from what seemed to Western Europeans excessive fermentation. Their reasons, though, varied. A. Sokolovskii, for one, suggested that the freshest, driest rye flour did not need to be soured, but older grain did; he described the rationale as being one of pure taste: the sourness (created by either vinegar or lactic acid) hid the strong taste of the rye.[53] A. Charukovskii, however, was more scientific in his description. He suggested that rye flour simply had to be treated differently from those flours to which Western Europeans were more accustomed; its gluten was "tougher than the gluten of wheat flour," and thus required additional leavening. In fact, even with that extra leavening via fermentation/souring, the resulting loaf was likely to be "dense, heavy, hard to digest for unaccustomed stomachs, but also quite nutritious."[54]

In addition, Russian authors were well aware of the foreign association of their bread with unpleasant, even off-putting tastes, and argued for a different interpretation of the line between "desirable" fermentation and "bad." An English description of Russian rye bread as "not nutritious, not healthy, and not tasty" was greeted with incredulity, and a strong argument in favor of Russian methods. In a published response to such negative foreign accounts, a Russian journalist described "pillowy, soft, tasty, and healthy" bread produced by Russian methods of bread baking, not the sour, unpalatable mess described by foreigners.[55] Others took issue with the very description of the sour, Russian rye bread; one author noted that properly baked rye bread ought not to have an "unpleasant odor," or be "too sour."[56] But of course, this brings up the role of acquired taste in defining the line between "just sour enough" and "too sour." For Russians, proper rye bread was "just sour enough." For foreigners, that same bread might be "too sour."

This line between "just sour enough" and "too sour" was further developed in discussions of kvas. Kvas was generally accepted as the "common" or "national" drink of Russia; one journal author even claimed "kvas was, is, and will be one of the most beloved and most consumed beverages of the Russian man."[57] Perhaps even more than the sour Russian rye bread, kvas represented the nation. Some claimed that Russian elites had switched their allegiance to white, wheaten breads, but almost all agreed that kvas still called to the Russian palate; as the Scottish traveler Robert Bremner put it, "this kvass is the thinnest, sourest, queerest kind of stuff ever concocted; yet the Russian could not live without it. It is patronized by all ranks and all denominations."[58]

As Bremner's description suggests, just as they found Russia's rye bread to have an unfamiliar and unpleasant taste, many foreign travelers also found kvas to be something of a shock. R. B. Paul claimed that when he "ventured to take a draught from a huge mug full of quass, the national drink, I thought for a moment that I was poisoned … when I tasted the composition of water, fermented flour, and liquorice, which my kind friends presented to me."[59] It, too, was most of all described in terms of its sour, fermented taste: "a fermented acidulated liquour," or "sourish but undecided" and one which was "to those unaccustomed to it, … not agreeable at first."[60] But this description hints at a major difference in descriptions of kvas and rye bread: where the rye bread was most often simply unpalatable and nothing more, a foreigner could acquire a taste for kvas, perhaps because fermented drinks of other sorts were more common than sour breads. Edward Jerrman commented "at first its taste is quite insupportable, but one soon gets accustomed to it and prefers it to any other beverage."[61] Many other travelers commented on the drink's acidity, or sourness, and agreed that it was an acquired taste.[62] Even J. G. Kohl, who had so disliked Russian bread, described kvas as "a light and wholesome beverage" and gave advice on how to make it.[63]

For Russians, kvas was simply the national drink. It was "used everywhere in Russia;" it was "the most healthy drink;" it even "protected from scurvy, sepsis, and inflammatory illnesses."[64] The idea of kvas as something particularly healthy appeared frequently. In 1839, the editor of the journal *The Friend of Health* commented, "nothing can be better to drink, in northern countries, than well prepared kvas."[65] One Russian writer agreed that a certain degree of sourness was appropriate, but it ought to have its limits: "The quality of every good kvas should be that its sourness is moderate and not artificial, that it is lightly spicy and aromatic, and that it has no sediment: the cleaner and more transparent the kvas, the healthier it is."[66]

But a problem lurked in the normal methods of kvas production. Although fermented, it was not a highly alcoholic beverage, which created problems when it came to storage. In other words, its fermentation only partially fulfilled the goal of most fermentation, to prolong edibility or potability. Kvas's fermentation was so limited that one traveler claimed that its low alcohol content meant that kvas would "only keep for a few days unless placed in an ice cellar."[67] To A. Jourdier, a French traveler and writer on agricultural topics, this characteristic made kvas not only unpleasant, but actively unhealthy. As he put it, "kvas is above all unhealthy because it is never like itself, not only from one day to the next, but even from one hour to another." Essentially, Jourdier argued, the process of fermenting kvas was less rigorously controlled than was the process of producing other fermented beverages, like wine, beer, or cider (which he proposed as a particularly useful alternative to kvas for Russians). The result was that three times in ten, a bottle of kvas was too young, two times it was just right, and five times it was too old and "more or less bad."[68]

This was a particularly harsh assessment of the national beverage, but even some Russian subjects agreed that the production of kvas had its dangers. Karl Geling believed that kvas was in general a good, healthy, national drink—but he also noted that "kvas that is still young, flat, cloudy, raw, containing within itself many unfermented particles of flour, continues to ferment in the stomach itself, and therefore inflates the stomach, hinders digestion, and causes pain and diarrhea."[69] Others agreed, noting that kvas was healthy (and, indeed "the very best drink after water") only if "it is well soured/fermented and has no rawness." Moreover, if kvas was under- or over-fermented, it could have consequences ranging from gas, distention, and diarrhea, to indigestion and "weakness in the stomach."[70] This was another variation on the fuzzy line between fermentation as "just enough" change and rot as "too much"—kvas could be "just right," but both under- and over-fermentation could turn it into something dangerous.

The third food in the trinity of the fermented was cabbage. It was, of course, widely recognized as the most typically Russian of all vegetables, widely consumed, and nearly indispensable.[71] And, too, the idea that Russians above all preferred soured cabbage was common. Furthermore, authors, both foreign and Russian, recognized that the Russian method of souring cabbage via fermentation was rather different from, say, the German method of producing sauerkraut; one traveler described it somewhat inaccurately thus: "instead of employing vinegar and juniper-leaves in the process, the Russians simply slice the vegetable very small, then pour water over it, and let the compound lie until the cabbage becomes sour by the fermentation that has taken place."[72] This author left out the centrally important role of salt in the process (salt retards the development of bad bacteria but allows good bacteria to flourish), but he was otherwise correct that Russia's sour cabbage was sour due to fermentation, not pickling.

Even wider claims were made in an anonymous article in the journal *The Russian Farmer*. Its author wrote of a new fad in France for "sour cabbage, long the favorite food of the Slavic tribes." Thrilled by the recognition of the "goodness and taste" of such cabbage, he explicitly linked it with Russian—or perhaps more generally with Slavic—identity:

> In French journals praising cabbage as an excellent popular food, they call it *surcroute* from the German Sauerkraut and take it as a native German dish. ... *The Russian Farmer* considers it necessary ... to affirm that cabbage moved to the Germans from the Slavs just like it now moves from the Germans to the French, exactly like an innovation; the proof of this is the fact that sour cabbage in Germany itself is not in general use; it is in general use only among the Slavs; it is a Slavic food.[73]

Fermentation in particular not only marked cabbage as uniquely Russian but also helped answer a major question faced by Russian medical authors: Western European medical knowledge suggested that cabbage was not particularly healthy, and might even be so difficult to digest that it caused problems. Russians faithfully reported on these foreign attitudes, which claimed that, for example, broccoli was the healthiest and most nutritious vegetable of the brassicas, cauliflower followed, and plain cabbage the least tender and the least nutritious.[74]

They also argued, however, that sour or fermented cabbage was something entirely different. Not only was it "our generally used, favorite food" but also it was "more pleasant and better" when "well made."[75] Another author was even clearer. Like foreign doctors said, plain cabbage was difficult to digest, "swells the stomach," and acted as a diuretic. But "that very same cabbage, when fermented, is only dangerous to those with weak stomachs, but otherwise is nutritious."[76] In other words, sour, fermented cabbage was not only the particular glory of Russian cuisine but also the particular key to Russian health. According to one writer on the medical requirements of soldiers, such cabbage was "as important to maintaining the health of Russian soldiers as all the preceding foods; and therefore always, whenever there is the least possibility, it must be tried that soldiers have not the least insufficiency [of it]."[77]

In these accounts, the very act of fermentation transformed cabbage from something possibly harmful to something actively healthy. According to one doctor, fermented cabbage could even act medicinally, as he reported on a successful course of treatment of a woman with mania, cured by constant consumption of fermented cabbage. (One sign she was cured? She requested shchi [sour cabbage soup] with black [presumably sour] bread.)[78] Similarly, in 1841, warnings against cabbage—which "little feeds the body, [and] is digested in the stomach with difficulty"—were amended with the note that fermented cabbage was not only healthy, but could serve a medicinal function—and that furthermore, "however strange these methods of healing are, their usefulness is confirmed by numerous experiences, even if theory has not yet managed to explain the beneficial strength of fermented cabbage."[79]

For all this favorable attention to fermented cabbage as national and healthy, a few voices did sound a note of doubt about its production and consumption, a note that echoed other concerns about the line between acceptable and unacceptable levels of transformation through fermentation. One journalist claimed that "cabbage and salted cucumbers should never be stored in the same cellar as other provisions; their acidic odor and emanations will create dampness in the cellar and can be harmful."[80] This was a minor problem, but hinted at the concept of putrefaction—the acidic odor and emanations might, particularly in a world in which miasma theory was still prominent, infect good provisions with the possibility of the bad.

As in the case of kvas, the process of fermentation, so difficult to control, could cause problems.[81] Karl Geling, who compiled a guide to medical oversight of food (and other things) attuned to Russian realities, particularly noted that the normal process of fermentation was good, but had potential problems: "if salted and fermented items are kept in a cold place they stay good a reasonably long time; in other cases, they easily move on to putrefaction, and then are not only unwholesome to eat, but even infect the air."[82] Others gave additional advice on keeping even sour/fermented cabbage good for longer. Katerina Avdeeva wrote that "sometimes at the beginning of summer [that is, more than half a year after it was first prepared] sour cabbage loses its firmness and color, becoming soft and moving towards putrefaction." She followed with a piece of doubtful advice: "in that case, one should thrust into the middle of the barrel with the cabbage a birch stake that reaches to the very bottom. From this substance the cabbage will take on its previous color and firmness."[83] This was perhaps overly thrifty advice, for more often, fermented cabbage leftover at the end of winter had spoiled; in one account, "every spring we see that the proprietors of corner stores throw out huge masses of rotted fermented material."[84]

Some sought to fix this problem by adding on an additional layer of preservation: drying. In 1850, one P. Davydov reported about recent experiments with drying fermented cabbage. He had been inspired, he wrote, by discussions of specially constructed drying ovens and had decided to investigate whether the traditional Russian stove could do just as well. He found the wife of a retired non-commissioned officer who had used the Russian stove for just this purpose, and reported her method: "well, sir, it was simple—take it and dry it." Davydov found this perfectly acceptable. An editorial comment on Davydov's article, however, found this method not quite right. Using a special oven, the editor argued, "saved all the worth of fermented cabbage, that is, a pleasant acidity, freshness, taste, savoriness, nutritiousness, and anti-scurvy properties." Even better, it could be kept for a long time, and "when dry has no scent at all, though when cooked it has the pleasant scent of warmed shchi." Davydov's experiments with the method of his Russian informant, however, "has an extremely unpleasant appearance and, more importantly, has an unpleasant odor, which is completely incompatible with the expected use of cabbage in sanitary contexts."[85]

There is and has long been a temptation to link sets of tastes like these to unconscious knowledge of nutritional needs.[86] Dr. Matthew Guthrie, born in Scotland, but practicing medicine in St. Petersburg in the late eighteenth century, found Russian tastes for things sour and fermented to be the key to their unexpected healthiness despite the limitations of their northern clime. As he put it:

> if nature had not taught these people habits, and given them a taste which galloping travellers treat with contempt, they most undoubtedly [would] have sunk under the scurvy, as they are, for the greatest part of the year, exposed to the influence of those predisposing causes to putrid complaints that make the body of the Greenland seaman livid; yet under all these disadvantages such seems to be the efficacy of the regimen they observe, that putrid diseases are strangers to their huts, and the Russian boor enjoys a state of health that astonishes an inhabitant of a country where the dreadful consequences are so well known of bad air within, excessive cold without, joined to a want of fresh vegetables for a length of time.[87]

What was this "taste which galloping travellers treat with contempt" but which provided the Russian peasant with abundant health? A taste for kvas, sour rye bread, and sour cabbage.

But nutritional concepts aside, these three foods generally stood in for the concept of a national, Russian taste. This idea was common not only in Western accounts of Russian eating habits but also in Russian responses. Ivan Boltin took particular offense at the French visitor LeClerc's statement that Russians ate bland foods. He argued instead that the most characteristic food of the Russian people was instead the notably sour *shchi*, and felt that this indicated LeClerc's total lack of understanding of the Russian people.[88] It is a bit unclear why this particular calumny affected Boltin so sharply, but he was far from alone in explaining Russian tastes in terms of their preference for the sour or acid, not the bland. Faddei Bulgarin explained Russian disdain for potatoes (this was in 1841, when the tuber had not yet fully entered into the culinary world of Russia) by noting that Russian peasants found potatoes to be "bland," and therefore against their normal palate. "The Russian man loves sourness," he wrote. "He prefers a piece of stale rye bread with kvas to any potato dish." Bulgarin's proposed solution? German potato salad! Or rather, a Russian variation: Bulgarin noted that the required "vinegar, oil, and pepper are luxuries, our Russian man could eat potatoes with kvas and onions, and I am sure that he will like this dish."[89]

In his 1823 account of "the character of the Russians," Robert Lyall spent some time analyzing earlier authors' descriptions of the country and its people, including the account of Dr. Edward Clarke. Among other issues, Lyall commented on Dr. Clarke's use of kvas/kvass/quass to indicate something particular about Russia. Lyall focused on Clarke's description of Russian nobles feasting on "raw turnips and drinking quass" as an indication of their low cultural (and by implication, low political) status. Lyall found this an inappropriate conclusion, for the raw turnips were really raw radishes eaten as part of the *zakuski* table, while "potations of kvass imply no more in Russia, than drinking porter, or beer in England." Furthermore, he noted, "throughout Dr. Clarke's work, the word *quass* (kvass), which he calls vinegar, is always put in italics, as if there was something very characteristic and barbarous in its use. The reason of this I cannot divine. Kvass, when well fermented, is an acidulous, pleasant, and healthy beverage."[90] Lyall is here actually being unfair to Clarke; although the doctor does equate kvas with "a pot of vinegar," he also says much the same thing as later travelers: "it looks turbid, and is very unpleasant to strangers; but, by use, we became fond of it."[91]

Lyall's goal, however, was to point out that there was a tendency among foreign travelers to equate Russia with barbarism, and furthermore that things like snacks of "raw turnips," and a taste for sour kvas or sour bread or sour cabbage were supposed indicators of their rough and uncultured essential nature. Foreigners used these tastes to emphasize Russian otherness, and it is perhaps because of this that later Soviet taste-makers emphasized very different concepts in their building of a new, modern, Soviet consumer, as Anton Masterovoy's chapter in this volume argues. At the same time, some nineteenth-century Russian authors read this same set of tastes as indicating a toughness, rather than a roughness, best encompassed by the saying "healthy to a Russian, death to a German." In both these variants, the foods discussed here—including the gastronomic ones that signified a foreign taste even wilder than the Russian—proved particularly useful at distinguishing between groups.

Furthermore, this basic idea, that lines between the "desirable" and the "bad," between the "pleasantly" sour and the "too," were based in part on individual taste and in part on cultural norms, has larger implications because they come up against the boundary of what can be considered food. Stepping outside the bounds of Russia, it is more generally foods like these, the rotten and the fermented, that give rise to visions of national cuisines, and most successfully mark their consumers as members of a united nation. As one modern food writer puts it, many fermented foods are acquired tastes, and "one culture's greatest culinary achievement is sometimes another's nightmare."[92] More than any other, it is these foods that lead those unaccustomed to them to feel a certain shiver of at least unease, and at most disgust at the thought of crossing that boundary between fermented and rotten, from food to non-food. They serve, as a result, as the ultimate barrier for acceptance, the perfect means of distinguishing insider and outsider.

Notes

1. On water cures: "Lechenie vodoi v Il'menauskom zavedenii, opisannoe Berlinskim d-om Zaksom," *Drug zdraviia* 7 (6) (1839): 43–5 (which noted that the first rule of water cures was perfectly clean, clear, odorless water); "Gidropatiia est, iskusstvo lechit' bolezni vodoi," *Drug zdraviia* 7 (27) (1839): 213–4; and "O vodolechenii," *Drug zdraviia* 11 (27), 29 (32) (1843): 209–10, 225–6, 250–2. On a new emphasis on the healthiness of water: Iv. Arngol'dt, "O vliianii vozdukha i vody na zdravie chelovecheskoe," *Zavolzhskii muravei* (1832): 711–25, 762–78, here 763; Parfenii Engalychev, *O prodolzhenii chelovecheskoi zhizni, ili domashnii lechebnik, zakliuchaiushchii v sebe: sredstva, kak dostigat' zdorovoi, veseloi i glubokoi starosti, predokhraniat' zdorov'e nadezhneishimi sredstvami i pol'zovat' bolezni vsiakogo roda, s pokazaniem prichin i lekarstv, pochti povsiudu pred glazami nashimi nakhodiashchikhsia, sostavlennyi iz luchshikh otechestvennykh i inostrannykh pisatelei Kniazem Parfeniem Engalychevem*, 6th ed. (St. Petersburg: Il'ia i Stepan Loskutovy, 1848), vol. 1, 65. On temperance movements in general, as well as explicit admonitions to drink water instead of vodka, see "Krest'ianskoe tovarishchestvo trezvosti v Rossii," *Zemledel'cheskaia gazeta* (April 12, 1838): 230–1; I. Leonev, "O broshiurke A. G., kasatel'no p'ianstva v Rossii," *Zemledel'cheskaia gazeta* (May 9, 1847): 290, and *Ruchnaia kniga dlia gramotnogo poselianina* (St. Petersburg: Aleksandr Iakobson, 1857), 271–3.
2. Arngol'dt, "O vliianii vozdukha i vody na zdravie chelovecheskoe," 764.
3. A. Charukovskii, *Narodnaia meditsina, primenennaia k russkomu bytu i*

raznoklimatnosti Rossii (St. Petersburg: Tipografiia Voenno-Uchebnykh Zavedenii, 1844), vol. 2, part 3, 212.

4 Jean-Pierre Goubert, *The Conquest of Water: The Advent of Health in the Industrial Age*, trans. Andrew Wilson (Princeton, NJ: Princeton University Press, 1989), 60–1.

5 Maguelonne Toussaint-Samat, *A History of Food*, trans. Anthea Bell (Oxford: Blackwell, 1994), 737–42; Rebeca Garcia and Jean Adrian, "Nicolas Appert: Inventor and Manufacturer," *Food Review International* 25 (2009): 115–25, esp. 117–18. Appert's methods were also reported on in Russia. See Ivan Dvigubskii, *Leksikon sel'skogo i gorodskogo khoziaistva* (Moscow: S. Selivanovskii, 1836–40), vol. 7 (1837), 82–4; Tikhvinianin, "Sokhranenie plodov i ovoshchei, po metode izvestnogo ekonoma—khimika Appera," *Zhurnal obshchepoleznykh svedenii* (1837): 134–5; and Doktor Puf, "Lektsiia XXIV", "Lektsiia XXV," and "Lektsiia XXVI," *Zapiski dlia khoziaeva* (1844): 190–1, 198–9, 206–7.

6 Garcia and Adrian, "Nicolas Appert," 122–3.

7 Lois N. Magner, *A History of Infectious Diseases and the Microbial World* (Westport, CT: Praeger, 2009), 32–3.

8 Mary Douglas, *Purity and Danger: An Analysis of Concepts of Pollution and Taboo* (London: Routledge, 2002), 3.

9 Alan Davidson, *The Oxford Companion to Food*, 2nd edn, ed. Tom Jaine (Oxford: Oxford University Press, 2006), 296. Others describe fermentation as "desirable" change, or suggest that fermentation helps "destroy undesirable components." See Geoffrey Campbell-Platt, "Fermented Foods—A World Perspective," *Food Research International* 27 (1994): 253–7 and A. Blandino et al., "Cereal-Based Fermented Foods and Beverages," *Food Research International* 36 (2003): 527–43.

10 Robert Scott and William C. Sullivan, "Ecology of Fermented Foods," *Human Ecology Review* 15 (1) (2008): 25–31.

11 One review of fermented foods suggests a wider range of "flavours (sweet, sour, alcoholic and meat-like) [that] appeal to large numbers of humans." Keith H. Steinkraus, "Nutritional Significance of Fermented Foods," *Food Research International* 27 (1994): 259–67, here 259.

12 For an overview of the development of the concept of umami, see Ole G. Mouritsen et al., "Seaweeds for Umami Flavour in the New Nordic Cuisine," *Flavour* 1 (4) (2012): 4.

13 Sandor Ellix Katz, *The Art of Fermentation* (White River Junction: Chelsea Green Publishing, 2012), 17, and more generally 33–4.

14 Claude Lévi-Strauss, "The Culinary Triangle," trans. Peter Brooks, in *Food and Culture: A Reader*, ed. Carole Counihan and Penny van Esterik (New York: Routledge, 1997), 28–35, here 29.

15 He is far from alone in thinking of cuisine as constructed, not purely biological (or microbiological). For other such accounts, see Claude Fischler, "Food, self and identity," *Social Science Information* 27 (2) (1988): 275–92, esp. 284–7; Igor de Garine, "Introduction," in *Cuisines reflets des sociétés*,

ed. Marie-Claire Bataille-Benguigui, Françoise Cousin (Paris: Sepia, 1996), 9–28. For a summary of some of the literature on national cuisines, in particular, see my "National Cuisines," in *The Oxford Handbook of Food History*, ed. Jeffrey Pilcher (New York: Oxford University Press, 2012), 444–60.

16 Yuri Lotman and Jelena Pogosjan, *High Society Dinners: Dining in Tsarist Russia*, trans. Marian Schwartz; ed. Darra Goldstein (Totnes: Prospect Books, 2014), 81–3.

17 See a similar discussion in the largely technical W. R. Stanton, "Microbial Processes in the Production of Food," in *Essays in Agricultural and Food Microbiology*, ed. J. R. Norris and G. L. Pettipher (Chichester: John Wiley & Sons, 1987), 345–67, esp. 346–8; or Jyoti Prakash Tamang, *Himalayan Fermented Foods: Microbiology, Nutrition, and Ethnic Values* (Boca Raton: CRC Press, 2010).

18 This is, of course, a variation on the sorts of different tastes enjoyed by different classes described in Pierre Bourdieu, *Distinction: A Social Critique of the Judgement of Taste*, trans. Richard Nice (Cambridge, MA: Harvard University Press, 1984).

19 On the uptick in agricultural journals, see http://individual.utoronto.ca/aksmith/research/agricultural_journals.tiff (accessed May 11, 2015). For more general discussion of such sources, see my *Recipes for Russia: Food and Nationhood under the Tsars* (Dekalb: Northern Illinois University Press, 2008).

20 "Nechto o lechenie sokami iz svezhikh rastenii i syvorotkoi," *Drug zdraviia* 7 (25) (1839): 194–5, here 195.

21 Iakov Zakharov, "O paliustrovskoi mineral'noi vode," *Umozritel'nye issledovaniia imperatorskoi Sanktpeterburgskoi akademii nauk* 5 (1819): 223–4, here 223.

22 Kondratii Grum, *Opisanie mineral'nykh vod, lechebnykh griazei i kupanii russkikh i zagranichnykh* (St. Petersburg: Tipografiia Departamenta vneshnei torgovli, 1855), vol. 2, 4.

23 Review of *O ustroistve i pol'ze vodochistitel'nykh kolodtsov*, "Bibliografiia," *Moskovskii telegraf* 8 (8) (1826): 337; Edward Tracy Turnerelli, *Russia on the Borders of Asia: Kazan, the Ancient Capital of the Tartar Khans; with an Account of the Province to Which It Belongs, the Tribes and Races Which Form Its Population, etc.* (London: Richard Bentley, 1854), vol. 1, 250.

24 Ivan Veltsin, *Nachertanie vrachebnogo blagoustroistva ili o sredstvakh zavisiashchikh ot Pravitel'stva k sokhraneniiu narodnogo zdorov'ia* (St. Petersburg: Imperatorskii Shliakhetnyi Sukhoputnyi Kadetskii Korpus, 1795), 45; K. I. Killian, *Domashnii lechebnik, ili obstoiatel'noe i iasnoe pokazanie kak vo vsekh opasnykh, skoropostizhnykh i khronicheskikh, kak naruzhnykh, tak i vnutrennikh bolezniakh pri otsutstvii vracha, mozhno podat' vazhnuiu pomoshch' posredstvom odnikh domashnikh sredstv i diety; vserkh togo, kak postupat' kasatel'no preduprezhdeniia boleznei i khraneniia svoego zdraviia,* trans. Petr Butkovskii (St. Petersburg: Ivan Glazunov, 1823), vol. 2, 174; Roman Chetyrkin, *Opyt voenno-meditsinskoi politsii, ili pravila k sokhraneniiu zdorov'ia russkikh soldat v sukhoputnoi sluzhbe* (St. Petersburg:

Iversen, 1834), 43; Karl Geling, *Opyt grazhdanskoi meditsinskoi politsii primenennoi k zakonam rossiiskoi imperii* (Vil'na: A. Martsinovskii, 1842), 334–5; Engalychev, *O prodolzhenii chelovecheskoi zhizni*, vol. 3, 239; *Noveishaia povarennaia kniga, zakliuchaiushchaia v sebe 1046 pravil, sostavlennaia russkim povarom N. V. G … m, po metode K. Avdeevoi*, 2nd ed. (Moscow: Katkov i Ko, 1864), vol. 1, xi.

25 "Zapiska o prichinakh, po koim Kazan' prinadlezhit k gorodam, zdorov'iu neblagopriiatstvuiushchim," *Zavolzhskii muravei* 3 (19–20) (1833): 1077–96, 1130–8, here 1130.

26 Charukovskii, *Narodnaia meditsina*, vol. 2, part 3, 159–60. Unpleasant smell and taste were also characteristic of spoiled butter: "Sposob prigotovliat' slivochnoe maslo, dolgo neportiashcheesia," *Zemledel'cheskaia gazeta* (February 8, 1855), 44.

27 Eggs were the prime example of smell associated with rottenness. See, for example, "O kukhonnoi provizii," *Zhurnal obshchepoleznykh svedeniia* 1 (3) (1847): 183–93, here 190–1.

28 A. Nikitin, "O iadovitom veshchesstve obrazuiushchemsia v kolbasakh. (Venenum botulinum)," *Trudy obshchestva russkikh vrachei* 3 (1843): 105–13, here 106.

29 Karl Geling, *Opyt grazhdanskoi meditsinskoi politsii*, 302.

30 "O dichi voobshche," *Ekonom* 3 (81) (1842): 231–2.

31 Jean-Anthelme Brillat-Savarin, *The Physiology of Taste*, trans. Anne Drayton (London: Penguin Books, 1994), 84.

32 Ibid., 332.

33 "Zadacha," *Ezhemesiachnye sochineniia k pol'ze i uveseleniiu sluzhashchie* (1764): 283–8, here 287.

34 Marquis of Londonderry, *Recollections of a Tour in the North of Europe in 1836–1837*, vol. 1 (London: Richard Bentley, 1838), 131. Others agreed. See Thomas Raikes, *A Visit to St. Petersburg, in the Winter of 1829–30* (London: Richard Bentley, 1838), 289. More generally on the frozen meat markets, see A. B. Granville, *St. Petersburgh. A Journal of Travels to and from that Capital; through Flanders, the Rhenish Provinces, Prussia, Russia, Poland, Silesia, Saxony, the Federated States of Germany, and France* (London: Henry Colbourn, 1828), vol. 2, 408–9; Sutherland Edwards, *The Russians at Home: Unpolitical Sketches, Showing What Newspapers They Read; What Theatres They Frequent; and How They Eat, Drink, and Enjoy Themselves; With Other Matter Relating Chiefly to Literature and Music, and to Places of Historical and Religious Interest in and around Moscow; Comprising also Four Russian Designs (on stone)*, 2nd ed. (London: Wm. H. Allen and Co., 1861), 295–7.

35 *Bagatelles. Promenades d'un désoeuvré dans la ville de St.-Pétersbourg* (Paris: J. Klosterman, fils, et Delaunay, 1812), vol. 1, 230.

36 "Potreblenie nekotorykh tovarov v Rossii," *Biblioteka dlia chteniia* 5 (1834): otd. 7, 80. This was considerably up from its late-eighteenth-century place among imports; in 1793–5, the amount was 121,300 rubles of imported cheese, according to Arcadius Kahan, "The Costs of 'Westernization' in

Russia: The Gentry and the Economy in the Eighteenth Century," *Slavic Review* 25 (1) (1966): 40–66, here 44. Articles on cheese production include N. P. Filippov, "O prigotovlenii syrov, Shveitsarskogo i Parmezana," *Biblioteka dlia chteniia* 4 (1834), otd. 4, 15–29; "Fiziologiko-istoricheskoe opisanie Parmezanskogo syra," *Ekonom* 7 (158) (1844): 49–50; and "Prigotovlenie syra, na podobie angliiskogo stil'tona," *Kazanskie gubernskie vedomosti* 37N (1856): 288-9.

37 Charukovskii, *Narodnaia meditsina*, vol. 2, part 3, 168.
38 Doktor Puf, "Lektsiia XXXVI," *Zapiski dlia khoziaeva* (1844): 286.
39 *Prikhotnik ukazuiushchii legchaishie sposoby imet' nailuchshii stol* (St. Petersburg: Iv. Glazunov, 1809), 5–6.
40 "Bifsteks," *Zhurnal obshchepoleznykh svedeniia* 4 (1) (1849): IV, 62–5, here 63.
41 "Obshchie kukhonnye neizmennye pravila," *Ekonom* 7 (158) (1844): 23.
42 "O fazanakh," *Ekonom* 5 (126) (1843): 173.
43 "Postnye kiseli vsekh vozmozhnykh rodov," *Zhurnal obshchepoleznykh svedeniia* 4 (3) (1849): 237–42, here 237.
44 Robert Bremner, *Excursions in the Interior of Russia; Including Sketches of the Character and Policy of Emperor Nicholas, Scenes in St. Petersburg, &c. &c.*, vol. 1 (London: Henry Colburn, 1839), 152.
45 And the bread was distinctly sour: "we, however, could not eat it at all ... [it] was as sour as vinegar, both to taste and smell." Paul of Aleppo, *The Travels of Macarius, Patriarch of Antioch*, trans. F. C. Belfour (London: Oriental Translation Fund of Great-Britain and Ireland, 1836), vol. ii, 40–1.
46 "Prodolzhenie pis'ma o zemledel'stve v Kazanskoi i Orenburgskoi guberniiakh," *Ezhemesiachnye sochineniia k pol'ze i uveseleniiu sluzhashchie* (1758): 483–524, here 484.
47 Smith, *Recipes for Russia*, 3–5.
48 Akim Charukovskii, *Voenno-pokhodnaia meditsina* vol. 1 (St. Petersburg: I. Vorob'ev, 1836), 46.
49 A cookbook author claimed that "the (sour) starter for dough for bread of rye flour is known to everyone who makes it" (*Domashnee i sel'skoe khoziaistvo* (Moscow: Stepanova, 1852), 5. See also V. B., "Russkoe khlebopechenie," *Ekonom* 3 (95) (1842): 337–40 and 5 (106) (1843): 11–4.
50 J. G. Köhl, *Panorama of St. Petersburg* (London: Simms and McIntyre, 1852), 145.
51 The Author of *Revelations of Russia* [Charles Frederick Henningsen], "To the Editor of the Times," *Times* (London) June 21, 1847, p. 3 col. b.
52 William Coxe, *Travels into Poland, Russia, Sweden, and Denmark* (London: T. Cadell, 1792), vol. 2, 205. For more comment on its unpleasantness to the visitor, tied to its sourness or acidity, see Robert D. D. Pinkerton, *Russia: or, Miscellaneous Observations on the Past and Present State of that Country and Its Inhabitants* (London: Seely & Sons, 1833), 70; Granville, *St. Petersburgh*, 415.

53 A. A. Sokolovskii, *Pitatel'nye veshchestva i napitki* (Kazan': Tipografiia Universiteta, 1859), 98.

54 Charukovskii, *Narodnaia meditsina*, vol. 2, part 3, 142–3.

55 "Russkie khlebopeki v Anglii," *Posrednik* 8 (27–28) (1847): 105–7, 109–10, here 105.

56 Chetyrkin, *Opyt voenno-meditsinskoi politsii*, 36. Similarly, another noted that properly soured bread was very nutritious, and only when it had "excessive sourness" might it trouble "some (but probably not Russian) stomachs," Sokolovskii, *Pitatel'nye veshchestva*, 99.

57 I. Starchikov, "Peterburgskii lavochnik," *Literaturnaia gazeta* 23–24 (1845): 391–3, 406–9, here 393.

58 Bremner, *Excursions in the Interior of Russia*, 240. On its ubiquity across social divisions, see also Granville, *St. Petersburgh*, 423; Edwards, *The Russians at Home*, 328. A few Russians did, however, claim that kvas was going out of fashion, and was less commonly drunk in places like fashionable St. Petersburg. "Kvas," *Zhurnal obshchepoleznykh svedeniiakh* 1 (1) (1847): 65–7, here 65.

59 R. B. Paul, *Journal of a Tour to Moscow, in the Summer of 1836* (London: Simpkin, Marshall, & Co. and Whittaker & Co., 1836), 44.

60 Pinkerton, *Russia: or, Miscellaneous Observations on the Past and Present State of that Country*, 71; Leitch Ritchie, *A Journey to St. Petersburg and Moscow through Courland and Livonia* (London: Longman, Rees, Orme, Brown, Green, and Longman, 1836), 210

61 Edward Jerrmann, *St. Petersburg: Its People; Their Character and Institutions* (New York: A. S. Barnes & Co., [1855]), 69.

62 Paul of Aleppo, *Travels of Macarius*, 41; Augustus von Kotzebue, *The Most Remarkable Year in the Life of Augustus von Kotzebue; Containing an Account of his Exile into Siberia, and of the Other Extraordinary Events Which Happened to Him in Russia*, vol. 1 (London: Richard Phillips, 1802), 75ftnt; William Rae Wilson, *Travels in Russia, &c. &c.* (London: Longman, Reese, Orme, Brown, and Green, 1828), vol. 1, 355. In another case, it was reported that French soldiers (presumably from the Napoleonic invasion) "felt at first some repugnance towards the use of quass, but they very soon became accustomed to it, and in the end loved it so much as to manufacture it themselves." See John Antony Chaptal, *Chymistry Applied to Agriculture* (Boston: Hilliard, Gray, and Co., 1836), 280.

63 Kohl, *Panorama*, 147. Similarly positive descriptions include John Barrow, *Excursions in the North of Europe, through Parts of Russia, Finland, Sweden, Denmark, and Norway*, New Edition (London: John Murray, 1835), 110 (kvas "is really a most delicious beverage, especially on a hot summer's day, when brought up iced from the cellars").

64 Chetyrkin, *Opyt voenno-meditsinskoi politsii*, 51.

65 Giuetan, "O pishche i pit'e, naibolee svoistvennykh liudiam pozhilym i v starosti," *Drug zdraviia* 7 (43) (1839): 338 note.

66 Geling, *Opyt grazhdanskoi meditsinskoi politsii*, 344.

67 Edwards, *The Russians at Home*, 328.
68 A. Jourdier, *Excursion agronomique en Russie* (St. Petersburg: Chez S. Dufour, 1860), 161–2.
69 Geling, *Opyt grazhdanskoi meditsinskoi politsii*, 345.
70 Prokofii Kuzhelevich, *Nachertanie ostorozhnostei, sluzhashchikh k zdorovomu i blagopoluchnomu prodolzheniiu zhizni, dlia vsiakogo sostoianiia liudei* (Moscow: Tipografiia 8go klassa bozhukovoi, 1825), 13. Others agreed, listing similar worries about under- or over-fermented kvas: Aleksandr Nikitin, *Populiarnaia dietetika, ili ukazanie sredstv v sokhraneniiu zdorov'ia* (St. Petersburg: Eduard Prats, 1851), 122.
71 For example, William Tooke, *View of the Russian Empire during the Reign of Catherine the Second, and to the Close of the Eighteenth Century* (Dublin: P. Wogan, 1801), vol. 3, 169.
72 Bremner, *Excursions in the Interior of Russia*, 152–3.
73 "Kislaia kapusta vo Frantsii," *Russkii zemledelets* 7 (3) (1839): 180–1.
74 Giuetan, "O pishche i pit'e," 186; "Promysl' kapustoi brokoli v Londone," *Posrednik* 15 (14) (1854): 55.
75 V. Dobronravov, *Rukovodstvo k sokhraneniiu zdorov'ia i vospitaniiu cheloveka* (St. Petersburg: Tipografiia departamenta vneshnei torgovli, 1858), vol. 1, 182–3.
76 Dvigubskii, *Leksikon sel'skogo i gorodskogo khoziaistva*, vol. 2, 231.
77 Chetyrkin, *Opyt voenno-meditsinskoi politsii*, 40.
78 Figurin, "Rvota, izlechennaia kvashennoi kapustoi," *Drug zdraviia* 6 (19) (1838): 148–9.
79 "Eshche o kushan'iakh i v oobshche o pitatel'nyh veshchestvakh otnositel'no vliianiia, kakoe imeiut oni na zdorov'e cheloveka," *Ekonom* 2 (29) (1841): 234, 234ftnt. The most common claim was that sour cabbage was an effective anti-scorbutic. See Iv. Reipol'skii, "Tsinga (Scorubuts)," *Drug zdraviia* 17 (1849): 97–8, 105–6.
80 "O kukhonnoi provizii," 190.
81 Even in the 1960s, a report on "Yugoslavian pickled cabbage" (again really fermented cabbage), noted that "there is so little standardization of methods of manufacture." Carl S. Pederson, Gordana Niketic, and Margaret N. Albury, "Fermentation of the Yugoslavian Pickled Cabbage," *Applied and Environmental Microbiology* 10 (1) (January 1962): 86–9.
82 Geling, *Opyt grazhdanskoi meditsinskoi politsii*, 305. Another article commented "everyone knows the unpleasantness of keeping sour cabbage at home in barrels, and what an unpleasant odor infects the air" ("Pripasi," *Posrednik* 14 (47) (1853): 185–6, here 185ftnt).
83 K. Avdeeva and A. Avdeev, *Ekonomicheskii leksikon, raspolozhennyi po azbuchnomu poriadku*, vol. 1 (St. Petersburg, K. Zhernakov, 1848), 71–2.
84 "Poleznoe izobretenie dlia prodovol'stviia armii, flota i naroda," *Ekonom* 20 (1849): 160.
85 P. Davydov, "Sposob susheniia kvashenoi kapusty v russkikh pechakh,"

Trudy Vol'nogo ekonomicheskogo obshchestva 1, otd. iii (1850): 56–9. The "useful invention" touted by the *Ekonom* article, above, also suggested drying as a way of keeping all the medicinal qualities of fermented cabbage intact.

86 Mary Douglas warns against this view in *Purity and Danger* and "Standard Social Uses of Food: Introduction," in *Food in the Social Order: Studies of Food and Festivities in Three American Communities*, ed. Mary Douglas (New York: Russell Sage Foundation, 1984).

87 "Part of a Letter from Matthew Guthrie, MD of Petersburg, to Dr. Priestly, FRS on the Antiseptic Regimen of the Natives of Russia," in *The Philosophical Transactions of the Royal Society of London, from Their Commencement, in 1665, to the Year 1800; Abridged, with Notes and Biographical Illustrations*, by Charles Hutton, George Shaw, and Richard Pearson, vol. XIV, 1776 to 1780 (London: C. and B. Baldwin, 1809), 395–400 (quote from 396). See also E. D. Clarke, *Travels in Various Countries of Europe Asia and Africa: Part the First: Russia Tartary and Turkey*, 4th ed. (London: T. Cadell and W. Davies, 1817), 117, for another description of the ways that the Russian taste for sour things "counteracted" the "scorbutic effects" of their larger diet. On the larger process of transferring medical knowledge about scurvy across national boundaries, see Matthew P. Romaniello, "Circuits of Knowledge: Developing Therapies for Scurvy between Russia and Europe," paper presented at Continuity and Change in Russian Therapy, St. Antony's College, University of Oxford, 2014.

88 I. [N.] Boltin, *Primechaniia na istoriiu drevniia i nyneshniia Rossii G. Leklerka, sochinennyia general maiorom Ivanom Boltinym* (St. Petersburg: Tipografiia gornogo uchilishcha, 1788), vol. 2, 408, 410.

89 F. B., "Samyi prostoi i legkii sposob vozdelyvaniia kartofelia, sredstava k ego sokhrananiiu i sovet, kak zastavit' russkogo cheloveka poliubit' ego," *Ekonom*, 1 (1) (1841): 4–5.

90 Robert Lyall, *The Character of the Russians, and a Detailed History of Moscow* (London: T. Cadell, 1823), xxiii.

91 Clarke, *Travels*, 45, 45ftnt.

92 Katz, *The Art of Fermentation*, 35.

CHAPTER FOUR

Market pleasures and prostitution in St. Petersburg

Abby Schrader

On May 9, 1848, Count Iakov I. Essen-Stenbock-Fermor's brilliant new structure, *Passazh*, which spanned Nevsky Prospekt and Italianskaia Ulitsa in central St. Petersburg, opened to considerable fanfare. The gala event included a ribbon-cutting by the Petersburg Military Governor General, a celebratory breakfast for the workers who erected the building, blessings over bread and salt, and a formal meal. The highest echelons of the Petersburg public toasted the count, whose genius had brought to St. Petersburg such "an excellent building, the likes of which has never been seen in all of Europe."[1]

Stenbock-Fermor situated his gigantic private arcade in central Petersburg as an antidote to the nearby slovenly Russian markets, Little Gostinyi Dvor, Apraksin Dvor, and Shchukin Dvor. These featured disorderly dilapidated wooden stalls, unseemly storehouses, and petty traders who laid out their wares in a haphazard and outmoded manner.[2] In particular, he wanted to set off *Passazh* from Gostinyi Dvor, located just across Nevsky.[3]

Stenbock-Fermor not only sought to make shopping more pleasant for the city's refined classes but also aimed to shore up the city's blurred boundaries. By the mid-nineteenth century, elite Russians expressed increasing concern about how messy market practices challenged social order in the capital. Canal embankments crowded with motley peasants hawking smelly livestock and foodstuffs whose noxious odor melded unappealingly with that of the water posed a sensory assault. Contemporary Russian elites' efforts to construct themselves as modern, which they nearly always equated with Western, transpired in part through their attempts to modulate the sensory world of the capital city that theoretically epitomized the Empire's European orientation.[4]

Traditional Russian markets were noisy, odiferous spaces: peddlers verbally and physically accosted their consumers; the food they sold emitted enticing and less enticing smells depending upon its freshness; and exchange spilled out of stalls and stores and into the streets and under the bridges in a disorderly manner. In the late eighteenth century and early nineteenth century, local officials placed a premium on the cleanliness of both the capital's market squares and the merchandise being sold on them, advocating for "special supervision" to "prevent slovenliness and a repulsive smell." In particular, they ordered that that sellers be prohibited from keeping "raw meat, fatback, innards, and horns, and ... bringing small cattle with them into their stalls," threatening to prosecute violators.[5]

Sanitizing traditional bazaars did not go quite far enough. In Petersburg, elites devoted material, fiscal, and discursive capital to marginalizing and containing the dank, dark, and smelly markets and reconstructing the city center around visually appealing and literally enlightened emporia that showcased the luxurious, cultured, and technologically avant-garde. The perfume of exotic tobacco, *eau de cologne*, heady wines, and fresh flowers would replace the stench of rotting meat and produce. The sounds of peasants hawking their wares would be exchanged for mellifluous tunes struck up by touring orchestras and singers visiting newly-opened theaters populated with select audiences who enjoyed the latest nighttime diversions featured in their newly-illuminated cosmopolitan city center.[6]

Authorities were not alone in advancing this position; like their European counterparts, cultural commentators from inside and outside official ranks associated filth and stench with incivility and the control or neutralization of odors with modernity. The authors of Petersburg's panoramic literature mined the wealth of medico-statistical data about the cosmopolitan center to analyze life in the city and offer up direct or indirect advice about how to improve it.[7]

Panoramic literature took as its subject the physiological, living processes of the urban center and invited readers to engage all of their senses in exploring the city. Occupying a literary middle ground between the ethnographic and the fictional, panoramas first became fashionable in Paris of the early nineteenth century and were later popularized by authors like Balzac and Baudelaire who sought to classify the Parisian population into "easily recognizable social types" in order to make "the social hierarchy of the city 'transparent,' or easily legible."[8] Using the Parisian prototype as a model, Petersburg's panoramists transported readers along cosmopolitan streets and bridges and through the ceaseless and ever-changing activity of the urban center's marketplaces and public spaces. The city, and particularly its main artery, Nevsky Prospekt, became a "broad field for observation for the writer about morals ... the lifestyle, the doings, the passions and the weaknesses of residents of practically all status groupings. ... Women, girls, maidens, soldiers, state officials, the old, the small, the worldly, the dandy, the journalist—all of them at the appointed hour rush along Nevsky Prospekt."[9] The readers who devoured this literature used more than their eyes. They conceived of themselves as consumers who traveled through and experienced the city, gathering "information by sensation" about it in their efforts to know the metropolis.[10]

Knowing a city or making it legible does not mean simplifying it. As historian Victoria Thompson has argued, such physiognomic sketches actually presented a "more complex vision of the city and its inhabitants" than commonly held, often focusing on the dualistic nature of both.[11] This certainly holds true in the case of Petersburg. For its panoramists, the urban sector embodied both progress and danger. It at once was the site and facilitator of technological breakthroughs in architecture and engineering and the source of anxiety about the moral and medical perils posed by modernity. The authors of panoramas highlighted both aspects.[12]

Petersburg's urban planners and social commentators deemed it essential to upgrade and modernize the capital's infrastructure by instituting projects to pave sidewalks, lay bridges, extend street lighting, ensure water safety, and clean courtyards if the progressive tendencies of urbanization were to win out in Russia, or at least in Petersburg.[13] Efforts to improve the city's markets by stripping away customary practices and layouts and replacing these with modern consumer infrastructure were part of this broader endeavor. They regulated stalls, storehouses, and bazaars and relegated their activity to the margins of the capital, preferably concealing it within controlled boundaries. They hoped this might shore up what they deemed to be a necessary division between the cosmopolitan environment that they wished to inhabit and the realities of contemporary Petersburg that called this into question.

City planners obviously understood that transforming the metropolis would have a salubrious impact on all. But the advance of the capital's "civilization threshold" also implicitly provoked anxieties because it brought various social groupings into greater proximity and increased their interdependence. In the meantime, Russia's official estate (*soslovie*) system was becoming blurrier and less descriptive of social realities. Nowhere was this more evident than in urban Russia. As Alexander Martin has shown in his analysis of urban life in the era of Nicholas I, "at home and on the street, Muscovites daily crossed paths in ways that promoted cultural hybridity and social mobility even as they reinforced a particularistic estate consciousness and traditional forms of authority"; the same, he suggests, held true of social relations in contemporary Petersburg.[14]

Urban planners, authorities, and panoramists believed that elevating the experience of shopping in the capital's elite districts would attract, and perhaps even create, a new kind of consumer with fresh expectations. Whether purchasing or just window-shopping, the modern customer would possess good taste and discernment. For the period under discussion, however, the point was not to open up the consumption of luxury items to the lower social rungs; indeed, quite the opposite. Writers and planners suggested that proximity to and the ability to see, smell, touch, and ingest rarefied European goods made Petersburg's elites distinct and set them apart from the masses.¹⁵ In their "pursuit of exclusiveness," as sociologist Pierre Bourdieu has termed it, upper-crust Petersburgers not only pursued innovative habits and forms of consumption, but through these reinforced their dominance over the vast majority of the city's residents who could not access such items, the appropriation of which "appear as the surest indications of the quality of the person."¹⁶ The opening of the *Passazh* shopping arcade was one means of enabling the urban elite to demarcate itself from the lower estate and establish its identity based upon consumption.

Less than two decades after the arcade's debut, sentiment about it had changed radically. As was true of its Parisian counterparts, the glass covered arcade of *Passazh*, which ostensibly provided elegant shelter from the climatic and moral discomforts of the outside world, quickly devolved into what cultural philosopher Walter Benjamin termed "a street of lascivious commerce … wholly adapted to arousing desires."¹⁷ As anthropologist David Howes argues, the "palace of consumption" created "consumer desires of all sorts in all people" and presented those who frequented it with "a variegated spectacle of goods to be viewed and occasionally sampled."¹⁸ This is what made *Passazh* and the upscale Nevsky Prospekt shopping district dangerous to men and women alike.

Faced with a world centered on commodity exchange and shopping, women took on new roles as store clerks, shop girls, and consumers of the fashions and experiences being sold in high-end establishments giving them potential economic independence from their patriarchal families by earning their own money and making consumer choices. But this newfound freedom also placed them in jeopardy as they navigated dark or unnaturally lit streets alone or were tempted with goods and services that were financially out-of-reach. Regardless of their actual status, their association with consumption "rendered female consumers more publicly visible than they had formerly been," turning them into "part of the display." This became a "means for women to market themselves as commodities for male consumption." As historian Sally West points out in her discussion of the experience of shopping in late Imperial Moscow, this was how some single women secured husbands.¹⁹ But women strolling through Nevsky's fashionable district also often attracted less well-intentioned attention from men who objectified them and perceived their bodies and their company to be as much for sale as the objects on display in the cases and windows that lined the avenue. *Passazh,* and the portion of Nevsky upon which it stood, constituted the epicenter of Petersburg's commercial sex trade. The commodification of daily life in this district was inherently threatening to city officials and social commentators.²⁰ Rampant consumerism promoted debauchery in the arcade and further blurred the lines between the legitimate and illegitimate in an increasingly complicated, post-Emancipation urban environment.

Artifice on the avenue

In the 1830s and the early 1840s, central St. Petersburg—especially Nevsky Prospekt—was becoming the preserve of well-heeled sophisticates who epitomized refinement. These cosmopolitan elites, whose voices rang out clearly "in all possible languages—except Russian!" frequented the "row of cafes, taverns, fashionable shops, and stylish shoe stores" that lined the avenue, outfitting themselves and their homes in the latest European mode by indulging in the "mountain of crystal, porcelain, bronze, diamonds, and gold" and "all of the refinements of luxury, elegant taste, wealth, splendor, and brilliance" that could be procured on Nevsky.[21] Nevsky was celebrated as the place to find "all the articles of good taste, whims of fashion, articles with enchanting adjectives attached to them: *English, Dutch, Italian, French.*"[22]

But taking a closer look at the allegedly modern city center, the authors who wrote panoramas, physiologies, travelogues, and feuilletons revealed much of this luxury to be ersatz. In 1839, one Petersburg panoramist, historian, and statistician, Ivan Il'ich Pushkarev, wryly noted: "Some call this long street a renowned district of fashion; others call it a large European market. But it seems to me simpler and more justifiable to say that this is the home of Russian petty industry, which crosses into here from Bol'shaia Sadovaia Street and dresses itself up in a foreign costume for the sake of

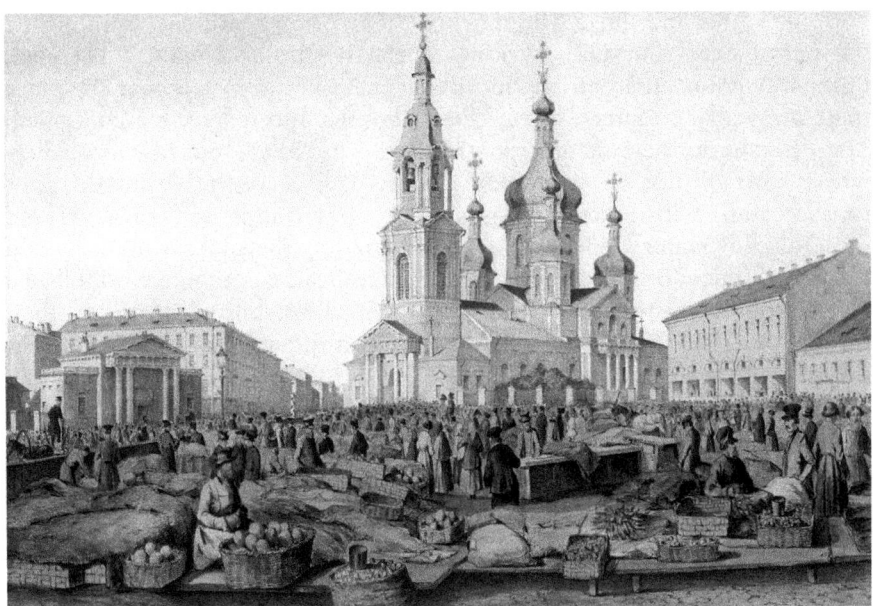

FIGURE 4.1 *Ferdinand Victor Perrot,* View of Sennaia (Haymarket) Square, *1841.*

blind imitation."[23] The unsuspecting shopper fell prey to an elaborate window-dressing scheme whereby deceitful traders passed off themselves, their products, and their city for something they were not. Petersburg's elite consumers not only fetishized luxury objects but also mistook the item that glittered in the avenue's shop windows for the real thing. The mirror reflected not reality but what the purchaser wanted to see. The plate glass windows of Petersburg's swank shops thus played a significant role in stimulating desire for new goods and experiences.[24]

Rather than condemn modern market practices, Petersburg's panoramists attributed the difficulty of shoring up Nevsky Prospekt's reputation as the preserve of elite Petersburg to its proximity to the underbelly of the capital city. The best sections of town, the Admiralty and Liteinyi districts, were where "the people of the highest circle, of the grand, tony and fashionable world" resided. Yet, as Aleksandr Pavlovich Bashutskii noted in 1834, disorderly Haymarket Square (Sennaia Ploshchad') and Gorokhovaia Street spilled over into these high-end districts: with "their dark bands," Haymarket Square and Gorokhovaia "stretch across such brilliance with their markets, with their filth and their dark cries, with their ceaseless motion and their incessant noise, with their dense, motley popular crowds ...with the dirty and sharp voices of their cabmen, traders, women, children, and workers. This is Nevsky Prospekt of the masses."[25]

The "ubiquitous nomadic industry" and "petty trade" that prevailed in these popular street markets led to sensory overload: spatial crowding was compounded by the disarray of goods and the rough, rural cast of both the wares and those who hawked them, often "casually" and outside the purview of the state. Writing at the height of Nicholas I's reign, Pushkarev commented at length: "Everywhere you turn, all over the place there are stalls, counters, cases, chests, booths and tents." He continued: "In Petersburg there is not a street, not an alley, not a passageway where you will not see petty stalls, either fruit or vegetable stands ... or tobacco stalls with boxes of cigars ... or meat stands with sausages and meatballs."[26] Major General Krol', nominated by the Chief Administration for Communications and Public Buildings to head a committee established to investigate the status of markets in St. Petersburg, confirmed that, throughout the city, "petty stalls have grown numerous to the point that they can no longer be counted."[27]

Although it was technically illegal to operate a business without documentation and paying fees, numerous sellers set up shop along the streets, under the bridges, and on the outskirts of markets, hawking their wares from carts and tables without permission or supervision.[28] This situation was particularly bad in the third Admiralty district, which was "the focal point of Petersburg's productive activity," and home to major commercial centers, among them Haymarket Square, Nikol'sk market, and Apraksin, Shchukin, and Gostinyi dvors, more taverns, bars, pubs, cafeterias, and food halls than in any other district in the city, and the greatest concentration of members of the middling and lower estates, "who carry out various forms of exchange." As Pushkarev recounted, "the internal order of the houses, and particularly the courtyards, which are hardly comfortable, are crowded here, and even repel one's eyes with their lack of cleanliness."[29] While some lauded the markets along Sadovaia as a gastronomical paradise, these stalls and especially the ones located at Haymarket Square, lured all sorts: they brought together "the rich and the poor, the bountiful and red-nosed Russian cook, the French chef, the housewife, well-known and famous gentlemen who reside in palaces, and the poor Russian who has but five rubles [in his possession] and hoped not to be taken for a beggar or a thief."[30]

This hubbub complicated authorities' efforts to control the urban environment. As Petersburg's Military Governor General remarked in the mid-1840s, the copious and ever-increasing number of peasants who sought to peddle the foodstuffs that they brought with them from the village lacked official places to trade on Haymarket Square. They therefore set out their wares along the embankments of Ekaterininskii canal and the adjacent side streets. The environs of the market were so congested that residents had difficulty getting to their homes, and "because of this crowding, the appearance of the city is blemished."[31] This contributed to the "sorry look" of the square and its surrounding blocks, where "hawkers bring out their trays and bast mats, place them on the ground, arranging a place to trade, as the peasants from the suburbs also do, who sell food items from their carts. It was, as it is still now," noted panoramist Peter Nikolaevich Stolpianskii, reflecting on the state of city in the late 1850s from the vantage point of the *fin de siècle*, "the belly of St. Petersburg, and entirely badly organized."[32]

Pushkarev, who harshly critiqued all traditional Russian markets, felt that Gostinyi Dvor warranted especial condemnation. Its primary liability was that it was sited at the nexus of elite and lower-class Petersburg. As such, Gostinyi Dvor functions as the:

> chief tributary of first-rate petty industry in Petersburg; the majority of ships arriving in this port bring their cargo here; long strings of sledges with goods arrive here from the Nizhegorod market; the Germans from Vasilievskii Ostrov bring the ordinary gloves they sew here, and so do the Russian haberdashers ... and from here petty traders drag off porcelain and bronze, broadcloth and linen, shoes and boots, and various other wares made by our manufactures and our craftsmen ... and often sell them in stores under magical names like: French and English products!

He elaborated: the ostensibly modern products sold in Nevsky's finest shops themselves originated in the lowly and slovenly Russian markets of Apraksin and Shchukin Dvor or Haymarket Square. From there, they made their way down the avenue, passing through the hands of cunning traders who reinvented their pedigrees, and ended up being sold in Gostinyi Dvor, the rows of market stalls that stood at the corner of Sadovaia and Nevsky: "In order to serve you up something *not Russian*," explained Pushkarev, "they bring here from the filthy Russian master-studios, things made by Russian hands ... various goods, which are later placed on mirrored glass shelves or on mahogany tables of luxuriously appointed shops."[33]

To compound matters, the facilities out of which merchants traded in Gostinyi Dvor were not up to European standards. Eduard Jermann, a German who visited St. Petersburg in 1841, depicted the building that housed the market stalls as "not very cheerful"; its dull and nondescript stone vaulted passages "have a damp and not very clean look." Gostinyi Dvor was even more ominous by night: merchants closed up shop at dusk, which was as early as three in the afternoon during the winter, "it being strictly forbidden to have lights in the building." He noted that "here and there burns a glimmering lamp, in the niche under the image of some saint, and by its feeble illumination of these gloomy vaults, only increases their dismal aspect." The sense of general foreboding posed by the structure was only exacerbated by the packs of fierce, howling and barking wolfhounds chained to the stalls. While Jermann readily conceded that "every conceivable object ... of necessity and luxury" was for sale in Gostinyi Dvor, the merchants did not display their wares attractively.[34] Johann Georg Kohl, who visited Petersburg a year later, had a more favorable impression of Gostinyi Dvor, but he observed the pall cast by the darkness, the brief hours that one could devote to commerce in the winter, and the "unmerciful cold" that confronted those who visited the open market stalls.[35]

Sensitive to these problems, Bashutskii, who worked in the State Council, devised a plan in 1843 to shore up the division between Nevsky's elite emporia and the popular bazaars contiguous to it. He recommended erecting a two-story building with room for sixty-four shops connected to the main corpus of Gostinyi Dvor by a "splendid gallery." This glass-enclosed, Parisian-inspired structure would "be lined with stores on both sides and present the public with an excellent enclosed place to walk at all hours of the day and in all kinds of weather."[36] As Bashutskii explained, this "magnificent line of luxurious shops," this "gallery, or a passage," would "beautify the capital" by altering "the aesthetics of Gostinyi Dvor, which is disgraceful for splendid Nevsky Prospekt."[37]

Closing off the mall from the street preserved proper social relations by eliminating not only the "filth and deleterious impact of our changeable climate" but also the "push of the customers who are members of the dirty masses" shielding the "public"—a term that Bashutskii reserved for Petersburg's high society—from the "popular crowd." The "division of society into circles," which was "the necessary consequence of a variety of proclivities, tastes, and in some respects, modes of life," was being assaulted by the metropolis' messy market culture, with its fluid lines and transgressed boundaries. Renovating Gostinyi Dvor would reserve Nevsky for the elites to whom Bashutskii felt the street rightfully belonged.[38]

Lighting the interior of Gostinyi Dvor was integral to Bashutskii's plan. St. Petersburg was the first Russian city to bask in the glow of artificial illumination; yet the lamps that lined the city center in the late 1830s and 1840s cast a relatively faint flicker over a small portion of the city's streets and failed to transform it.[39] Even less well-lit were building interiors. Appalled that the inside walls of the neoclassical shopping center designed by Vallin de la Mothe "completely eclipse the light in the stalls, which even without their obstruction would not have been sufficient," Bashutskii advocated that the merchants raise funds to run gas pipelines into Gostinyi Dvor. Potent lighting would brighten the "dark and gloomy" stalls and enable elite consumers to discern between "true luxury items and those goods whose splendor was based on a trick of the eye."[40]

That such renovations might inflate prices was no cause for concern; after all, Gostinyi Dvor should be the preserve of high-end clientele, asserted Bashutskii; pricing the "popular crowd" out of the market would be a desirable side effect. Wealthy consumers would realize that everything here that was "according to their taste and their comfort:" "the cleanliness, order, and safety" afforded by the new construction "would keep out the dampness, the wind, the cold, the filth, and the darkness" and enhance the lives of Petersburg's "best public."[41]

It was easier for Bashutskii to draft this plan than it was for him to secure its implementation. Gostinyi Dvor's merchants took issue with the project immediately upon its presentation by the City Duma. The capital investment and assessments needed to finance construction would bankrupt current merchants and prevent new merchants from opening stalls. Only the rich might benefit from the new building.[42] Authorities and merchants feared the dangers posed by the interior use of gas lighting. Even if it were possible to assure that the interior could be safely lit, such artificial illumination might obscure the true color and richness of their fabrics, which would "spoil completely under gas lighting" according to the merchants.[43]

A passage to modernity

Although the merchants resisted implementing Bashutskii's plan, several years later, Petersburg did acquire a modern, gas-lit emporium in the form of a glass-enclosed *Passazh* funded by Stenbock-Fermor.[44] Echoing Bashutskii, the count deemed that his *Passazh* would serve as an alternative to undisciplined Russian bazaars like Gostinyi Dvor, located just across the street. Noting that the "obsolete" trade in Gostinyi Dvor "was set up in a way suited to the needs, lifestyle, habits and rules of exchanges of another century," Stenbock-Fermor scoffed at its merchants who had refused to foot the bill for renovations and the installation of "lovely window displays" that "enticed the public." This was short-sighted: Petersburgers' tastes had grown more refined and so had their desire for shelter from the popular crowd and filth endemic to the characteristically Russian markets that featured dilapidated wooden stalls, unseemly storehouses, and petty traders who relished defrauding customers.[45]

Stenbock-Fermor's *Passazh* sought to provide Petersburgers transit into modern European consumer culture. This was expressed in the building's architectural features. The majestic interior was innovatively lit by both natural and artificial means: covered by an iron-framed roof enclosed with glass, the building's upper-level balconies and central arcade were illuminated by daylight. The glass arcade would be a beacon to passersby on the dark streets outside: 800 gas lamps—equivalent in number to the lamps then installed along the capital's streets—set aglow the interior of shops, apartments, and walkways at night and the vast underground shopping tunnel throughout the day.[46] *Passazh* also boasted indoor running water at a time when this was practically unheard of in the city; R. A. Zheliazevich's design included pipes to supply water from the count's private baths in the Liteinyi section to the building's modern plumbing, which also offered fire protection.[47] Thus, *Passazh* afforded those who frequented it a new experience of their environment: the increased and altered visibility furnished by a skylight and gas lamps; climate control that allowed fashionable Petersburgers to shed their streetwear when strolling the arcade in the dead of winter; and creature comforts that marked the space as distinctive.

While similar in form, *Passazh* served a different purpose than its Parisian counterpart, which constituted a shortcut between two avenue blocks. As the feuilletonist for *The Saint Petersburg Record* put it, "among us, no one walks; we only stroll."[48] Only the poor or members of the middling strata were pedestrians; in contrast, the elites, for whom *Passazh* was the target audience, disembarked from carriages at the door and promenaded the fashionable arcade—to see and be seen—in much the same way as they ambled through the gardens surrounding imperial palaces. In this respect, *Passazh* constituted an extension of elite social spaces.

Stenbock-Fermor's *Passazh* altered this experience in a fundamental and peculiarly modern way by focusing strolling around consumption. The amusements concentrated under the arcade's roof were rarefied and seductive: the tunnel contained wine cellars and beer purveyors, tobacco humidors, and shops selling fresh flowers and exotic fruits and vegetables; the building was home to a state-of-the-art concert hall that held a thousand; there were exhibition spaces for curiosities from near and far and restaurants and coffee houses where shoppers and pleasure-seekers could take refreshments.[49] As one commentator writing in the fashion press put it in 1851, "*Gostinyi Dvor* is a Russian bazaar, a memorial to older times, an episode from Moscow life. The *Passazh* is a European commercial street, a copy of foreign customs, a scene from foreign morals and manners."[50]

Although the count was unable to secure tenants for many of *Passazh*'s shops by the time the arcade opened, one feuilletonist optimistically proclaimed that "there is no doubt that … from now on *Passazh* will be a meeting place (*rendez vous*) for the entire Petersburg public, and where there is a crowd of people, there trade is always successful!"[51] He later elaborated:

> [I]t seems … that, in the approaching fall and winter, our social life … will center around *Passazh*: in the morning—walking in the bright, warm, graceful gallery … among the educated society that gathers here to inspect the new products made in Russia and abroad that are attractively arrayed in the glass windows of stores … later, a walk around the stores. … to buy something, or to enjoy some *fantasie du moment* … At that moment, you by chance meet up with friends or acquaintances and eat a nice lunch. … Having hardly finished eating … you take pleasure in a little cup of coffee and a Havana cigar—by then it's seven o'clock—and you prepare to hear Gil'man play music. … At ten o'clock … a ball starts up … where you give yourself over to dancing, taking hold of a young beauty in a waltz. … In a word, from morning until deep into the night you spend every minute in *Passazh* … We are certain that our wondrous, elegant, and gigantic *Passazh* will not only be a place of trade and production, but also a place of pleasure, uniting these two functions in a way that is useful and satisfying.[52]

By the 1860s, the "trade in *Passazh*" that grew "more lively with every passing day" and the nature of its pleasures turned out to be very different.[53] This decade was "the heyday of the Passage"; however, the changes wrought in contemporary Petersburg altered how *Passazh* was used, perceived, and represented.[54]

Sex and the city

The Emancipation of 1861 and the subsequent Great Reforms complicated the Russian social order. A more fluid society made possible the emergence of phenomena like mass migration to the urban center; mass-circulation newspapers with a much more popular, diverse general readership than that of the thick journals of a generation earlier; and a new mass consumer culture. This, in turn, reinforced a relatively freer exchange of ideas and people.[55]

Even as fluidity fostered vibrancy in the capital city, it heightened anxieties. This played out along the pages of the newspapers' feuilletons, which "regularly profiled public displays of all kinds." The anonymous authors struck an intimate tone with their readers, served as guides to the city, and provided not only information, frequently embellished, but also examined the quandaries posed by modern commercial relationships in cosmopolitan Petersburg.[56] Functioning in their own way as *flaneurs,* feuilletonists conceived of their columns as edifying. In their ethnographic explorations of the city, they exhibited less interest in extolling the virtues of Petersburg's physical grandeur than in assessing its moral quality.[57] The capital's boulevard press therefore regularly featured critiques about all aspects of urban street life, many of which contained lurid details about public lewdness, prostitution, men who preyed on women, women who invited such advances wittingly or otherwise, and the seemingly impossible task of controlling the underbelly of modernity.[58] The boulevard newspapers' reporters and feuilletonists approached the topics of commodity exchange in the fashionable emporia and the circulation of women's bodies in public from a multisensory perspective, highlighting not only the visual and olfactory but also touch, and particularly that of an overtly or implicitly sexualized nature.

Everyone—regardless of status or gender—was engaged in the vibrant commerce along Nevsky. This opened up legitimate opportunities for women to locate positions as seamstresses, shop clerks, and other pink-collar jobs that enabled them to more or less support themselves by working in the public rather than domestic sphere. Likewise, this allowed women to construct themselves as consumers: female shoppers moved through the bright modern world of department stores, checking out the luxury merchandise that purveyors artfully displayed. Work and shopping brought women into the money economy and thus at least to some extent extricated them from the direct patriarchal control of fathers, husbands, or those who oversaw their domestic service.[59]

That St. Petersburg was a city more focused on the public than the domestic sphere also explains its attraction to men. St. Petersburg was by design and tradition a masculine milieu: established by Peter the Great in 1703 as the headquarters of his navy and merchant marine, the city continued to be marked by a noted imbalance between the sexes even once it became the capital half a century later. As the bureaucratic hub of the Russian Empire and base of several of its most important military and naval garrisons, Petersburg was the destination for the elites for whom service was a requirement. Even once Catherine the Great abrogated this obligation, the city remained appealing to men because it afforded unique opportunities, particularly for those of high birth and the middling ranks of society.

At mid-century, there were 100 men for every seventy-eight women in St. Petersburg; therefore marriage was less prevalent in the capital than it was in other European and Imperial Russian cities, and a world that "demanded the participation of the male sex" predisposed the population toward "materialism and egoism" according to a *Petersburg Leaflet* article.[60] In turn, this excessive focus on individualism, rather than on the collective, meant that it was unsurprising that "[f]amily ties were not well developed" in the city center, which instead was "chiefly the place of traders who bring to it all sorts of commodities." Here, the emphasis was on "street life" and not domestic relations.[61]

Urban amusements and depravity went hand in hand for journalists in the boulevard press. As *Petersburg Leaflet*'s feuilletonist remarked sarcastically in an 1865 installment of the "City Diary":

> [o]ver the past four or five years, vice has made some very successful inroads in Petersburg. There was a time, and not very long ago, when it was absent ... you could count the number of depraved females strolling along Nevsky on your fingers. Those days are gone. Russia is embarking with swift feet upon the path of progress, and depravity is quickly propelling her forward.

The author related this sharp increase in immorality to the city's "many institutions of pleasure," particularly its musical, theatrical, and café culture.[62] *Passazh* was the hub of this debauched "culture"; bands of "young *dzhentel'men* dressed in the latest French mode and speaking French ... tormented numerous women and girls on the street in front of *Passazh* and *Gostinyi Dvor* and went drinking and carousing in *Passazh*."[63] There they found so-called "shop girls" and "seamstresses" eager to peddle themselves and not just their wares.

The proliferation of prostitution in the city's bustling commercial center indicated to journalists the crass commodification of the relationship between the sexes that had supplanted normal familial ties. Men who were not interested in marriage found it easy to satisfy their needs through "commercial transactions" with all sorts of women. Like other merchandise peddled in Petersburg's markets, the capital's prostitutes were arranged according to value and status. Poorer ones walked the streets of downtrodden neighborhoods such as Haymarket Square as registered prostitutes. Their more elite counterparts eluded regulation, passed themselves off as shop clerks or seamstresses, or pretended to be society women doing errands along Nevsky. The "brilliant Camelias"—unregistered courtesans whose nickname derived from the 1848 novel by Alexandre Dumas, fils, *La Dame Aux Camélias*, whose heroine forged liaisons with Paris' powerful and wealthy scions—frequented Nevsky's vibrant club scene.[64] The north side of Nevsky, where *Passazh* was located, was a particularly notorious haunt of both registered prostitutes and "secret" Camelias; stores closed down early, but bars, hotels, dance halls, and restaurants stayed open late and were a focal point for women eager to lure in drunken men with their seductive can-cans.[65]

The boulevard press expressed especial anxiety about elite women in and around *Passazh*. This was largely attributable to the fact that observers could not determine the identity of these women based upon their appearance or activities. Moreover, there was a great deal of fluidity between categories—a seamstress could make ends meet by selling her own body if needed or a female shopper could provide sexual favors to a gentleman suitor in exchange for a costly bauble that she had seen on display earlier. That they could readily pass from one category to another was problematic in Imperial Russia, where authorities strove to ascribe a fixed identity to each of the empire's subjects.[66]

Those who wrote for the boulevard press certainly acknowledged that marriage and legitimate job prospects for young women were dim. One observed that this made it hard to hold accountable impoverished girls who descended into debauchery. After all,

> everyone knows that women nowadays, and especially those who are poor, find it difficult to enter into marriage; after age twenty, wedlock becomes increasingly unlikely. At that stage ... a girl becomes a burden for destitute parents, and she seeks out decent labor to achieve self-sufficiency; but, given that the sphere of honorable undertakings for women is quite circumscribed, she succumbs to the oppressiveness of her everyday needs and involuntarily falls into prostitution.

Nonetheless, he also saw women as contributing to the problem: they increasingly sought husbands "practically only for economic advantage." What made this any different from prostitution, he wondered? Both conditions involved women exchanging their bodies for material benefit.[67]

This theme played out in a long, cautionary tale recounted in *Petersburg News* in 1868. "Natasha in Petersburg" revolves around a penniless young Petersburg migrant supporting her widowed mother. While homesick, Natasha nonetheless was initially optimistic about her prospects: "'I am capable of work: I am young, strong, not lazy, and I have a head [on my shoulders],' she said." Her first impulse was to locate a position in domestic service. Yet she soon grew dejected; none of the bureaus that she visited could find her a governess position. Her small, cold, and dank rented room was expensive and her supply of rubles was running perilously low; the one family in the city whom she knew denied her assistance because it feared that she would steal an eligible bachelor away from their own daughter.

Natasha had no recourse but to seek employment in the public sphere. After pounding the pavement and being turned away by shopkeeper after shopkeeper, Natasha received a note from a purveyor of trendy wares in the venerable *Passazh*. Amazed at her luck, she ran off to the store to take the position. But "[i]t happened that the owner ... was not in. Natasha turned to the milliners and began to converse with them. Not a quarter of an hour passed before they felt sufficiently familiar with her that they were unashamed to inquire whether she had a 'sweetheart' and informed her that they were wanting for nothing: in the evening, they strolled along Nevsky and in *Passazh*," and "sometimes formed liaisons with guests, with young men." Natasha quickly grasped the true nature of their labors and ran from the store without waiting for its matron. But how long could she subsist without employment? A girl on her own in the big city was in a perilous position, counseled the author of this piece.[68]

This was not the only risk that a single girl faced. Journalists reported that women walking alone in the evening, particularly along Nevsky, were constantly in danger of being mistaken as ladies of the night. One feuilletonist overheard a Staff Captain from the Gatchina Lifeguards Regiment propositioning a modestly dressed young woman. When the reporter inquired about the "insolent language" he was using, the captain replied that, "it was always his habit [to say such things] to women who were out walking alone."[69]

Authorities expected single men to act in a boorish manner toward unaccompanied females and frequently looked the other way when they did. In an 1865 installment of the "City Diary," *Petersburg Leaflet's* feuilletonist described how he was returning home one night when he witnessed a group of men on the sidewalk in front of *Passazh* catcalling women "for whom walking the street was not a craft" right under the nose of a policeman. "We did not think that the police tolerated such disorder along one of Petersburg's main thoroughfares," the journalist exclaimed. It was "high time to pay attention to the nighttime disorders perpetrated along Nevsky by both men and women, to those filthy, cynical gestures that we cannot help but perceive with disgust."[70]

These and similar outcries went unheeded. In one November 1868 incident, a well-bred woman headed home along Nevsky from a tutoring gig. "She had not quite passed *Passazh*," reported the feuilletonist, "when a young man flew out at her, declaring: "'Madame, allow me to take your hand!' The girl looked at him with disbelief and continued along her way, utterly silent. 'Don't stand on ceremony, *madame*!' persisted the predator, seizing her by the hand. 'Where would you like to go, to Palermo, to Nice?'" Fed up, the girl screamed at him to stop and began to "run in the direction of Anichkin Bridge. But the gentleman hardly felt the sting of this reproach" and caught up with her near the Fontanka, where he embraced her and declared, "'here, take this, you slut (*shliukha'*)', kissing her unceremoniously." The feuilletonist who reported this horrific—but hardly extraordinary incident—lamented that no one, including the police, took notice. "It is vile … vile … a thousand times vile," he declaimed, "that such abuses can take place on Nevsky, our best street, which is situated so that women who work somewhere or another practically always have to return home from their labors via it late in the evening. To go home along [Nevsky] is to invite abuse upon oneself."[71]

There is a deep relationship between hapticity and ownership embedded in the "politics of touch." This is evident in the stories concerning the assault of women along Nevsky. In a world where tactility and sex were increasingly associated with one another, it is not surprising that men used the gaze to colonize and express their ownership of women. By grabbing, embracing, and manhandling women they perceived as single and of a lower social status, Petersburg's male predators reinforced the patriarchal order and their preeminence within it. While journalists expressed sympathy toward the female targets of unwanted advances, they blamed them for "inviting abuse" by circulating in public without a male chaperone.[72]

Journalists acknowledged that some women did "earn their bread on the streets." But the majority were "women and girls who have to return home late, sometimes even after midnight, from [legitimate employment at] printing works, publishing houses, and workshops." Since "most Petersburg residents of the middle classes lack the means to hire a lackey or coach, most return home alone, without an escort." Writers expressed outrage that young ladies "who walked modestly along Nevsky" were not only subject to the hoots, whistles, and insults hurled at them by the capital's Don Juans and Lovelaces, but also were targeted by undercover agents of the Medical Police Committee who hauled them off to the station for questioning and registration as prostitutes.[73]

One 1868 incident near *Passazh* particularly riled the press. Alfimov, a Medical Police Committee inspector operating undercover, encountered three young ladies heading home along Nevsky around eleven o'clock at night.[74] When they got to the corner of Nevsky and Sadovaia, the inspector—who was disguised as an elderly man—approached one of the girls, suggesting that she accompany him to a hotel. She rebuffed his advances, so he propositioned one of her companions. At this point, the three took flight, racing off toward *Passazh* in tears. Upon turning the corner at Karavannaia, they were seized by a policeman who cited them for prostitution. The girls, now all in tears, begged to be released, but the cop refused, instead heeding the now-authoritative voice of the inspector who insisted on dragging the young women down to the police station. A crowd formed, and many of its members volunteered to accompany the girls to the precinct house. As it turns out, the three girls were laborers in one of *Passazh*'s workshops and their boss provided documentation to secure their release. The matter was brought before the Justice of the Peace who exonerated the inspector because he was merely "following the instructions given to him" when he attempted to entrap the women.[75] The press decried subjecting innocent women to such treatment; even though women who could prove their virtuousness would be freed, the presumption of guilt amounted to "defamation, threats, and even violation."[76]

The press accused private security firms hired to police upscale galleries such as *Passazh* of similar offenses. In 1867, *Petersburg leaflet* profiled a misguided attempt undertaken by *Passazh*'s administrators to clamp down on prostitution. Proprietors fretted that the sex trade conducted by "'fair creatures'" on or near their premises was eclipsing legitimate business and cutting into sales revenues because it led "well-behaved female consumers" to avoid *Passazh*.[77] Taking matters into their own hands, they raised 2,400 rubles to hire private guards. Posted at the entrances and landings to the upper gallery, they were authorized to monitor "the behavior of the women who stroll there" and eject young women suspected of being "fallen but fair creatures."[78]

The success of this system was predicated on the guards being able to distinguish between Camelias and innocent shoppers, which proved to be impossible. Both dressed in the same *au courant* manner. Moreover, there was fluidity between the two groups: an otherwise upstanding woman might opt to compromise her virtue and "treat" a man to acquire unaffordable finery, reverting to her chaste ways after her desire was satisfied.[79] Predictably, this led to considerable confusion. In one case, private guards nabbed a young lady and cited her for disorderly conduct; their chagrin was palpable when her father, an army captain who had been walking a few paces behind her, intervened on her behalf. In another case, a married woman stopped in to make a purchase at a kiosk and was detained by a policeman who "humiliated [her] in a very beastly manner" right in front of her husband. In a third instance, guards blocked access to an unaccompanied woman—the respectable wife of an official. While they were interrogating her, a group of "precisely the kind of women whom they were supposed to bar from the premises" entered *Passazh,* accompanied by "a group of drunken merchants" whom they were entertaining for the evening.[80] Only the accompaniment of husbands and fathers spared female consumers the embarrassment of being labeled public women. Journalists considered that women who lacked the intervention of patriarchal forces had "abandoned appropriate 'female' behavior emphasizing modesty, restraint and self-sacrifice to participate in the world of commerce."[81]

Journalists claimed arrests were "preventing upstanding shoppers from frequenting their stores" for fear "of being mistaken [for prostitutes] and the ensuing scandal." After a year of experimenting with this system, the *Passazh* merchants admitted that they were unable to distinguish between upstanding women engaged in commercial transactions and women who frequented shopping emporia to sell themselves and abandoned the program.[82]

While the press deplored sting operations and expressed sympathy for impoverished girls forced into prostitution to make ends meet, it nevertheless sought to rid the metropolis of high-end courtesans who circulated in and around *Passazh*.[83] Registering prostitutes was not working. One feuilletonist exclaimed: "And who gave 'public women' the right to take over Nevsky Prospekt, and lead commercial establishments to incur losses in the evening? Why don't we consider moving this 'trade in livestock' to some other place, to some street, where this sort of disorder would be less evident and not as alluring and have a less corrupting influence?"[84] The press blamed the Camelias for making matters "worse for those unfortunate women who stroll along Nevsky in the evening and at night. Most of Petersburg's residents are familiar with the brazen tone of such women:

"they are embarrassed by nothing; they fear nothing; they pace the streets (often staggering to and fro), laugh and converse loudly, and brush against all passersby. They have no reason to be modest ... and engage in their industry openly, flaunting it in front of everyone."

The presence of Camelias along Nevsky and in the cafes, restaurants, and arcade of *Passazh* not only led men to believe that every woman had a price tag attached to her but also corrupted the morals of honest women. They invited official oversight and led police to ensnare and shame the innocent. Indeed, some of these good girls, journalists suggested, were provoked by such cruelty into registering.[85]

But why would a good girl do this? As I have already suggested, journalists writing in the boulevard press implied that young ladies were tempted by the spectacle of the high-end prostitute enjoying sumptuous goods and services. As historian Marjorie Hilton has concluded in her profile of the late Imperial Russian retail landscape, "as the popular dailies depicted the situation, simply being in the proximity of buying and selling posed dangers. ... The message was that all who entered the retail sphere became vulnerable to the lure of luxury, as well as to criminals masquerading as respectable men and women."[86] The availability of indulgences allegedly fueled the commercial sex industry by providing male profiteers with a new way of "living off of women." Profiteers lent women money "to buy the luxury goods." When the women could not repay "in an honest way," procurers used clever tactics to transform them into "pieces of living meat" who staffed the brothels of "landladies" with whom the pimps worked.[87]

Journalists expressed ambivalence about the autonomy of both men and women in St. Petersburg at mid-century, and how this altered the relationship between the sexes. In their exposés, they portrayed men as predators or protectors and women as victims or victimizers. In the process, they suggested that male agency could be good or bad: men could torment the women whom they encountered or they could be heroes who interceded on behalf of the female targets of assault. In contrast, journalists implied that there was something inherently dangerous about female agency: regardless of whether they were out shopping, working for a living, or selling their bodies, the women in the narratives of the boulevard press potentially corrupted the metropolis' socio-sexual fabric.

This brings us back to the story of Natasha that appeared in *Petersburg News*. As it turns out, Natasha ultimately could not resist the commodities whose brilliance assaulted her from the shop windows, stimulated her imagination, and beckoned her to reach out, touch, and find some way of acquiring them. She was unable to restrain herself in the face of their allure.[88]

Unable to find a job that paid the rent, Natasha was strolling along Nevsky and bumped into a friend from the provinces, a lovely brunette named Olia, who was ambling down the avenue on the arm of an elderly man. Embarrassed, Olia made plans to meet Natasha the next evening at a fashionable hotel where Natasha recounted her woeful experiences in the capital and wondered how Olia managed to get by in the big city. Her friend responded, "'Don't ask, Natasha … if I told you, you would run from me. … It's better if you figure it out for yourself. …You saw that old guy, right?" Natasha was shocked. Olia continued: "'Yes … what can I do? Fate … Need and hunger brought me to this … Meanwhile, don't think that it's so horrible… it isn't in the least … I have arranged things so that everyday life gets better and better.'"

Olia informed Natasha that this choice made of necessity now allowed her to live well. Olia even suggested to Natasha that she would help set her up as an unregistered courtesan. After all, she knew how "to take care to sort out things properly and with caution." Horrified and offended, Natasha stood up from the table, and exclaimed: "'What's with you, Olia! I'd sooner starve to death than deviate from the path of righteousness!'" Reluctantly accepting the calling card that Olia pressed into her palm "in case she ever needed it," Natasha fled the hotel.

Two more weeks passed. Although Natasha kept setting her sights lower and lower, she still could not find gainful employment. With two rubles left in her pocket, her landlady threatening to evict her if she could not make the rent, and deep hunger gnawing at her belly, Natasha sought out Olia to borrow ten rubles. That night, Olia was entertaining several men. Everyone seemed merry and Natasha was enticed by the bright lights and the girls' attractive toilette. Stimuli aroused all of her senses and Natasha proved unequal to resist them: donning one of Olia's gowns, Natasha sat enveloped in the sights, sounds, smells, and tastes of the luxurious things she so desired. She partook in the sumptuous meal, tasting every delicious morsel, and enjoying herself more than she had in a long time. She went to bed happy, but was not alone for long; soon enough, she was joined by a "young, handsome man" who made advances upon her. This assault was the price she paid for the pleasurable touches, tastes, sights, and smells earlier in the evening. Natasha skulked away in shame, but had nowhere left to go. The tale concludes on an ambiguous note: the author asserts that Natasha, who was unable to return home to her mother in the provinces after these events, "abandoned Petersburg."[89] Given her lack of options, it is not far-fetched to interpret her departure from the city as suicide, which, like prostitution, threatened the late imperial cultural order.[90]

While the era of the Great Reforms had made life in St. Petersburg more dynamic, an unintended consequence was lack of control. The success of a modern shopping arcade like *Passazh* was predicated on its openness; yet, if it remained accessible to the public, then all people—including Camelias and their paying customers—could frequent it. And if it proved impossible to control decadence at *Passazh*, which was, even with its incorporation of glass and natural lighting into its architecture, still set off from the street, then this was even truer of the avenue upon which this emporium was situated.

Nevsky Prospekt embodied that which was perilous about life in Russia's capital. Both Nikolai Gogol—who wrote about the illusory nature of the avenue in an 1835 short story named after the thoroughfare—and his literary and journalistic successors sounded the same cautionary note: the goods and people who inhabited Petersburg, that most intentional of cities, and passed along Nevsky, that most deliberate of avenues, might be passing themselves off as something other than what they truly were. As Gogol laments:

> Oh, do not trust this Nevsky Prospekt! ... All is deception, all is a dream, all is not what it seems! ... This Nevsky Prospekt lies at all hours, but most of all when the thick pall of night descends upon it ... when the whole city turns into noise and glitter, when myriad carriages pour from the bridges, when postilions shout, leap up and down on their horses and when the devil himself lights the street lamps, only to show everything in an unreal guise.[91]

Lamplights made the streets accessible, yet their alluring radiance was as much a source of deception for the feuilletonists of Petersburg's Great Reforms-era boulevard press as it had been for Gogol in his 1835 story.

In an effort to prevent the city from telling such lies and wreaking havoc with those who lived, worked, and took pleasure in it, writers of panoramic literature and urban planners (who were sometimes the same people) sought, unsuccessfully, to shore up the boundaries between Petersburg's elite and European features and its déclassé and Russian ones. Neither increased lighting nor architectural advances could eliminate urban artifice. Indeed, the construction of *Passazh* failed to provide a space where elites would promenade and instead ended up constituting a place where prostitutes, criminals, and other suspect types congregated and sought out intercourse of one sort or another.[92] Strollers along the gas-lit streets poured into and melded with those promenading within the gas-lit arcade; the two crowds were indistinguishable.[93]

Interpolating themselves into the modern world of commerce in multiple ways—as shopgirls, customers, and commodities—female consumers and courtesans purchased the luxury goods they enjoyed—exchanging sometimes money and sometimes their own bodies. Girls working in legitimate and illegitimate professions both mingled in *Passazh* and along Nevsky and neither the Don Juans of the street nor the authorities could discriminate between them. These girls not only were on display—by choice or against their will—but they became livestock that men evaluated through gaze and touch. As the Natasha story suggests, women seeking jobs in the city easily slipped from regular employment into prostitution when need or temptation arose.[94] Like Olia, they were not eager to formalize their new status as prostitutes, even if regulations mandated it. This made pinning down their identities even more problematic.

Surely, harsh realities deprived Petersburg's women of access to decently paying jobs and the potential for marriage, forcing some of them to turn tricks. Ever realistic about the world in which they lived, journalists called for containing this traffic in women. But they understood the limitations. Police might crack down on procurers who lured the girls into prostitution with fashion they could not afford, but it was the commodification of the modern urban center itself that seduced both men and women. The boulevard press's own focus on this titillating dialectic of modernity only served to intensify and multiply the experience of sex in the city without offering an antidote to it.

As historian Mary Louise Roberts has noted, in the "'specularized' urban culture of arcades, boulevards, and department stores, woman was inscribed as both consumer and commodity, purchaser and purchase, buyer and bought."[95] This phenomenon was evident in post-Emancipation Petersburg, where a new cosmopolitan culture was taking shape. Changing economic conditions increased women's opportunities but also their need to work, and many traversed the unavoidable Nevsky in the search of chances, some legitimate and some illegitimate, to make money. Woman moved from simple objects of consumption to a more complicated position as both consumed and consumer and in the process further destabilized gender identities in the late imperial period. Some women succumbed to desires for fine clothing and baubles; others merely attempted to mitigate poverty. Increasingly, women were entering into the world of circulation, commodity exchange, and consumption; this made it harder for everyone involved—officials, polite society, and passersby—to tell a girl who worked from a working girl.

Notes

1   Rossiiskaia Gosudardstvennaia Istoricheskii Arkhiv (RGIA), f. 218 op. 3, 1846–1847, d, 774, ll. 1–2ob, 4–5, 6–6ob, 7–9ob, 15–18. The press's claim that this building was innovative is an exaggeration. See Patrice Moncan and Christian Mahout, *Le Guide des passages de Paris: Guide pratique, historique, et littéraire* (Paris: SEESAM-RCI, 1991).
2   For a contemporary critique of Petersburg's traditional markets, see Ivan I. Pushkarev, *Opisanie Sanktpeterburga i uezdnykh gorodov S. Peterburgskoi gubernii* (St. Petersburg, 1839), Kniga III, 5–11.
3   RGIA, f. 218, op. 3, 1843, d. 71, ll. 14–5, 31–4.
4   On this process more broadly, see Alexander M. Martin, *Enlightened Metropolis: Constructing Imperial Moscow, 1762–1855* (Oxford: Oxford University Press, 2013).

5   For example, in the 1840s, authorities ordered that the city's popular Haymarket Square "be scrubbed every Saturday, and the sidewalks and the alleys behind them should be washed down every day before trade begins" and enhanced regulations to "guarantee the city's outward hygiene and the provisioning of fresh products, to the greatest possible extent, for domestic consumption." RGIA, 218, op. 4, 1848, d. 1871, ll. 16ob, 19ob–20, 23–23ob. On renovating and cleaning markets, see Tsentral'nyi gosudarstvennyi istoricheskii arkhiv Sankt-Peterburga (TsGIA SPB), f. 253, op. 4, 1844–1848, d. 16, ll. 12–12ob. Foreign and domestic travelers frequently remarked upon the city's smell. Martin, *Enlightened Metropolis,* 43–51. For the unsanitary conditions at customary Russian markets in general, see Marjorie L. Hilton, *Selling to the Masses: Retailing in Russia, 1880–1930* (Pittsburgh, PA: University of Pittsburgh Press, 2012), 27–8. Urban smells and marketplace stench were hardly unique to St. Petersburg. On filth, stench, and germs elsewhere in Europe, see for example Alain Corbin, *The Foul and the Fragrant: Odor and the French Social Imagination* (Cambridge, MA: Harvard University Press, 1986) and David S. Barnes, *The Great Stink of Paris and the Nineteenth-Century Struggle Against Filth and Germs* (Baltimore, MD: Johns Hopkins University Press, 2006), especially 189–90, 222–6.

6   On retail marketing in Russia in the broader European context, see Hilton, *Selling to the Masses,* 16–24.

7   On this project in Russia, see Martin, *Enlightened Metropolis,* 261–93. On the French context, see Corbin, *The Foul and the Fragrant,* 111–60.

8   Walter Benjamin, "Paris: The Capital of the Nineteenth Century," in *The Writer of Modern Life: Essays on Charles Baudelaire,* 30–45.

9   Alexander Pavlovich Bashutskii, *Panorama Peterburga,* Kniga III, 85–6. On resemblances between Bashutskii's work and Gogol's "Nevsky Prospekt," see Donald Fanger, *The Creation of Nikolai Gogol* (Cambridge, MA: Harvard University Press, 1979), 112. For more on Bashutskii's background and career, see Alexander Martin, *Enlightened Metropolis,* 278–84.

10 On the public's sensation of the city through the consumption of print media see Walter Benjamin, "On Some Motifs in Baudelaire," in *Illuminations,* ed. Hannah Arendt, trans. Harry Zohn (New York: Shocken Books, 1969), 159, 166–7.

11 Victoria E. Thompson, "Urban Space and Bourgeois Identity in Early Nineteenth-century Paris," *The Journal of Modern History* 75 (3) (2003), 523–5.

12 Walter Benjamin, "Paris Capital of the Nineteenth Century," in *Reflections,* ed. Peter Demetz, trans. Edmund Jephcott (New York: Shocken Books, 1978), especially 146–51, and Walter Benjamin, *Charles Baudelaire: A Lyric Poet in the Era of High Capitalism,* ed. Michael W. Jennings, trans. Howard Eiland et al. (Cambridge, MA: Harvard University Press, 2006) 35–9, 66–8; here 35.

13 The perception that machine-made goods were cleaner and purer than handcrafted ones persisted into the era of factory production. Sally West, *I Shop in Moscow: Advertising and the Creation of Consumer Culture in Late Tsarist Russia* (Dekalb: Northern Illinois University Press, 2011), 107–8.

14 Alexander L. Martin, "The Estate System in Everyday Life in 1820s Moscow," *Cahiers du Monde Russe* 51 (2) (2010), 340.

15 On how the experience of shopping in the new urban arcades and department stores resembled being a spectator at and taking pleasure in an urban exhibit, see Erika Diane Rappaport, *Shopping for Pleasure: Women in the Making of London's West End* (Princeton, MA: Princeton University Press, 2000), 28.

16 Pierre Bourdieu, *Distinction: A Social Critique of the Judgement of Taste*, trans. Richard Nice (Cambridge, MA: Harvard University Press, 1984), 281–2.

17 Walter Benjamin, *The Arcades Project*, trans. Howard Eiland and Kevin McLaughlin (Cambridge, MA: Harvard University Press, 1999), 42.

18 David Howes, "HYPERESTHESIA, or, The Sensual Logic of Late Capitalism," in *Empire of the Senses: The Sensual Culture Reader,* ed. David Howes (London: Bloomsbury, 2014), 284–5.

19 West, *I Shop in Moscow,* 142–3.

20 On the corrupting consequences of the new consumer culture in the West, see Elaine S. Abelson, *When Ladies Go A-Thieving: Middle-Class Shoplifters in the Victorian Department Store* (New York: Oxford University Press, 1989), 32, 46–7.

21 Bashutskii, *Panorama Peterburga*, Kniga III, 86; V. Bur'ianov, *Progulka s det'mi po S. Peterburgu*, chast' 2aia (St. Petersburg, 1838), 160–1.

22 Pushkarev, *Opisanie Sanktpeterburga*, Kniga III, 12–4.

23 Ibid.

24 On this, see Howes, "HYPERESTHESIA," 284–99.

25 Bashutskii, *Panorama Peterburga*, III, 85–6, 137–9.

26 Pushkarev, *Opisanie Sanktpeterburga*, Kniga III, 11, 16.

27 RGIA, f. 218, op. 4, 1848, d. 1871, l. 20ob.

28 RGIA, f. 218, op. 4, 1848, d. 1871, ll. 14–14ob.

29 Pushkarev, *Opisanie Sanktpeterburga*, Kniga I, 74.

30 Bur'ianov, *Progulka s det'mi, chast' 2aia,* 140–4. On Sennaia Ploshchad's reputation as a lively and crowded center of village trade in the city, also see F. Shreder, *Noveishchii putevoditel' po Sankt-Peterburgu s istoricheskimi ukazaniiami* (St. Petersburg, 1820), 22.

31 TsGIA SPB, f. 253, op. 4, 1844–1848, d. 16, ll. 1–1ob.

32 Petr Nikolaevich Stolpianskii, *Peterburg 50 let tomu nazad. Istoricheskaia spravka* (St. Petersburg, 1909), 8–9.

33 Pushkarev, *Opisanie Sanktpeterburga*, Kniga III, 5.

34 Eduard Jermann, *St. Petersburg its people; their character and institutions*, trans. Frederick Hardman (New York: Barnes, 1853), 145–7.

35 Johann Georg Kohl, *Russia and the Russians, in 1842* (London: Henry Colburn, 1842), 127–8. For a comparison with Moscow, see Hilton, *Selling to the Masses*, 36–9.

36 RGIA, f. 218, op. 3, 1843, d. 71, ll. 14–15ob. For more on Parisian passages, see Christopher Rollason, *The Passageways of Paris: Walter Benjamin's Arcades Project and Contemporary Cultural Debate in the West,* http://www.wbenjamin.org/passageways.html#fn9 (accessed November 3, 2014); Benjamin, *The Arcades Project.*
37 RGIA, f. 218, op. 3, 1843, d. 71, ll. 14–19ob.
38 Bashutskii, *Panorama Peterburga,* Kniga III, 102–3, 108–10.
39 According to a report published in *Sankt Peterburgskie Vedomosti* in 1848, of the 4,726 streetlamps in the city, only 455 burned gas. The rest burned lamp or hempseed oil. Alexander Matveichuk, "At the dawn of the Kerosene Era," *Oil of Russia* 1 (2006), http://www.oilru.com/or/26/464/ (accessed September 29, 2011); Matveichuk, "Pioneer of Russia's Gas Business," *Oil of Russia,* No. 3 (2011), http://www.oilru.com/or/48/1030/ (accessed November 7, 2011). Alexander Yefimov and Lyudmila Volkhova, "Pioneers of the Methane Age," *Oil of Russia* 2 (2005), http://www.oilru.com/or/23/389/ (accessed November 7, 2011); "Statisticheskii ocherk S. Peterburga. Stat'ia 2," *Sankt-Peterburgskie Vedomost* 99 (5 May 1848), 396; Milica Banjanin, "Where Art the Street Lights Running To? The Poetics of Street Lights in Russian Modernism," *New Zealand Slavonic Journal* 38 (2004): 88 n.4; Bashutskii, *Panorama Peterburga,* Kniga III, 166; M. I. Pyliaev, *Staryi Peterburg: Rasskazy iz byloi zhizni stolitsy* (St. Petersburg: Paritet, 2003), 344.
40 RGIA, f. 446, op. 12, 1843, d. 1, ll. 132–133; RGIA, f. 218, op. 3, 1843, d. 71, ll. 13, 15ob, 18.
41 RGIA, f. 218, op. 3, 1843, d. 71, ll. 18–20ob.
42 RGIA, f. 218, op. 3, 1843, d. 71, ll. 31ob–32ob.
43 Pyliaev, *Staryi Peterburg,* 343–4; RGIA, f. 218, op. 3, 1843, d. 71, ll. 40–40ob.
44 RGIA, f. 218 op. 3, 1846–1847, d, 774, ll. 1–2ob, 4–5, 6–6ob, 7–9ob, 15–18.
45 Pushkarev, *Panorama Peterburga,* Kniga III, 5–11; RGIA, f. 218, op. 3, 1843, d. 71, ll. 14–15, 31–34.
46 *Vedomosti Sankt Peterburgskoi gorodskoi politsii* 50 (112) (May 22, 1848), 2; K., "Fel'eton: Peterburgksaia letopis'," *SPB Vedomostii* 35 (February 12, 1848), 137–8; V. M. "Fel'eton politseiskoi gazety 5ogo Iuniia. Proshedshaia nedelia. Peterburgskaia i vsiakiia novosti," *Vestnik Sankt--Peterburgskoi gorodskoi politsii* 9 (123) (June 5, 1848), 2.
47 RGIA, f. 218 op. 3, 1846–1847, d, 774, ll. 1–2ob, 4–5, 6–6ob, 7–9ob, 15–18.
48 The author uses the word "*guliat*'" which suggests strolling, rather than walking. K., "Fel'eton: Peterburgskaia letopis'," *Sankt Peterburgskie vedemosti* 35 (February 12, 1848), 137.
49 *Vedomosti Sankt Peterburgskoi gorodskoi politsii* 50 (112) (May 22, 1848), 2; K., "Fel'eton: Peterburgksaia letopis'," *SPB Vedomostii* 35 (February 12, 1848), 137–8; V. M. "Fel'eton politseiskoi gazety 5ogo Iuniia. Proshedshaia nedelia. Peterburgskaia i vsiakiia novosti," *Vestnik Sankt-Peterburgskoi gorodskoi politsii* 9 (123) (June 5, 1848), 2.

50 "Gostinyi Dvor i Passazh," *Moda: Zhurnal dlia svetskikh liudei* 8 (April 15, 1851), 61, cited in Christine Ruane, "Clothes Shopping in Imperial Russia: The Development of a Consumer Culture," *Journal of Social History* 28 (4) (Summer 1995), 767.

51 "Fel'eton politseiskoi gazety 22ogo Maia. Proshedshiia nedelia," *Vedemosti Sankt Peterburgskoi gorodskoi politsii* 50 (112) (May 22, 1848), 2.

52 V. M., "Fel'eton politseisko gazety 21ogo Avgusta, Proshedshaia nedelia," *Vedemosti Sankt Peterburgskoi gorodskoi politsii* 9 (185) (August 21, 1848): 1–2. Also see V. M. "Fel'eton politseiskoi gazety 25ogo Sentabria. Proshedshaia nedelia. Peterburgskaia i vsiakiia novosti," *Vedemosti Sankt-Peterburgskoi gorodskoi politsii* 9 (212) (September 25, 1848): 1–2; "Fel'eton politseiskoi gazety 23ogo Oktiabria. Proshedshaia nedelia. Peterburgskaia i vsiakiia novosti," *Vedemosti Sankt-Peterburgskoi gorodskoi politsii* 9 (234) (October 23, 1848): 1–2.

53 "Fel'eton politseiskoi gazety 23ogo Oktiabria. Proshedshaia nedelia. Peterburgskaia i vsiakiia novosti," *Vedemosti Sankt-Peterburgskoi gorodskoi politsii* 9 (234) (October 23, 1848): 2.

54 Katia Dianina, "Passage to Europe: Dostoevskii in the St. Petersburg Arcade," *Slavic Review* 62 (2) (Summer 2003): 244.

55 Louise McReynolds, *The News Under Russia's Old Regime: The Development of a Mass Circulation Press* (Princeton, NJ: Princeton University Press, 1991), 20–32; Louise McReynolds, "V. M. Doroshevich: The Newspaper Journalist and the Development of Public Opinion in Civil Society," in *Between Tsar and People. Educated Society and the Quest for Public Identity in Late Imperial Russia*, ed. Edith Clowes, Samuel D. Kassow, and James L. West (Princeton, NJ: Princeton University Press, 1991), 233–4; Abbot Gleason, "The Terms of Russian Social History," in *Between Tsar and People,* 15–27; Daniel Brower, *The Russian City Between Tradition and Modernity, 1850–1900* (Berkeley: University of California Press, 1990), 1–6, 22–8, 188; Ruane, "Clothes Shopping in Imperial Russia," 770–1.

56 Katia Dianina, "The Feuilleton: An Everyday Guide to Public Culture in the Age of the Great Reforms," *Slavic and East European Journal* 47 (2) (2003): 187–210; quotation from 188.

57 On Petersburg feuilletonists as *flaneurs*, see J. A. Buckler, *Mapping St. Petersburg: Imperial Text and Cityshape* (Princeton, NJ: Princeton University Press, 2006), 99–108.

58 Hilton discusses negative portrayals of merchants and retail trade and how these stories transmitted "the message that the retail sphere provided the space and enticements for various kinds of social transgression." Hilton, *Selling to the Masses*, 27–30, here 29.

59 See Barbara Alpern Engel, *Breaking the Ties that Bound: The Politics of Marital Strife in Late Imperial Russia* (Ithaca, NY: Cornell University Press, 2011), 80–100.

60 Between 1856 and 1865, 1/125 Petersburgers were married, compared to 1/115 Berlin residents; 1/109 Parisians; 1/105 Brussels residents; 1/110

Kievans; 1/107 Odessans; 1/93 Rigans; and 1/91 Kazan' residents. "Koe chto iz statiski Peterburga," *Peterburgskii listok* 6 (63) (May 3, 1869), 1; Mikhail Kamentsev, "Peterburgskiia devushki. (e) zakliuchenie," *Peterburgskii listok* 6 (45) (March 27, 1869): 1–2.

61 Aleksandr S., "Peterburgskiia prostitutsiia. (Ocherk prostitutsii v Peterburge. N. B—skago. *Arkhiv sudebnoi meditsiny*, 1868, g. kn. 4)," *Peterburgskii listok* 5 (175) (December 5, 1868): 1–2.

62 "Gorodskoi dnevnik: Lestnitsa razvrata," *Peterburgskii listok* 2 (149) (October 21, 1865): 2–3.

63 "Feuilleton: Peterburgskoe obozrenie," *Peterburgskii listok* 1 (17) (April 12, 1864): 1.

64 Laurie Bernstein, *Sonia's Daughters: Prostitutes and Their Regulation in Imperial Russia* (Berkeley: University of California Press, 1995), 1–2, 30–4; Aleksandr S., "Peterburgskiia prostitutsiia," 1–2.

65 Aleksandr S., "Peterburgskiia prostitutsiia (Ocherk prostitutsii v Peterburge. N. B—skago. *Arkhiv sudebnoi meditsiny*, 1868, g. kn. 4)," *Peterburgskii listok* 5 (177) (December 10, 1868): 1–2; also see "Khronika: Prostitutsiia v Peterburge," *Peterburgskaia gazeta* 2 (183) (December 21, 1868): 2; F. Sh. "Gorodskoi dnevnik: Esche novyi sposob prosit' milostyniu," *Peterburgskii listok* 2 (144) (September 28, 1865): 3; S., "Khronika: O molodikh prostitutskiakh," *Peterburgskii listok* 6 (52) (April 8, 1869): 1–2. On this also see Bernstein, *Sonia's Daughters*, 86–93.

66 Gregory Freeze, "The *Soslovie* (Estate) Paradigm and Russian Social History," *American Historical Review* 91 (1) (1986): 11–36; Elise Kimerling Wirtschafter, *Structures of Society: Imperial Russia's "People of Various Ranks"* (DeKalb: Northern Illinois University Press, 1994). On the *soslovie* system, see Alison K. Smith, *For the Common Good and Their Own Well-Being: Social Estates in Imperial Russia* (Oxford: Oxford University Press, 2014).

67 Vasilii Pertsev, "Zaiavlenie: Prakticheskiia zamechanii po povodu zhenskago voprosa," *Peterburgskaia gazeta* 2 (14) (January 28, 1868): 3–4.

68 D. Z...skii, "Natasha v Peterburge. (Ocherk)," *Peterburgskaia gazeta* 2 (54) (April 25, 1868): 1–3.

69 "Khronika: Oskorblenie zhenshchiny sredy belago dnia," *Peterburgskii listok* 5 (137) (September 29, 1868): 1.

70 "Gorodskoi dnevnik: Net prokhodu ot zhenshchin," *Peterburgskii listok* 2: 46 (March 28, 1865), 3.

71 "Khronika: Eshche i eshche o lovelasakh," *Peterburgskii listok* 5 (163) (November 14, 1868): 1–2.

72 As Mark Smith has demonstrated, during the modern era, tactility became increasingly "commodity-laden" and "property-riddled." For more on the link between hapticity and gender relations, Mark M. Smith, *Sensing the Past: Seeing, Hearing, Smelling, Tasting, and Touching in History* (Berkeley: University of California Press, 2007), 99–102, 114–16.

73 "Khronika: Eshche i eshche o lovelasakh," *Peterburgskii listok* 5 (163)

(November 14, 1868): 1–2. The boulevard press devoted considerable attention to decrying the activities of Lovelaces—named after the villain in Richardson's *Clarissa*—who preyed on innocent women in Petersburg. See for example, "Khronika: Molodye bul'varnye lovlasy," *Peterburgskii listok* 5 (151) (October 24, 1868): 2; "Ulichnye zametki," *Peterburgskii listok* 5: 87 (June 23, 1868): 3; "Khronika: Nenakazannye lovlasy," *Peterburgskii listok* 6 (38) (March 15, 1869), 2–3; "Khronika: Iunye lovlasy Peterburgskoi storony," *Peterburgskii listok* 6: 161 (November 1,1869): 1; S., "Khronika: Ulichnye Don-khuan v klube," *Peterburgskii listok* 6 (181) (December 6, 1869): 2; Dim—ov, "Feuilleton: Nashe zhit'e-byt'e," *Peterburgskaia gazeta* 2: 141 (October 6, 1868): 1–2.

74 The Medical-Police Committee (*Vrachebno-politseiskii komitet*) regulated prostitution; see Bernstein, *Sonia's Daughters*, 20–84.

75 "Khronika: Vozmutitel'nyi zakhvat," *Peterburgskii listok* 5 (139) (October 3, 1868): 1–2; "Khronika," *Peterburgskii listok* 5 (148) (October 19, 1868): 2; "O vrachebno-politseiskom nadzore," *Peterburgskii listok* 6 (82) (June 7, 1869): 1.

76 "Khronika: Vozmutitel'nyi zakhvat," *Peterburgskii listok* 5 (139) (October 3, 1868): 1–2. The police were notorious for abusing suspected prostitutes. See Bernstein, *Sonia's Daughters*, 30–1.

77 "Osobaia politsiia," *Peterburgskii listok* 5 (33) (March 10, 1868): 2.

78 Ibid.; "Raznyia izvestiia," *Peterburgskii listok* 3 (42) (March 19, 1867): 3.

79 Ruane, "Clothes Shopping in Imperial Russia," 765–88, esp. 772.

80 "Osobaia politsiia," 2.

81 Ruane, "Clothes Shopping in Imperial Russia," 774.

82 "Govoriat," *Peterburgskii listok* 5 (45) (April 7, 1868): 3. Also see "Raznyia izvestiia." The problems posed by hiring private detectives to keep emporia under surveillance were not unique to Russia; on how the "dilemma of detection" played out in late nineteenth-century America, see Abelson, *When Ladies Go A-Thieving*, 120–47.

83 Aleksandr S., "Peterburgskie prostitutsiia" (Ocherk prostitutsii v Peterburge. N. B—skago. *Arkhiv sudebnoi meditsiny*, 1868 g., kn. 4)," *Peterburgskii listok* 5 (175) (December 5, 1868): 1–2; 177 (December 10, 1868): 1–2; 178 (December 12, 1868): 1; 188 (December 31, 1868): 1–2.

84 "Khronika: Eshche i eshche o lovelasakh."

85 "O vrachebno-politseiskom nadzore."

86 Hilton, *Selling to the Masses*, 29.

87 A. I. B—ov, "Torgovlia zhivym miasom," *Peterburgskii listok* 3 (19) (February 3, 1866): 2–3.

88 For a British comparison, see Abelson, *When Ladies Go A-Thieving*, 46.

89 D. Z ... skii, "Natasha v Peterburge."

90 On journalists' preoccupation with suicide, see Irina Paperno, *Suicide as a Cultural Institution in Dostoevsky's Russia* (Ithaca, NY: Cornell University Press, 1998), esp. Chapters 2 and 3.

91 Nikolay Gogol, "Nevsky Prospekt," in *The Diary of a Madman, The Government Inspector, and Selected Stories*, trans. Ronald Wilks (London: Penguin Press, 2005), 78–112; here 111–112.
92 Thompson, "Urban Space and Bourgeois Identity," 551.
93 Walter Benjamin, "The Paris of the Second Empire in Baudelaire," in *The Writer of Modern Life*, 81–5.
94 On the movement of women from legitimate employment in into prostitution, see Barbara Alpern Engel, "St. Petersburg Prostitutes in the Late Nineteenth Century: A Personal and Social Profile," *Russian Review* 48 (1) (January 1989): 22–3, 27–31.
95 Mary Louise Roberts, "Gender, Consumption, and Commodity Culture," *The American Historical Review* 103 (3) (1998): 818.

PART TWO
Revolutionary Russia

CHAPTER FIVE

The taste, smell, and semiotics of cigarettes

Tricia Starks

The 1863 manual *The Art of Tobacco* pronounced, "the taste of tobacco may only be truly valued by smokers. No type of language may express that pleasure. That sensation will never be completely defined."[1] Not only could the taste of tobacco be appreciated only by the smoker, but sensory historians argue it could only be experienced in a certain body, time, place, and culture. Many factors work to individualize our experience of taste: age, diet, heredity, and habit can affect mucous composition. The taste buds themselves change during the course of a life cycle, replenishing every seven to ten days, and some dying out entirely with age. In youth sweetness is alluring, but as years and dietary routines deaden the taste buds, we become more inured to, and even craving of, bitterness.[2] Taste is not situated only in the mouth, but is colored by scent. Tobacco impacts the body on all these levels—affecting the saliva of the smoker and damaging taste buds, rising through the nose, journeying through the brain, and traveling into the lungs.

The production of tobacco assures further contingencies. Very few smokes are composed of just one tobacco type, and different varieties have subtly different tastes. Cigarettes are packed with blends of tobacco that bring together the sweet, high-nicotine Virginia leaf with the buttery burley and the aromatic Oriental. These blends help to mask the burning nicotine itself, which smacks of burning rubber.[3] Manufacturing practices leave their own residue. Drying tobacco, either in the open air or in barns, takes away its sweetness; a soak in a complex "sauce" of aromatics and flavorings restores it.

Personal biology, choice of leaf, the method of curing, and the sauce in which the blend is marinated are not the only contributing factors to the final taste of a cigarette. The flavor of tobacco in late imperial Russia was a mix of not only leaves, sugars, and spices, not just the spark of flame that brought them all to life, but also convoluted intersections of cultural meaning, political understandings, and social associations. As Mark M. Smith cautions, historians must be careful "to distinguish between the production and consumption of the senses" since consumption is "hostage to the context in which it was produced."[4] Emotions and the mental state influence the palate. Intellectual nuances and emotions temper our experience, allowing a bitter taste to be sweetened by a pleasant memory or recollections of past revulsions to engender long-lived distastes.[5] Russian smokers inhaled intellectual concepts alongside a Virginia or an Oriental variety. They imbibed associations with these areas—luxury, class-consciousness, sex, the Orient, and the Western world; and they were transformed physically for the experience. In effect, the taste of tobacco was a complex cultural bricolage. Anthropologist Claude Lévi-Strauss posited the idea of bricolage—the reworking of existing materials and concepts into a new object of cobbled meaning—as a way of developing and displaying identity.

Yet, still, biological and psychological issues sway the cultural and emotional associations of tobacco smoking. As historian Martin Jay notes, the senses are "situated at the unstable crossroads of nature and culture" and cannot be fully taken out of one for the other.[6] Just as contemporary psychology addresses tobacco dependency as a complex "biopsychosocial" phenomenon, historians must include all of these concepts in their reconstructions. The body of the smoker must be brought under examination. For instance, the languor often attributed to a smoke, which might seem only a cultural association, can have biological underpinnings. In the established smoker, nicotine withdrawal can cause feelings of diffused panic and anxiety. Delivery of nicotine gives a "fix" and thus, smoking is linked with relaxation even as it is both cause and cure of the smoker's disquiet. At the same time, the comforting camaraderie of smoker society is often cited as both a reason for starting and a barrier to quitting. The relaxation associated with cigarettes comes as a complex, biological reaction to the chemical dependency of smoking but is tied to social comforts as well. The socially and biologically driven aspects of addiction assure that a purely cultural construction of taste will be incomplete.

The taste of tobacco is a mass of different, yet interconnected, considerations—it is at once biological and social, chemical and cultural, generational and historical. To fully embrace the total experience of the consumer, a history of the taste of Russian tobacco must be more than biology and botany, extend farther than commodities networks, and address more than consumer identities and scientific theories; it must be, as this chapter outlines, a sensory history of Russian tobacco as well.

Historiography

The sensory has not been central to tobacco histories. Literary works concentrate on culture and the semiotics of smoking, missing out on the biological experience as well as the social, economic, and medical understandings of the habit.[7] Concentrating on the art, the studies neglect the sensory realities—both positive and negative—of smoking. Historians of tobacco have focused on trade, manufacture, or cessation campaigns producing rich industrial, commodity, and public health histories, but dealing with taste unsystematically. When taste is explored, it is as part of the deceptive practices of marketers and manufacturers rather than as a part of smoking culture.[8]

This sensory gap in tobacco studies mirrors the general distancing of the entire field of history from the body and the sensory. The senses most involved with smoking are both considered ephemeral and highly individual—smell and taste.[9] Since the foundations of sensory inquiry in the Platonic era, taste and smell have been discounted as "lower" senses, more bestial and less capable of transcendent "aesthetic" enjoyment. According to historian Priscilla Parkhurst Ferguson, taste is generally seen to lie "in the company of touch and smell, well below the much less aggressively sensual faculties of sight and hearing."[10] Some sensory theorists even argued that by the heyday of smoking in the nineteenth and twentieth centuries, taste and smell were less honed than in pre-modern societies as a consequence of enlightened privileging of sight.[11]

While smell in particular has been denigrated as less relevant in a "deodorized" modern environment, Mark M. Smith contends that it is a fallacy that certain senses are less modern and civilized or that one sense was supreme "at the expense of the other senses."[12] Historian Mark S. R. Jenner similarly argues against a post-Enlightenment sensory world where certain senses are lost. Instead he maintains that modern cityscapes are not deodorized but re-odorized by industry and science with specific meanings of race and class attached to smell. He urges historians to determine "not whether odors matter more in the past, but how and where *particular* odors mattered or were said to matter."[13]

Alexander M. Martin has identified just such a contextualized attention to odor in nineteenth-century Moscow. Although the smells of the city probably did not change appreciably over the century, the attention paid to them, and the articulation of disgust over scent, was modulated by political, social, and cultural circumstances. He details a transition over the course of the nineteenth century. When Catherinian policies focused on the backwardness of the lower classes, stench became a marker of their social danger. As the century progressed, and the well-ordered police state became more embedded and entrusted, this perception of the malodorous city was tempered, until the debacle of the Crimean War reanimated concern.[14]

Historians have also been relatively neglectful of taste. According to philosopher Carolyn Korsmeyer, the general denigration of taste in the West comes from misgivings over the moral implications of its sensual dimensions as "both touch and taste figure as the senses that require the most control, since they can deliver pleasures that tempt one to indulge in the appetites of eating, drinking, and sex."[15] She notes that the less "bodily" senses of sight and hearing are seen as more capable of rational and aesthetic enjoyment but taste, physically connected to the lower body through digestion, is given as a metaphor for aesthetic sensibility (to have good taste) but is excluded from aesthetic senses (appreciation for music or the visual arts).[16]

Looking to the definition of aesthetics from Immanuel Kant where disinterested enjoyment (i.e., not good, useful, or sensual) was the marker of non-gustatory taste, tobacco would seem a candidate for this type of artistic appreciation since it is neither a necessity nor useful. Like wine, tea, or liqueur, it sits at a mid-way point between regular consumables and fine art—connoisseurship. The taste associated with the gourmet developed at different levels and speeds across Europe in the nineteenth century as class differentiation required further distancing of the bourgeois from the other. Historian Robert Jütte argued that in Europe, for instance, taste was an issue for the French, but less so among the Germans and English.[17] As Alison Smith illustrates in this volume, the development of national cuisines often intersected with discussions of nationalism and national identity. Literary scholar Darra Goldstein has shown the ways in which Russian rulers from Peter the Great to Catherine the Great have attempted to Europeanize the population by changing diet, while in this volume, Aaron Retish and Anton Masterovoy identify the peculiar Russian and Soviet attempts at developing and even managing a national palate.[18]

The problem of recovering taste and smell in the past is made even more problematic for historians of tobacco who must confront the horrific consequences that come from use of the product. According to a 2013 World Health Organization report about 400,000 Russians die every year from smoking-related illnesses.[19] To discuss the sensory experience of tobacco as anything other than a negative in the face of such high mortality rates might be interpreted as playing into the hands of the merchants of death and giving credence to the manipulations they have perpetrated on consumers. But to fully reconstruct the past habit, histories of manufacture, prevention efforts, and medical investigation must be viewed alongside the odes, enticements, and pleasures that smokers and marketers detailed.

Reconstructing the taste and smell of tobacco

The cigarette is a modern method of tobacco delivery for mass consumption. Cigarettes differ from pipes and cigars in that the smoke is acidic, smoother, and more easily inhaled. The Russian-style cigarette (the *papirosa*—a hard-paper tube attached on one end to a fine paper, tobacco-stuffed cartridge) first appeared in Russian administrative documents in 1844.[20] By the early nineteenth century, an established import system had primed Russians to tobacco use and an already sophisticated snuff and pipe-tobacco industry in Russia had created methods of blending and flavoring tobacco that allowed subtle mixtures and the rise of differing tobacco houses as preferred suppliers for aficionados.

Blends of tobacco that combined leaf from around the world that were then marinated in complicated sauces allowed distinct tobacco experiences beyond the simple choice of pipe, snuff, or cigarette. The foundation of the blend is leaf. Even though species are very similar genetically, their flavor can vary widely because of disparities in soil, climate, and curing.[21] Like wine, tobacco can carry a sense of place through taste—*terroir*.[22] The most common tobacco varieties—Virginia, Burley, and Oriental—each has a distinctive palate related to regional agricultural and production differences. Virginia, also called "bright tobacco," is primarily associated with the United States, but is also grown in Argentina, Brazil, China, and India. Flu-cured in barns with charcoal fires, it exudes fruity and grassy notes. Its flavor is sweet and light, but it is saturated with deceptively high levels of nicotine. Burley tobacco, grown in South America and the Mediterranean, is cured over months in open-air barns. The leaf is light to dark brown and possesses earthy, buttery flavors. Both Virginia and Burley have a good burn quality, which gives a quicker reaction because the nicotine is more rapidly delivered, and they are easier to enhance with aroma and sauce allowing for more flavor variants. They are more chemically addictive.[23] Oriental tobaccos, sometimes called Turkish and more prevalent in Eastern Europe and Russia, are sun-cured in the open air. Lower in nicotine and sugar than other varieties, their taste is still strong because of their highly aromatic yet tiny leaves.

Russians, particularly of the upper classes, used primarily Oriental leaf.[24] This was a result not only of proximity or from their extensive contacts in the region but also nearly two centuries of war and their own cultivations in Ukraine. This preference extended well into the twentieth century because of trade relationships, in particular between Russia and Bulgaria. As historian Mary Neuburger details, Bulgaria became the largest exporter of tobacco in the second half of the twentieth century as a result of the Bulgarians being the key suppliers to the Soviet Union's smoking market.[25]

While these varietal distinctions are clearly drawn today, it is not evident that such definitive typing of tobacco held true before the twentieth century. Historian Barbara Hahn argues in her history of the American tobacco industry that standards for cultivation and controls for curing in the United States were still in flux in the 1800s.[26] Even though the exact taste of leaf from the period cannot be resurrected, this does not mean the historian cannot recover, at the very least, ideas about trade, the world, and

Russia's place from the complex recipes for tobacco products available.[27] Mid-century home recipes for cigarette blends indicate that leaf from around the world, or cultivated from seed from around the world, was available for purchase in Russia and that exotic aromatics were considered attainable and necessary to good tobacco blending.[28] Further, Russians of the nineteenth century recognized tobacco types and flavors according to regions, indicating that even if the technology was inconsistent, the associations of geography and taste were developed.

By the turn of the century in Russia, firms like Bogdanov and Laferm mixed foreign and domestic tobacco for an increasingly sophisticated market willing to pay more for high-grade Turkish tobaccos over domestic Ukrainian stock.[29] These blends indicate a global vision of tobacco consumption that incorporated all three of the major tobacco types and even many sub-variants, but also expressed itself in the primacy of expensive and elusive over domestic and accessible.[30]

The distinctive scents of different varietals of smoked tobacco were evident to those around, allowing for individuation that created markers for inclusion in a community of consumers of a similar brand or style of leaf.[31] The smell of tobacco connected to conceptions of the urban population—working man, urban danger, and productivity. Western anxiety over the transgressive powers of odors, especially in the urban environment, appeared as early as the sixteenth century but by the nineteenth century, as theorist Alain Corbin has articulated, urbanites assumed an association of scent with issues of class.[32] Just as smell could mark the other, appreciation of scent could be seen as a mark of class distinction as elites were believed to have heightened sensitivity or the presence of the aroma of certain tobacco brands and blends could signal membership in a certain milieu.[33] The positive associations of tobacco's smell, with exotic lands and precious spices, delicate flavors and refined tastes, became also a marker for inclusion with certain groups. Priscilla Pankhurst Ferguson argues that while social theorists like Pierre Bourdieu might emphasize taste in theory, historians look to practice and the ways in which taste does more than buttress the bourgeoisie but also creates "taste communities" that bring people together in a shared identity.[34]

Russian tobacco blend and sauce recipes indicate the global vision of consumers. The 1852 volume *On the Cultivation and Fabrication of Tobacco* educates the Russian small manufacturer on the history of tobacco, the methods for growing, the sorting and preparation of leaf, and the fabrication of cigarettes, cigars, snuff, and chewing tobacco.[35] The book includes a great many blend recipes, each beginning with a standard 100 pounds of various leaves, conforming to American industry standards at the time.[36] Each batch would produce roughly 80,000 cigarettes according to current tobacco measures (200 cartons of twenty packs each consisting of twenty cigarettes). The average nineteenth-century smoker consumed thirty to forty cigarettes a day (a pack and a half to two packs) and they were sold in groups of ten or even as singles.³⁷ These recipes would thus produce enough for roughly five to seven average smokers for a year.

These cigarettes may have been meant for sale but not necessarily. Tobacco can be stored for long periods. Some pipe tobacco is kept for decades if left in good moisture and proper temperature. The recipes could have been either multiplied or divided in size, but the language of the book and its set-up as a primer on tobacco all give an air of the do-it-yourselfer rather than established manufacturers. Until the invention of the Bonsack machine in 1880, cigarettes required hand-rolling, and most were produced by a limited number of skilled rollers in small workshops until the consolidation of Russian tobacco firms began in the mid-1800s. Larger firms would employ dozens of rollers, mostly women, in cigarette production until mechanization took hold.³⁸ Given the small size of cigarette manufactures, the likelihood that a household would have multiple male (and a few female) smokers, and the lengthy storage-life of tobacco, these recipes could very well have been intended for personal use or for the production of excess for minor household sales. Even later in the century, as cigarette tube production mechanized, the aficionado continued to pack cigarettes at home where he or she had control.³⁹

The Russian recipes in the book all begin with mixtures conceptualized on a global scale. Formulas call for leaf from Havana, Santo Domingo, Virginia, Puerto Rico, and Louisiana to join tobacco from Ukraine, the Palatinate, and Hungary indicating a vast trading empire of global tobacco, which Russians expected to connect to easily. The blends themselves are named for equally distant and exotic locales: Maracaibo Basin Canaster⁴⁰ Blend (a pipe tobacco named after an area between the Columbian and Venezuelan coast), Best Puerto Rico, or Varina Farms (after a Virginia Plantation).⁴¹ The presence of such distinctive tobacco blends and glamorous names indicates an assumed access to varied tobacco and a knowledgeable clientele regarding international options. Matthew Romaniello argues that Russian tobacco imports came from around the world from the seventeenth century onward. As Russians expanded their vision of empire, so did their trade routes extend outward. Russian smokers would have had longstanding familiarity with global variants of tobacco.⁴²

Recipes address more than just blend of leaf. Tobacco, when cured, loses its sweetness. The additional steeping in "sauce" restores the "natural" taste of tobacco and supplements the flavor. Additives can also accelerate burn in ways that heighten the potency of nicotine. For instance, today's American sauces include ammonia additives, which were recognized in the twentieth century as valuable for giving smoke a "richer, smoother, 'chocolate-like' taste reminiscent of a burley blend" as well as allowing for higher nicotine yields by replicating a "freebasing" experience.⁴³ According to the entry from Brokgauz's 1896 Russian encyclopedia, tobacco sauce could include: "saltpeter, table salt, potash, honey, sugar, spirits, raisins, chicory coffee, coffee grounds, incense, anise, and dill."⁴⁴ A host of ingredients, humble and exotic, joined this basic set and created a mass of different flavors while influencing burn and the feel of the inhalation. *On the Cultivation and Fabrication of Tobacco* gave not just leaf blends but also some of the most detailed sauce recipes available. These included rare and expensive substances, as well as general household items.[45] Recipes featured saltpeter and alcohol alongside flavorings such as sugar, nutmeg, cinnamon, clove, vanilla, cardamom, anise, bergamot (sweet lemons), Spanish raisins, kubebi, fresh lemon peel, hard candies, licorice, and dill.[46] While many would certainly add sweetness, other items seem more important to enhancing aroma or burn. All three elements—taste, scent, and burn—are essential to a satisfying smoke.

Sauce formulas included more than just dry ingredients. Aromatics that would seem more suited to perfumes joined the stew such as ambergris, violets, incense, orange blossom, lavender, amber, and rose petals.[47] Finally, a diverse category of unusual woods—rosewood, Sassafras wood, violet wood, and cascarilla—enhanced the brew and perhaps influenced the burn.[48] In addition, tea, "good cognac" "best tea," Muscat, rose water, and wine joined the herbals and sweets.[49] The specificity of the herbals does not carry through to identifying the liquids where generic categories of tea, alcohol, and wine are given rather than particular products, varieties, or blends. Given the distinctions associated with each one of these commodities, such generalist categories seem intentionally vague. Perhaps this reflected an assumption by the guide's author that the tobacco connoisseur would already have educated tastes in the field of established gourmet products like tea, wine, and liqueurs.

The cascade of flavors and scents, when combined with the aromatic Oriental leaf most associated with Russia, would indicate that nineteenth-century Russian tobacco blends had a quite heady, if not overwhelming, flavor and smell that would be easily contrasted by both consumer and bystander with the lighter aromas and more delicate flavor associated with Virginia leaf. The differences of the smell of Russian smokers were quite evident to foreign travelers according to memoir literature.[50] Just as Matthew Romaniello and Alison Smith describe with cold and fermented food, foreigners saw a specific national character in the sensory experience of the Russian smoker.

For Russians, images and tastes associated with foreign locales accompanied leaf blends, and sauces associated cigarettes with aromas and flavors that further broadened the image and appeal of tobacco as cosmopolitan. While, as Smith notes, sourness might be associated with Russian cuisine, the blends of Russian tobacco and their sauces depended instead upon international styles with notes of sweetness combined with smells of comfort to evoke luxury and elegance. Nineteenth-century Russian smokers distinguished between a "strong Turkish" and a "light Maryland" smoke, even as the cigarette itself remained a consistent five inches long and sold at five for ten kopecks.[51] Advertisers might, at times, blur distinctions. A

Nevskii firm in 1888 marketed their Turkish tobacco as possessing a "mild and pleasant taste" and beneficial to those with "complaints of cough, bitterness, and heartburn from smoking."[52]

Much like the tobacco leaf blends, the mixtures of aromatics, herbs, and essences for creating the sauces speak to a Russian consumer intimately connected to world trade and to tobacco users with educated and sophisticated palates who envisaged themselves part of an interconnected global economy. Cascarilla, the aromatic bark of a West Indian shrub, and kubebi, tailed peppers from Java, joined equally exotic and undoubtedly expensive flavors. Ambergris, the stone produced in the digestive system of sperm whales, is quite rare.[53] This singular commodity is avidly hunted and averages a price near its weight in gold, though at times it has fetched triple that.[54] Cascarilla, kubebi, and ambergris, all undoubtedly precious in the nineteenth century, are here listed in an ostensibly humble set of home craft instructions.

Expensive ingredients brought luxury even more to the forefront of the tobacco experience, and the odor released in the smoke allowed this bricolage to penetrate not just through the inhalation into the lungs but also into the skin and hair. In this way, the mixture became an experience not just for the individual smoker but also for all those around. In the sauce, even more than the leaf choice, the complex interplay between scent and taste played out. The scarcity of ingredients became a means of class differentiation, even as it softened the taste. The cigarette became a cultural construction of ideas, flavors, and perfumes that connected consumer choice to social status and a philosophical stance, which could then be fully embodied. Rather than just displaying worldly proclivities on their person or in their product choice, smokers internalized difference—weekly, daily, hourly—through the taste of tobacco and then exuded the marker of their cosmopolitanism through their exhalations and sweat. In as much as scent can evoke flavor, the companion of the smoker became a taster of the world as well.

Advertising the meaning of tobacco's taste and smell

Cigarettes united users in more than a swirl of scent and smoke. As Bourdieu argues, in both its cultural and political dimensions, consumption, especially educated consumption, allowed for the expression of class differentiation, the creation of the self, and a legitimation of the bourgeois worldview.[55] Historian Christine Ruane demonstrates that for the emerging Russian urbanites, with more money available to them for discretionary spending, a growing base of industrial goods, and less tolerance for traditional mores and class barriers, consumption became a way to express modernity, to challenge tradition, to practice individualism, and to join with like-minded buyers.⁵⁶ In her history of Russian advertising, Sally West adds radical political dimensions to Russian, urban consumer society. She contends that buying choices promoted individual and group identities that created consumer communities and a bourgeois worldview, which ultimately undermined the power of the autocratic state.⁵⁷ Consumption, if properly trained and engaged in, could be a sign of cultivation—a key means of marking status. Like other shoppers of the late nineteenth century, Russian smokers conveyed important indications of their class and political aspirations through their choice of products.⁵⁸

Recent histories of the culture of tobacco use in turn-of-the-century Canada and Britain focus on the relationship between the cigarette and increasing class distinctions, the advent of consumer culture, and liberal conceptions of the individual. The historian Matthew Hilton details how smoking became integral to Britain's middle-class and individual identity over the course of the nineteenth and twentieth centuries and argues that this incorporation of smoking into middle-class culture was rooted in liberal notions of independence and individuality.⁵⁹ The historian Jarrett Rudy transfers the theory on liberal smoking identity to turn-of-the century Canada to find similar methods of differentiation through consumption.⁶⁰ For Russians, consumption likewise allowed individuation, and the product itself had political meaning.⁶¹ By purchasing leaf from these various localities then scenting and flavoring it with precious additives, the Russian smoker expanded their worldview into the broad imperial boundaries of Russia and even farther afield, to embrace the globe and foreign concepts.

Russian tobacco advertisements underscored the international associations of blend, sauce, and product in their visuals and evoked concepts of the exotic, worldly, and luxurious in their appeals to buyers. As historian David Howes detailed, despite the theories of Karl Marx that capitalism alienated the senses, sensory appeals are deeply embedded in consumer capitalism and marketing of goods.⁶² Russian cigarette brand names reflected the cigarette flavors—Sweetness, Dessert, and Cream.⁶³ Cream brand tobacco advertisements used visuals of sophisticated smokers alongside an evocative slogan—"It's not tobacco! It's CREAM!"—to appeal to the palate as well as imply the bourgeois tastes of their users. Given the rough inhalation associated with Russian tobacco blends today, in comparison to Western smokes, the "smooth" nature of any nineteenth-century Russian tobacco seems debatable, but the slogan, and the strong popularity of the brand at the time, would indicate that the appeal resonated.

Advertisements spoke to not just the most basic concepts of sweet or strong but also to the global scope of the cigarette in an appeal to the discernment of the smoker, the expansionist pretentions of the Russian Empire, or the political airs of a Western-leaning elite. Kolobov and Bobrov, a tobacco factory out of St. Petersburg, could have chosen to market itself with the allure of the capital city or its manufacturing prowess. Instead,

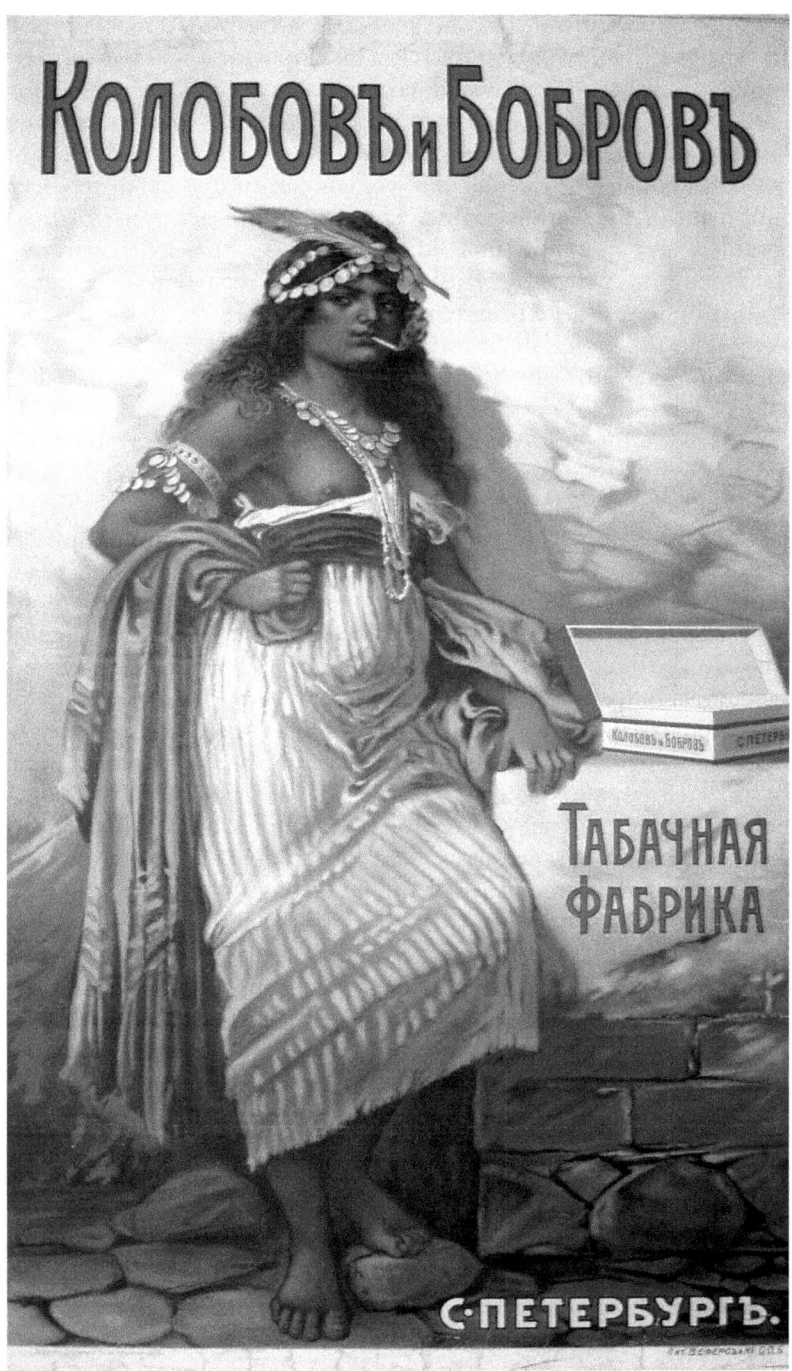

FIGURE 5.1 *Kolobov i Bobrov tabachnaia fabrika. Courtesy of Russian State Library.*

they chose an orientalist vision of an enticing, scantily-clad woman for their brand. The poster shown in Figure 5.1, a bit risqué for a street advertisement available to not just the cultivated gaze but also the flaneur's leer, shows a woman, barefoot and bare breasted on a cobble stone street leaning against a plaster wall. The umber tones evoke a warm climate and the draped fabrics and coined necklaces of the woman call to mind the stereotypical accouterment of the Turkic people. The visual implies the use of fragrant Oriental leaf and an exotic sauce to highlight a Turkish-style cigarette.

The globalism of the leaf blend and the sauce recipe are here joined by imperialist designs on the primitive colonial female—ready for possession. Smoking, and the materials flavoring the cigarette, thus becomes an act of domination. While the advertisement is undated, the Russo-Turkish wars served as backdrop to most of the late imperial period.[64] In these conflicts, Russia gained a foothold on the Black Sea, the Crimean peninsula, and moved deeper into the Caucuses. Here a Turkish maiden is a symbolic stand in for Russia's pretension for conquest in the Great Game.

The advertisement held multiple possible meanings for the nineteenth-century Russian viewer. On its most basic level, the promise of pleasure is given the viewer in the unspoken invitation of the half-naked, barefoot, and brazenly staring female. The warmth, languor, and sensual indulgence of tobacco are all communicated in her gaze. Further, the advertisement invites the viewer to indulge yet another sensual pleasure—touch. The nude torso and glowing shoulder and breast all invite the viewer's eye to glide over the skin of the smoking woman. At the same time, her slightly tensed hands and bare feet imply rough surfaces to contrast with the silken fabrics and warm skin. The evocation of rough and smooth mirrors the feel of tobacco's inhalation and the conflicted haptic pleasures associated with smoking.[65] The use of the nude female, alongside consumable items, links sexual appetites to other fleshly cravings. Carolyn Korsmeyer remarks of a woman similarly posed with food, she is "delectable visually, but she is also devourable, consumable" a pairing of "images of gustatory and sexual hunger with deliberately sensual effect."[66] This seems equally applicable to the pairing of woman with cigarette.

Especially popular in posters were images of the "other" as representative of tobacco.[67] The Bogdanov factory's poster for their Cigar[68] brand cigarettes (Figure 5.2) featured a black male holding bright yellow tobacco leaf (Virginia) out to the viewer. American tobacco was often depicted with African-American or golliwog images in the global market, but the smiling tobacco worker would have had a strange resonance in Russia, where earlier political allegory had often employed the American slave as stand in for the Russian serf. Certainly emancipation in both Russia and the United States had tempered that relationship but had not obliterated it.[69] In the post-emancipation, post-Civil War world of which this poster was part, the African-American male, here as producer and dealer of bright leaf, brought to mind both economic and political freedom, aligning tobacco with liberation as well as Western production and American ideology.

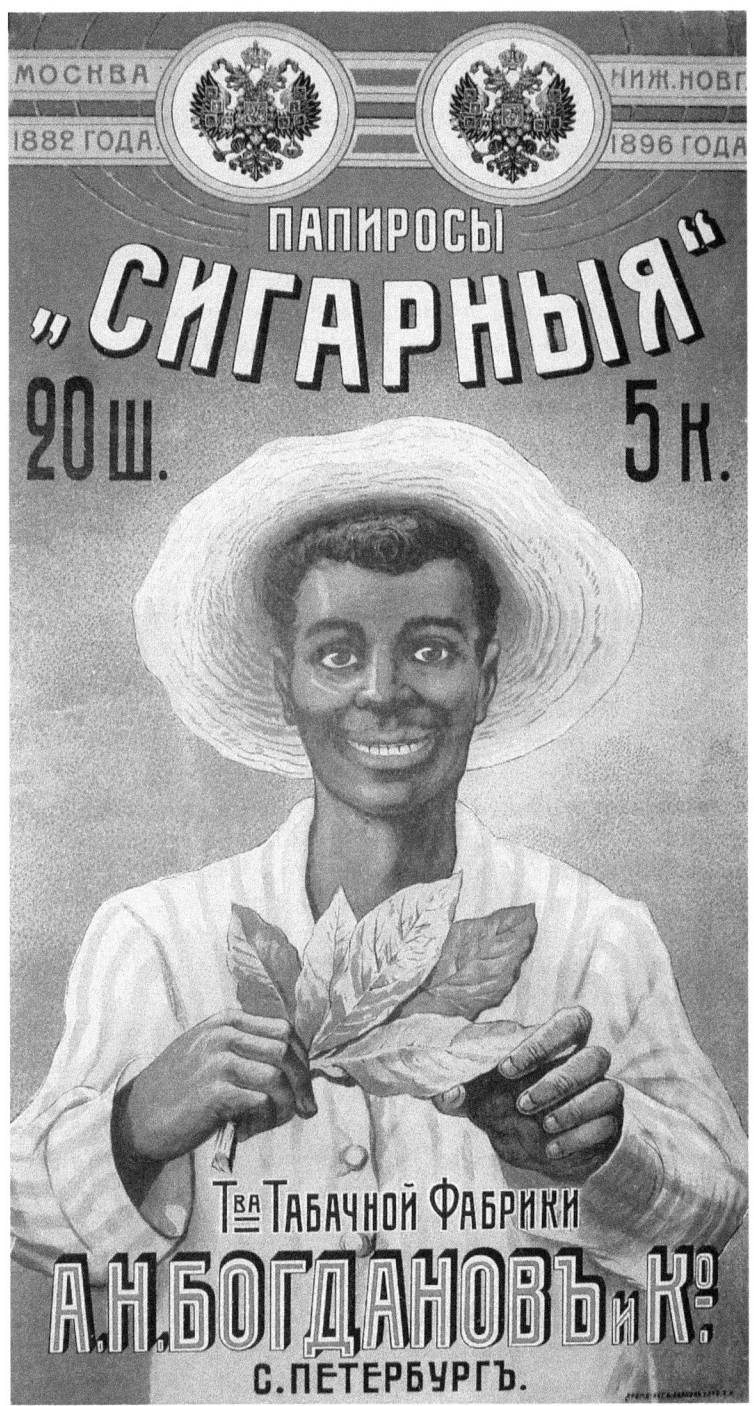

FIGURE 5.2 *Papirosy "Sigarnyia." Courtesy of Russian State Library.*

The advertisement is not a wholesale adoption of American imagery, but like the cigarette itself—a blend. The name itself transgressed the boundaries between different tobaccos and styles of smoking—a cigarette that was a cigar?—but there were other subtle changes as well. The borrowing of an American image is made Russian in three ways—the poster nods to the St. Petersburg base of the Bogdanov concern; the name of the cigarette implies the use of oriental tobaccos, to impart a cigar-like flavor; and the top of the poster features seals gained from Russian national manufacturing competitions (Moscow, 1882, and Nizhnyi Novgorod, 1896). These cigarettes are thus a foreign and domestic product, emerging as a mixture of associations that the consumer could purchase. This blending of leaf from around the world echoed in advertising posters of the period, which mixed promises of foreign flavors with images of exotic locales and alien names with connections to local producers and markets.

The taste of the cigarette

The modern cigarette is a poor approximation of its nineteenth-century predecessor. Growing and processing tobacco leaf has gone from a cottage industry to the concern of international agribusiness allowing for little variation in the quality of tobacco. The growth of the chemical industry generally over the course of the century, and cigarette additive research in particular, has resulted in stronger, dramatically-more-addictive smokes. Even the paper surrounding the cigarette has been engineered and improved to allow for smoother, better burn and faster conveyance of addictive substances. From industry advances, one can guess that the flavor of the past was rougher than today's cigarette, but the experience of that flavor may have been smooth. Indeed, the popular brand name Cream implied a mellow, comforting smoke. To recover the "taste" of the nineteenth-century Russian cigarette is nearly an impossible task.

The modern smoker is different from his predecessor as well. Medical advances and public health campaigns against both smoking and the resulting smoke transformed these from bad habits and occasional nuisances to major societal dangers and breaches of not just etiquette but law. From this a modern smoker associates very different concepts with their habit. For the smokers of the nineteenth century, however, medical and societal opprobrium of tobacco was not so strongly drawn and the smell and taste of smoking held different meaning. As literary scholar Constantine Klioutchkine argues, the cigarette held explicit connections to liberation among literary and cultural figures in nineteenth-century Russia.[70] Sally West similarly notes the association of smoking with foreign ideas and modernity in turn-of-the-century Russian advertising.[71] And these associations led smokers to endure sensory suffering of other kinds. Alexander

Martin even details how seminary students were willing to exchange an "hour or two" in a stinking outhouse "for the sake of a furtive smoke that also symbolized their autonomy."[72]

For the nineteenth-century Russian smoker, their cigarette was a mash of Western and Oriental products tasting of materials both familiar and extravagant, which then became the flavors of liberation. Further, the taste and scent could become an indicator of connoisseurship and class differentiation. The consumption of a product itself composed of materials associated with areas of liberation, democracy, and freedom carried strong meanings. The composition of the cigarettes became material manifestation of intangible political concepts—liberty, liberalism, and cosmopolitanism. The cigarettes' mix of tobaccos allowed the smoker to inhale and internalize the international. The blend was cosmopolitan, and when the smoker inhaled it, they by ingestion became worldly as well. By smoking Virginia tobacco or Western blends a Russian consumer imbibed the West and made it part of them.[73]

The flavor and scent it produced for both the user and for those surrounding the smoker would be unique in a land where Turkish blends predominated. Brand choice made a statement that was also a sensory performance. The scent of incense, rosewater, or sassafras in their tobacco did not just temper the taste; it also penetrated flesh and saturated clothing. The smoker created a modern identity through consumption of a blended product that actually became a part of the body and its presentation. The Russian smoker consumed the world, bringing it physically into their very person, and steeped in its smoke, they embodied a global, imperial vision of Russian identity. Enlivened by these many flavors, the smoker became tobacco's emissary to the outside world and allowed others to taste secondhand the imperial project and the modern.

Notes

1   Funding for this project came from the Kennan Institute for Advanced Russian Studies, the National Council for Eurasian and East European Research, the National Institutes of Health, National Library of Medicine, and the Fulbright College for Arts and Sciences. S. B., *Torzhestvo tabaku fiziologiia tabaku, trubku, sigar, papiros, pakhitos i tabakerki* (St. Petersburg: Tip. Sht. otd. korp. vnutr. strazhi., 1863).

2   Diane Ackerman, *A Natural History of the Senses* (New York: Random House, 1990), 138–43.

3   Robert Proctor, *Golden Holocaust: Origins of the Cigarette Catastrophe and the Case for Abolition* (Berkeley: University of California Press, 2012), 362.

4   Mark M. Smith, "Producing Sense, Consuming Sense, Making Sense: Perils and Prospects for Sensory History," *Journal of Social History* 40 (4) (2007):

841. See also his *Sensing the Past: Seeing, Hearing, Smelling, Tasting, and Touching in History* (Berkeley: University of California Press, 2007).

5   Ackerman, *Natural History*, 138–43.

6   Martin Jay, "In the Realm of the Senses: An Introduction," *American Historical Review* 116 (2) (2011): 309. The ephemerality of taste is also crucial to the analysis of Gerald J. Fitzgerald and Gabriella M. Petrick in "In Good Taste: Rethinking American History with Our Palates," *Journal of American History* 95 (2) (2008): 396–7.

7   Igor Bogdanov, *Dym otechestva, ili kratkaia istoriia tabakokureniia* (Moscow: Novoe literaturnoe obozrenie, 2007); A. V. Malinin, *Tabachnaia istoriia Rossii* (Moscow: Russkii Tabak, 2006); Iain Gately, *Tobacco: The Story of How Tobacco Seduced the World* (New York: Grove Press, 2001); Sander L. Gilman and Xhou Zun, eds., *Smoke: A Global History* (London: Reaktion books, 2004); Matthew Hilton, *Smoking in British Popular Culture, 1800–2000* (Manchester: Manchester University Press, 2000); Richard Klein, *Cigarettes are Sublime* (Durham, NC: Duke University Press, 1993); Jarrett Rudy, *The Freedom to Smoke: Tobacco Consumption and Identity* (Montreal: McGill-Queen's University Press, 2005).

8   Carol Benedict, *Golden-Silk Smoke: A History of Tobacco in China, 1550–2010* (Berkeley: University of California Press, 2011); Allan Brandt, *The Cigarette Century: The Rise, Fall, and Deadly Persistence of the Product that Defined America* (New York: Basic Books, 2009); A. K. Demin, ed., *Kurenie ili zdorov'e v Rossii* (Moscow: Fond Zdorov'e i okruzhaiushchaia sreda, 1996); A. K. Demin et al., *Rossiia: Delo tabak, rassledovanie massovogo ubiistva* (Moscow: RAOZ, 2012); Jordan Goodman, *Tobacco in History: The Cultures of Dependence* (New York: Routledge, 1994); Barbara M. Hahn, *Making Tobacco Bright: Creating an American Commodity, 1617–1937* (Baltimore, MD: Johns Hopkins University Press, 2011); Richard Kluger, *Ashes to Ashes: America's Hundred-Year Cigarette War, the Public Health, and the Unabashed Triumph of Philip Morris* (New York: Alfred A. Knopf, 1996); Mary C. Neuburger, *Balkan Smoke: Tobacco and the Making of Modern Bulgaria* (Ithaca, NY: Cornell University Press, 2012); Cassandra Tate, *Cigarette Wars: The Triumph of "The Little White Slaver"* (New York: Oxford University Press, 1999).

9   Priscilla Parkhurst Ferguson, "The Senses of Taste," and Mark S. R. Jenner, "Follow Your Nose? Smell, Smelling, and Their Histories," *American Historical Review* 116 (2) (2011): 371 and 337, respectively.

10 Ferguson, "The Senses of Taste," 371.

11 Marshall McLuhan and Walter Ong, who argued that there is great divide between pre-modern "oral" society and modern "visual" culture, are credited with this innovative and incendiary theory.

12 Here, Smith is arguing against the influential work of McLuhan and Ong. Smith, *Sensing the Past*, 1–2.

13 Jenner, "Follow Your Nose?" 346.

14 Alexander M. Martin, "Sewage and the City: Filth, Smell, and Representations of Urban Life in Moscow, 1770–1880," *The Russian Review* 67 (April 2008): 243–274.

15 Carolyn Korsmeyer, *Making Sense of Taste: Food and Philosophy* (Ithaca, NY: Cornell University Press, 1999), 1–2.
16 Ibid., 3–5.
17 Robert Jütte, *A History of the Senses: From Antiquity to Cyberspace*, trans. James Lynn (Cambridge: Polity, 2005), 172.
18 Darra Goldstein, "Gastronomic Reforms under Peter the Great. Toward a Cultural History of Russian Food," *Jahrbücher für Geschichte Osteuropas* 48 (4) (2000): 481–510.
19 World Health Organization, *WHO Report on the Global Tobacco Epidemic* (Luxembourg: World Health Organization, 2013).
20 F. A. Brokgauz and I. A. Efron, eds., *Entsiklopedicheskii slovar* vol. XXXII (St. Petersburg: I. A. Efron, 1901), 421–3.
21 Hahn, *Making Tobacco Bright*, 5–6.
22 Ferguson, "Senses of Taste," 373.
23 Neuburger, *Balkan Smoke*, 209.
24 "Tabachnaia pormyshlenost' v Rossii: Stat'ia vtoraia i posledniaia," *Otechestvennyia zapiski: Ucheno-Literaturnyi zhurnal* XXVIII (1843): 32.
25 Ibid.
26 Hahn, *Making Tobacco Bright*, 2–7.
27 Smith argues that smell, and other senses, are accessible to historians because "written descriptions of smells from the past tells us what smells smelled *like*." In "Producing Sense," 849.
28 *O razvedenii i fabrikatsii tabaka* (Moscow: Tip. Aleksandra Semena, 1852); "Tabachnaia pormyshlenost' v Rossii," 26–32.
29 Bogdanov, *Dym otechestva*, 132–4.
30 *Kratkii ocherk*, 5–6.
31 Smith, *Sensing the Past*, 67.
32 Ibid., 27. Alain Corbin, *The Foul and the Fragrant: Odor and the French Social Imagination* (Cambridge, MA: Harvard University Press, 1986).
33 Smith, *Sensing the Past*, 66.
34 Ferguson, "Senses of Taste," 381.
35 *O razvedenii*.
36 Hahn, *Making Tobacco Bright*, 6–7.
37 Bogdanov, *Dym otechestva*, 78.
38 Tate, *Cigarette Wars*, 14–15.
39 Bogdanov, *Dym otechestva*. 59; *Kratkii ocherk tabakokureniia v Rossii, v minuvshei 19-m stoletii: Za period vremeni s 1810 po 1906 god* (Kiev: Petra Varskago, 1906), 8.
40 "*Knastera*" is a German blend that was popular in Russia. It is now used for a pot-tobacco blend.
41 *O razvedenii*, 125–53.

42 Matthew P. Romaniello, "Customs and Consumption: Russian Tobacco Habits in the Seventeenth and Eighteenth Century," in *The Global Lives of Things: Materiality, Material Culture and Commodities in the First Global Age*, ed. Anne Gerritsen and Giorgio Riello (London: Routledge, 2015), 183–97.

43 Terrell Stevenson and Robert N. Proctor, "The Secret and Soul of Marlboro: Phillip Morris and the Origins, Spread, and Denial of Nicotine Freebasing," *American Journal of Public Health* 98 (7) (July 2009): 1185.

44 Brokgauz and Efron, *Entsiklopedicheskii slovar*, 421–3.

45 *O razvedenii*, 132, 152.

46 Ibid., 126, 130, 131, 143, 145, 146, 150.

47 Ibid., 127, 130, 133, 138.

48 Ibid., 128, 134.

49 Ibid., 127, 136, 137, 149, 151.

50 For instance, Bertrand M. Patenaude recounts the reactions of numerous Americans to Russian tobacco odor in *The Big Show in Bololand: The American Relief Expedition to Soviet Russia in the Famine of 1921* (Stanford, CA: Stanford University Press, 2002), 579–80.

51 Bogdanov, *Dym otechestva*, 59. The two types had been in Russia for nearly a century with strong class connotations embedded in their very introduction. Catherine the Great secured seed for production in Russia with Maryland and Virginia aimed at the elite market; Malinin, *Tabachnaia istoriia*, 72–74.

52 Bogdanov, *Dym otechestva*, 135.

53 A stone of just over a pound was found by a British boy on a beach in 2012 and was valued at approximately $63,000.

54 Christopher Kemp, *Floating Gold: A Natural (and Unnatural) History of Ambergris* (Chicago: University of Chicago Press, 2012).

55 Ferguson, "Senses of Taste," 381.

56 Christine Ruane, "Clothes Shopping in Imperial Russia: The Development of a Consumer Culture," *Journal of Social History* 28 (4) (Summer 1995): 765–82.

57 Sally West, *I Shop in Moscow: Advertising and the Creation of Consumer Culture in Late Tsarist Russia* (DeKalb: Northern Illinois University Press, 2011), 4–8; Barbara Alpern Engel, *Breaking the Ties that Bound: The Politics of Marital Strife in Late Imperial Russia* (Ithaca, NY: Cornell University Press, 2011), 4.

58 Engel, *Breaking the Ties*, 170.

59 Hilton, *Smoking in British Popular Culture*, 3–5.

60 Rudy, *Freedom to Smoke*, 6, 14–5.

61 Dick Hebdige argues that these constructed items are one of many parts of the display of identity and often their meaning comes from their contrast to or combination with other cultural items. *Subculture: The Meaning of Style (New Accents)* (New York: Routledge: 1979).

62 David Howes, "HYPERESTHESIA, or, the Sensual Logic of Late Capitalism," in *Empire of the Senses: The Sensual Culture Reader*, ed. David Howes, reprint edn (Bloomsbury: London, 2014), 281–96.
63 Sweetness (*Sladkiia*), Dessert (*Desertniya*), and Cream (*Krem*).
64 Russia and Turkey battled in 1676–81, 1687, 1689, 1695–6, 1710–12, 1735–39, 1787–91, 1806–12, 1828–9, 1853–6, and 1877–8.
65 Elizabeth D. Harvey employs artistic visions of hard and soft in her exploration of hapticity in history in "The Portal of Touch," *American Historical Review* 116 (2) (2011): 397.
66 Korsmeyer, *Making Sense of Taste*, 169, 170.
67 *Gadalka* (fortune teller) papiros from Kharkov featured a golliwog in one of their posters and the Kolobov factory of St. Petersburg features a Turkish or gypsy woman on their factory advertisement for papiros.
68 *Sigarniia*.
69 See for example a study of the Russian reception of the American book post-1850—John MacKay, *True Songs of Freedom: Uncle Tom's Cabin in Russian Culture and Society* (Madison: University of Wisconsin Press, 2013).
70 Konstantine Klioutchkine, "'I Smoke, Therefore I Think': Tobacco as Liberation in Nineteenth-Century Literature and Culture," in *Tobacco in Russian History and Culture: From the Seventeenth Century to the Present*, ed. Matthew P. Romaniello and Tricia Starks (New York: Routledge, 2009), 83–101.
71 Sally West, "Smokescreens: Tobacco Manufacturers' Projections of Class and Gender in Late Imperial Russian Advertising," in *Tobacco in Russian History*, 102–19.
72 Martin, "Sewage and the City," 272.
73 Megan Ward, "Feeling Middle Class: Sensory Perception in Victorian Literature and Culture" (PhD Diss., Rutgers, 2008).

CHAPTER SIX

The sounds, odors, and textures of Russian wartime nursing

Laurie S. Stoff

Upon the outbreak of war in 1914, N. Chelakova, a young St. Petersburg socialite, was sent to the front to serve as a sister of mercy. Her first assignment was to perform triage on a trainload of wounded. She was immediately and strongly repelled, not only by the unfamiliar and terrifying sights she encountered but also by the sounds and smells that struck her as she came into contact with war-damaged bodies. Dozens of wounded were crammed into the freight cars of the train, lying on the dirty, blood-stained floor of the dark, dank wagons. Chelakova's description of this experience is laden with multiple, interwoven sensory perceptions:

> Late that night a long group of freight car wagons stopped on the side track. Around them, everything was empty and quiet, and the train itself could not be distinguished from other freight trains, slowly moving through the countryside. But every wagon of this train was filled with human cargo, mutilated, bloody, human bodies, moaning and suffering ... An orderly with a flashlight, ladder, and bucket of hot tea went with me. He placed the ladder before each wagon and together we entered. Inside was hot, humid, and fetid. It took some time for one's eyes to become accustomed to the darkness and take in the strange scene inside. On the floor the wounded lay close to one another in their grey overcoats, with bandaged heads and blood-soaked hand wraps, with arms and legs in crudely fashioned splints ... The sounds of heavy breathing, wheezing, and muffled groans were heard. The air smelled of blood and pus ... "Sister, this one is already ..." someone pointed to his neighbor. With great difficulty, the orderly removed the dead from the wagon. A cold horror filled my heart.[1]

Russia's sisters of mercy of the First World War were bombarded with numerous dramatic, indeed traumatic, sensory perceptions. Despite this, little attention has been paid to the impact of these sensations on wartime nurses.[2] In fact, most analyses of wartime experience focus primarily on visual observation. This is not surprising or even unwarranted. The images associated with war have such significant effects on participants, indelibly forged in their memories, that they often make comment such as, "I saw things I can never forget" or "no one should ever have to see the horrors that I witnessed." The use of photography and film to record the activities and experiences of the war is particularly useful to historians. Even Chelakova, despite being overwhelmed by other impressions once at the front, indicated vision as the primary way she believed she would experience the war when she purposefully chose to pack her camera.

The focus on sight has been argued by some scholars as characteristic of the modern era, with its concomitant rise in visual culture made possible by the advent of mass printing and technology such as photography and film. Certainly, the First World War highlighted this, with its large-scale mechanization and military innovations, as well as the prevalence of visual propaganda. The effects of mechanized weaponry on human bodies created evocative visual images, particularly for civilians conscripted and recruited into service. The experience of encountering damaged and deceased human bodies was especially harrowing. Samuel Hynes asserts that "the first sight of the dead is a fundamental part of the soldiers' tale, being as it is the extreme case of war's unfamiliarity for civilian soldiers."[3] German officer Ernst Jünger confirmed this idea in his recollections:

> And now at our first glance of horror we had a feeling that is difficult to describe. It was too entirely unfamiliar. We looked at all these dead with dislocated limbs, distorted faces, and the hideous colors of decay, as though we walked in a dream through a garden full of strange plants, and we could not realize at first what we had all round us.[4]

Hynes' assessment could easily be rewritten with the words "soldiers" replaced by "nurses." Jünger's remarks were echoed by those of Russian sister of mercy Lidiia Zakharova, whose encounters with corpses had similarly jarring effects. When she came across bodies in the trenches, she described the visual scene in haunting terms:

> They laid on their backs or with their faces to the ground, their arms and legs entangled together. Many sat in positions like living people, looking out over the parapet or at the back wall of the trench. The strangest ones were those who had not fallen after they died, but remained standing, shoulder to shoulder, with their rifles in their hands and their glassy eyes open ...[5]

Similar to the horror that Chelakova felt when she saw her first dead body, the psychological impact of this sight on Zakharova was dramatic. "I was astonished by what I now truly understood as humanity expressing its capriciousness and multifarious nature."[6]

Although what participants saw in war is certainly very poignant, privileging sight has led to the unfortunate disregard of other sensory perceptions and the neglect of important elements of wartime experiences. Technological warfare was not just registered through visual encounters: the sounds of aerial bombardment, the smell of gas, the feel of wounds created by artillery shrapnel were equally profound. Indeed, sight rarely functioned independently in the war zone. What was seen was coupled with, and at times even overshadowed by, other senses that affected individuals intensely. The importance of addressing other sensory experience has been promoted by a number of scholars such as Mark M. Smith, who has argued that "histories of the senses promise to rescue us from an Enlightenment conceit with visuality that is not only pernicious in its silent effect on historical writing but also responsible for a sometimes misleading, partial, and distorted 'view' of the past."[7] Adding auditory, olfactory, tactile, and gustatory perceptions to analysis of wartime experience is significant because often these senses were vital in shaping wartime experience and memory in ways beyond mere visual recollection. They function, as Martin Jay has argued, as "portals of vital information about the world, opening us to stimuli from without."[8]

This chapter seeks to integrate multiple sensory perceptions into descriptions of the war experience. In so doing, it works to create a more holistic understanding of what participants endured, as part of a "web of sensory relations" that David Howe has labeled "intersensoriality."[9] The experiences of nurse Chelakova related in the opening paragraph are demonstrative of this kind of inextricable intertwining. Attentiveness to other senses in war allows a richer, more complete understanding of wartime experiences and their impact. This approach is particularly useful for social history, which strives, as Smith indicates, "to consider the breadth, depth, and interlaced aspects of the human experience" and "go beyond an unwittingly visualist representation of the past" by "no longer simply assess[ing] past experience through the eyes of historical actors but now also consider[ing] hearing, smell, touch, and taste."[10] Wartime nurses experienced new, unfamiliar sensations, entirely strange when compared with the kinds of things that they were accustomed to seeing, hearing, smelling, touching, and tasting. The physical and mental impressions of these participants highlight the extent to which the war was a transformative experience, indicating the incongruity between life during peacetime and that at the front. Indeed, Chelakova's first encounter with the sights, sounds, and smells of wounded and dying men catalyzed a change in her from her initial romanticized notion of war. Thrilled by the prospect of joining the conflict, she had been overjoyed when she received a summons from the Red Cross to enlist as a nurse.

When she departed for the front, she excitedly packed her camera to document what she believed would be an historic experience. Faced with the violence of modern warfare, her attitude changed markedly. After just a few weeks in service, she described this transformation through a bombardment of brutal, visceral experiences. "Very recently, perhaps yesterday or even that very morning," she remarked on the wounded men, "they all had been strong, healthy, fully alive ... But now they lay in this freight car like carcasses of animals after the slaughter. It was impossible to determine individual faces from among this mass of mangled humanity, from among the bandaged heads, arms, legs, from the smell of clotted blood, sweat, and pus, from their groans of pain and misery."[11] The sensations Zakharova experienced similarly altered her thinking about war, from a form of escape from personal sorrow (she had enlisted in nursing service as a result of her depression and loneliness following her husband's conscription) to a loss of faith in humanity as a result of its violent excesses. She "felt as if she had been 'swallowed up' in a new life," "carried away in a powerful stream," as if the war was changing her into an entirely different being.[12]

I argue that the experiences of Russian wartime nurses move sense history beyond description of purely physical perceptions. As such, we should consider those that operated exclusively in the realm of the mind, including illusory perceptions such as hallucinations. Not only were these hallucinations highly significant for those who took part in wartime medical service but also these reveal the extent of psychological trauma caused by war experiences. Examining the sounds, odors, textures, and tastes, as well as illusory perceptions of Russian wartime nursing enriches our understanding of what the individuals who took part in war endured.

What emerges is an analysis that highlights the extent to which participation in war was a transformative act for women, one that shared significant similarities with male combatants, but simultaneously was shaped by and upset gendered expectations and social divisions in Russia. Despite the stark contrast with peacetime life, female nurses' experiences were actually quite similar to those of male combatants.[13] Combat and medical personnel recorded similar impressions when entering into strange, unfamiliar territory and confronted with the realities of the warzone. Simultaneously, while in many ways female nurses' sensations indicate strong parallels with male combat experience and thus diminish the perception of war's exclusive masculinity, gender figures prominently in their impressions. Nursing in early twentieth-century Russia was shaped by conventional, essentialist ideas of women as naturally caring and nurturing and thus particularly well-suited for medical service. The sounds, odors, textures, and tastes Russian sisters of mercy encountered often demonstrated the fallacy of seeing nursing as a feminine activity. In a similar vein, these impressions reveal both the ways that class and social status continued to operate as a determinant of experience despite the chaotic upheaval of war, while signaling noteworthy shifts in the structural landscape of Russian society.

The Russian war experience

Although Russian women engaged in a wide variety of activities during the First World War, from munitions manufacturing to ditch digging and combat, nursing was undoubtedly the most popular form of female service.[14] Thousands of women entered wartime medical service at the outbreak of the conflict. By 1917, the number of women serving as sisters of mercy was approximately 31,000.[15] These women were essential, as Russian military medical services were woefully unprepared for total war, unable to treat the millions of soldiers and civilians that were wounded and sickened by the hostilities and their ancillary effects. They came from nearly every social stratum of Russian society, from the imperial family and aristocracy to the peasantry and working poor. The majority, however, possessed middle- or upper-class backgrounds as a result of literacy requirements in many of the agencies responsible for deploying wartime nurses.

Although women engaged in medical services for nearly all of the other belligerents, and nursing across borders shared a number of common features, the Russian wartime nursing experience was different in several important ways. Unlike countries such as Great Britain, Russia lacked a developed professional cadre of nurses. Instead, nursing was part of the quasi-religious communities of the Russian Society of the Red Cross (thus the religiously-suggestive designation "sisters of mercy"), which operated independently of the International Red Cross, as well as part of other civilian organizations such as the Union of Towns and Union of Zemstvos (local government organizations). Prior to the war, very few women possessed nursing skills—there were only approximately 4,000 qualified sisters of mercy in the Russian Red Cross by the summer of 1914. This meant that the nation was forced to draw upon civilian women, train them perfunctorily, and send them to the front to perform medical service as quickly as possible to satisfy the tremendous demand.[16] Thus, most nurses, like soldiers, were not professionals. Not only was the war something worlds apart from their everyday lives but so was medical care.

Even more significantly, in contrast to the oft-stagnant trench warfare of the Western Front, combat on the Eastern Front was extremely mobile. While most Western nurses were assigned to stationary hospitals behind the frontlines, Russian medical personnel were required to move with the troops, so rapidly that medical units sometimes arrived at a location one day only to evacuate the next. Some sisters worked with fixed medical facilities, but many others were part of mobile units that operated alongside the armies on the front. Unlike most of their West European counterparts,

Russian nurses often served close to the fighting. Procedural regulations that restricted female medical personal to rear service were impractical on the Eastern Front where distinguishing between "front" and "rear" became virtually impossible. Many women served in mobile dressing stations, ambulatory transport units, and "flying columns," which moved along the frontlines. As a result, Russian sisters of mercy were not shielded from the ordeals of war; they experienced extreme cold, constant fatigue, contagious diseases, artillery fire, and aerial bombardment. They encountered death and destruction in the closest possible proximity.

Disquieting sounds

Russian nurses' first impressions of war often came through sound. Before they were able to see artillery explosions, aerial bombardment, machine-gun fire, or rifle shot, they could hear them. Many times they experienced these aspects of warfare aurally, never actually seeing the shells, bombs, or bullets. The importance of aurality is particularly significant in war, when the listener is often unable to connect sounds to a visual locus. "In modern warfare," commented futurist poet Luigi Russolo, "mechanical and metallic, the element of sight is often zero. The sense, significance, and the expressiveness of noise, however, are infinite."[17] The noises of war became a common means of interaction with conflict for wartime nurses since few participated directly in the fighting. This war was a different kind of conflict from those that preceded it and a different kind of experience from peacetime; new military technologies made new kinds of sounds.

Although the aurality of Russian urban life had undergone significant changes as a result of industrialization and thus included the clamorous noise of factories, automobiles, and other harbingers of modernization, the sounds of war were distinctly different—not only ubiquitous and loud but also dangerous and unnerving. Sister Sofia Bocharskaia remembered that the "sounds of the guns were deafening" and her fellow medical personnel found it "difficult to hear each other speak, so muffled was everything in the sound of the firing."[18] Chelakova recalled that from her hospital the sounds of war were clear: "day and night we listened to the unending fire of the cannons, reminding us that the enemy was extremely near … The constant booming of weapons, got closer and louder, then somehow faded and became quieter, but never grew completely silent."[19] She described how everyone in her military hospital, soldiers and medical personnel, men and women alike, reacted to hearing a German airplane bombarding them:

> The aircraft was now immediately above the barracks, even though the roof was painted with a large red cross. There was a large explosion and a column of black smoke went up over the fence. "Lie Down! Lie

Down!" someone yelled. But people just stood there, still, as if they had been turned to stone, with their eyes fixed on the airplane, like magnets. Another explosion—and again, another column of smoke rose above from the earth, like a black cloud... This was followed by two more explosions. One bomb fell on a cart with two horses, tied up to the fence. The soldier standing next to it was killed immediately. And yet, still no one stirred. A deathly silence prevailed.[20]

Countess Olga Putiatina recalled the boom of an explosion that left her and her fellow hospital workers "groveling on the bandage-room floor in a most undignified way—the combined shock of the air and noise and instinct for self-preservation," one which similarly affected the soldiers being treated there, who were "frightened out of their wits." She described the attempt to evacuate the patients as "a miserable performance with most bewildering and piteous cries all around."[21]

As disquieting as they were alone, the aural perceptions of war often came with other sensations. Bombs, shells, and bullets created loud and disturbing noises that were not only heard but also felt. Indeed, as scholars such as Steve Goodman have argued, it is problematic to understand sounds as sensations limited exclusively to what is audible without considering their resonances on structures and human bodies. In particular, the vibrations caused by military acoustics often "contribute to an immersive atmosphere or ambiance of fear and dread."[22] Bocharskaia described how she "heard the reverberation of masses of men marching," and "the rattle of machine guns."[23] She recalled that her unit sat for days listening to the bellowing of the guns and feeling their impact:

> We began to hear the sound of heavy artillery. At first one deep, rumbling discharge ... Then another, and each seemed an individual death. They came more quickly, the sound overlapping. It went on like a storm that lasted day and night. We became oppressed, and the cold seemed more intense... For days, the earthen floor shook with the reverberation of the guns, the windows rattled.[24]

Florence Farmborough, a British woman serving with the Russian Red Cross, recounted the sounds of war combined with physical sensations that she was unable to locate as external or internal:

> when an angry hiss was heard, grew louder and louder, and then the explosion! The roar was deafening, the room shook and there were frightening noises of splintering, slicing masonry and of glass breaking and falling. A great silence followed, but the room continued to shake and tremble; or was it, perhaps, our own limbs?[25]

The din of war would have been a stark contrast to the "quiet life" of peacetime for women of the upper and middle classes, from which many of Russia's sisters of mercy hailed. These women would have been accustomed to lives led primarily in the private sphere, indeed, in the privacy of the home, where as Sophia Rosenfeld has argued, "inescapable noise increasingly registered as a source of auditory distress."[26] Hearing the sounds of mechanized warfare from within medical facilities, which though not exactly private domestic spaces, were supposedly safe from military attack, could be particularly disconcerting.

Russian wartime nurses, unlike most of their Western counterparts, spent considerable time outside the limited protection of medical facilities. For some, the sounds of war were so unfamiliar that at first, they could not recognize them. In attempts to process them, they subconsciously identified them as familiar noises. As Bocharskaia traveled with her unit along the front, she was struck by the "sound of a great many bees buzzing" around her, but when she looked around to see where the bees were, she could not find them. The "bees" were actually bullets. "We were being shot at," she recalled with some embarrassment, "and I had not known."[27] Never having been fired upon, Bocharskaia could not process the sounds as bullets, and instead transformed them into something that she had heard before. Sound is often noted as a primary way for humans to orient themselves to their surroundings, as Claire Shaw indicates in this volume. In the strange setting of war, however, unfamiliar noises often did little to aid in assisting nurses in situating themselves in the zone of combat. As Russolo commented, "noise, which conquers the blackest gloom and the densest fog, can betray as well as save."[28]

War, and the horrors associated with it, transformed mundane and innocuous sounds into strange and menacing ones. Soldiers like German officer Ernst Jünger mistook innocent sounds for incoming shells, which induced "the habit of jumping at any sudden and unexpected noise. Whether it was a train clattering past, a book falling to the floor, or a shout in the night—on each occasion, the heart would stop with mortal dread."[29] Nurses at the front had similar experiences. Lidiia Zakharova's commentary regarding her first visual encounter with the dead is made all the more poignant by her inclusion of sound. The doctor traveling with Zakharova and her fellow nurses, Aleksei Petrovich S., sensing their emotional distress at seeing a dead German soldier, tried to comfort them with what were intended as soothing words: "It is nothing, nothing, sisters, hold on to your nerves. At first it is terrible, but then you get used to it." Instead of comforting the nurses, the doctor's words only seemed to make things worse. "We tried to smile," Zakharova wrote, "but the sound of a live human voice had an unsettling effect," as if accentuating the contrast between the living and the dead.[30] A familiar, non-threatening, even consoling sound in peacetime conditions, the human voice, was transformed by the war into something eerie and disconcerting.

War forced nurses, like soldiers, to grow accustomed to sounds in order to work effectively. Florence Farmborough was surprised at how quickly she adjusted to the gruesome sights and the harrowing wails of wounded men:

> We are very raw recruits, and it is not surprising that we sometimes wince, even shrink into the background, when an unusually ugly wound is bared for dressing, or when a man's cry of anguish follows an awkward attempt to alleviate an excruciating pain, it is, however, astonishing how quickly even a raw recruit can grow accustomed, though never hardened, to the sight and sound of constant suffering.[31]

Farmborough became convinced that nurses must ignore the cries of pain and fear from wounded soldiers, walk away from hopeless cases to tend to those who had a chance of survival, and leave behind immobile patients during unplanned retreats despite their begging exhortations. Becoming accustomed to, even ignoring, sensations that would, in other conditions, cause distress, was a necessary part of the job of wartime nursing. Ironically, the caring and nurturing characteristics conventionally assumed to make women better nurses were those that had to be suppressed for them to function effectively.

The sounds of the damage done to men's bodies by the violence of war were equally evocative and had similar psychological impacts on nurses as they did on soldiers. Sister of mercy Mary Britnieva, an Anglo-Russian nurse, described a haunting scene in a field, where she both watched and listened to the sounds of soldiers who had been exposed to gas convulsing, choking, and gasping, while coughing up bloody, frothy pieces of their lungs.[32] Her language is reminiscent of Wilfred Owen's poem "Dulce et Decorum Est," in which he wrote, "And watch the white eyes writhing in his face ... If you could hear the blood / Come gargling from the froth-corrupted lungs."[33] Britnieva's and Owen's depictions indicate the importance of the sounds associated with gas attacks for both nurses and soldiers, on both the Western and Eastern Fronts. The horror of this experience, Britnieva commented, continued to make her shudder many years after the war.[34] Farmborough recalled treating a wounded man who had a hole in his back large enough for her to insert her hand and which had severely damaged his lung, causing his breath to emerge from the hole "in gurgling, bubbling sobs."[35]

Wartime nurses frequently noted sounds as extremely prominent in the provision of medical care. Sister Khristina Semina remembered that after an intense battle "the wounded continued to be brought in and brought in, without end," she stopped seeing the patients, but only heard them. Again indicating the disorienting cacophony, she remarked, "You only heard— 'Sister! Sister!'—coming from all sides ... You did not know where to go, who to offer help to first!"[36] Farmborough described the operating room of her mobile unit as "filled with agonising groans, stertorous breathing, the rustle of moving arms, the murmur of voices, the clink of surgical instruments, the slash and click of surgical scissors, and always the deeply-drawn breathing of men performing a task of intense importance."[37] Those involved in surgical amputations commented on the harrowing noises: the sawing and cracking of bone, the clink of digits hitting the bottom of a metal bucket after being cut away, the thuds that replaced the clinks as the bucket filled with increasing numbers of appendages. Sofia Bocharskaia recalled hearing "the thin scrape of the saw" as she assisted a doctor perform a leg amputation.[38] While assisting in the operation, Bocharskaia recalled that "a frantic protest rose in me that to do such a thing to a man's leg was butchery. It was unnatural. The flesh looked firm and healthy. You could not turn a human body into a dreadful, lopped fragment of a man."[39] Her auditory perceptions served to heighten the impact of the violence perpetrated on male bodies, contributing to a great sense of the dehumanizing effects of the war.

Stench and sensibility

The odors of men's wounds disturbed women as much as the sounds of warfare and the sights of damaged bodies. Aleksandra Tolstaia, youngest daughter of famous writer Leo Tolstoy, remarked that she would never forget not only the sight but also the ghastly smell of one wounded man. "A shell had almost completely torn away both of his buttocks," she recalled, and "a terrible stench emanated from his wound. In place of his buttocks, there were two gaping dirty-grey wounds. Something swarmed within them, and bending over him, I saw ... worms! Thick, fat white worms!"[40] She was haunted not only by the sight of his decomposition but also by the putrid smell, which lingered in her memory and affected her ability to sleep and eat for a long time after.[41] Chelakova wrote about another experience when, despite the strong visual perception of a man reduced to a mere torso, smell figured equally prominently:

> I remember one soldier who had his leg amputated up to the knee ... Soon, he had developed gangrene in his other leg, which needed to be removed as well. Then, one after another, it was also necessary to amputate his arms, and he lay in his bed like a log. He was slowly rotting, and a terrible smell emanated from his body. At the request of the other wounded men, he was moved to the very end of the room.[42]

While one can imagine the smells of pus, blood, and dirt, the descriptions of the "smell of death" lack such tangibility and blended emotion with perception. Bochkarskaia remembered that she "felt dizzy as the smell of death" hit her as she entered a factory that had been converted to a hospital at the front, where the lower level was being used as a mortuary. "It filled the entire basement of the building and the odor rose up through all the floors," she recalled with revulsion.[43] Farmborough similarly highlighted the odor she encountered while walking through a field before she *saw* the corpse. "As I walked, I suddenly became aware of a nauseating smell," she recalled. Intending to avoid its source, she hurried away, only to unexpectedly stumble upon it. "A dead soldier lay at my feet. Swollen and blackened by exposure, his features had disappeared. He was lying on his back, with arms extended, and his uniform had burst with the pressure of his swollen, decaying body." To her horror, she noticed something moving in his chest, "a mass of crawling, writhing worms. Sickened, terrified, I turned and ran."[44] The sight of the corpse was secondary to the odor that first drew their attention and precipitated a physical reaction.

Touching war

Santanu Das has argued that touch is the most "intimate" and "elusive" sense because unlike sound or sight (but perhaps similar to smell) it cannot be recorded or preserved.[45] Tactile sensations disconcerted wartime nurses and worked to shape their experiences in salient ways. Distinct from women's pre-war lives, war involved significantly damaged, even dead, human bodies heightening the trauma associated with war. Touch often evoked shock and emotional tension, particularly when nurses experienced the feeling of human flesh in entirely alien contexts, such as on the battlefields or in the trenches, that stood in stark contrast to those associated with civilian life.

On one occasion, Lidiia Zakharova became separated from her unit after nightfall. She attempted to make her way through a field in the dark, but as she walked she noticed that the ground felt very strange, soft and spongy under her feet, but unlike mud or slush. She experienced a haunting combination of sensory perceptions, crystallized by the realization of just what she was treading upon:

> Brrr … that is one of the creepiest impressions that I took away from those difficult times. Darkness. Rain. Severe cold. Under my feet there was some kind of mush, the composition of which allowed for all kinds of assumptions; it was silent all around, but it was tangible in my every nerve that it was a population of corpses… . The first natural inclination was to call for help, but what came out was a terrifying shout, a frightening sound of a voice lurking in the darkness and the silence.[46]

Later, Zakharova had a similar experience when, on a foggy day while attending to wounded men on a river bank, her foot hit upon something hard in the marshy ground. She looked down to discover that she had stumbled over the severed, rotting head of a German soldier and she screamed "desperately and loudly," in such a way that once again she did not immediately understand the voice to be her own, as it took on completely unknown and frightening dimensions.[47]

Touch was no less important within the context of the medical facility. Sofia Bocharskaia recalled her first experience assisting in surgery, in which the feel of the patient's pulse steadied her through the procedure. "Far away inside me was a girl, frightened at the responsibility that had been given her," she recalled, "but she seemed small and vague, and I felt about me the movement of quick, decisive work, keeping time with the throb of the soldier's life beating his pulse."[48] While this perception proved stabilizing, others had the opposite effect. On another occasion, Bocharskaia held a man's hand tightly while the surgeon removed a bullet, and as she did, the flesh of her arm began to tickle. When she looked down she saw lice crawling from the man's arm up her sleeve, and although she was repulsed, there was nothing she could do; she had to remain absolutely still while the doctor worked.[49] Other nurses found touch similarly destabilizing. Aleksandra Tolstaia commented that she had particular difficulty growing accustomed to the experience of assisting in surgical amputations. She was unnerved by the sensation of holding the leg or the arm of a wounded soldier during amputation, wherein suddenly, after the limb was removed, "one felt a dead mass. A part of a human body remained in one's hands."[50]

Das argues that nurse's experience of touch in treatment on the Western Front evoked gendered reactions. Focusing on the helplessness that female nurses felt when touching the damaged bodies of men, he contends that this created an "impotence of sympathy" unique to women's experiences in war because of their lack of active combat. He asserts that, "called upon to serve the shattered remnants of the body, the subjectivity of the nurse is doubly eroded—first, through the gap with the male trench experience, and second, through the sheer magnitude of suffering, an experience that can never be owned by women either historically or ontologically."[51] The dichotomies created between active/passive and male/female by theorizations such as Das do not hold in the Russian context, wherein nurses experienced war in ways very similar to soldiers, or even in the context of mechanized and trench warfare, wherein soldiers often felt as helpless as nurses, and nurses did feel useful in the provision of care through their touch.

Despite addressing both Owen's poetry and Britnieva's memories about gas attacks, Das overlooks the striking similarity of their comments and thus misses the fact that both medical workers and soldiers had these reactions. Sensory perceptions led to feelings of guilt, remorse, and lack of control for soldiers who watched helplessly as their comrades in arms were wounded or killed. Men felt a distinct lack of individual agency in this war, with its heavily technological emphases and the use of trenches that led them to believe that they were unable to control their circumstances. Jan Plamper explains:

> Modern war exposes soldiers to drastically longer periods of rifle and machine gun shooting, shelling, and air bombardment. It makes the source of the attack difficult to locate. Trench warfare, a major feature of World War I, immobilizes soldiers, thus incapacitating the reflex to flee from the source of danger; by contrast, a premodern open battlefield and one-on-one bayonet combat offered the—shame-free—option of forward attack as an outlet for fight-or flight reactions ... All of these factors amount to a real and significant increase in psychological stress that had to spill over into the ways soldiers felt—and sometimes wrote—about what they endured.[52]

Literary scholar Margaret Higonnet found that in treating soldiers suffering from mental disorders caused by the war, "doctor after doctor remarked that the devastating 'sight of dead comrades' or 'the sight and sound of his lacerated comrades' was sufficient to arouse morbid agitation, nervous breakdown, with paralysis, cramps, or even delirium."[53]

Furthermore, Russian sisters of mercy expressed considerable agency through their ability to effect soldiers through their touch, part of the nurses' presumed natural, feminine ability to provide solace and comfort for wounded or dying men. Indeed, in this way, women not only did *not* feel impotent but also both they and many men believed female medical personnel had distinct advantages, able to provide relief when scientific measures failed. Sisters often talked about holding men's hands as they lay suffering. For men close to death, in particular, for whom other sensations had become dulled or deadened, the feeling of a nurse's warm hand was particularly valuable. Florence Farmborough recalled sitting with a fatally wounded man who could no longer see, who clenched her hand tightly with cold, clammy fingers, imploring her to stay. "'Don't go, don't go,' he gasped piteously, 'don't leave me in the dark'."[54] His tactile connection to the nurse was the last source of comfort. Dying men sometimes asked nurses for a last kiss prior to expiring, and sisters of mercy often complied. Although under normal circumstances such intimacy with virtual strangers would have been completely unacceptable, the exigencies of war transformed an act of sexual danger to sisterly or motherly love.

Providing succor to male patients made female nurses feel useful, even if they could not save them from impending death. This was conventionally believed to be one of the most important roles that wartime nurses carried out. Men and women alike spoke of the positive psychological, even "spiritual," impact that the mere presence of women had on the wounded and dying soldiers. As one Russian journalist commented, in the role of caring nurturers, sisters of mercy were seen as not only healing wounds but also "uplifting souls."[55] Like the passive, supportive role of wife and mother, providing uplift was often held in higher regard than her medical treatment. One head doctor expressed this view when he became overwhelmed with the numbers of seriously wounded men for whom he could do little. "How do I know how to make a man live? I'm not God," he rued. "You should know better than I, you should *feel* [italics mine] it with your heart."[56] In this context, the sensation of a sister's warm hand against the increasingly cold skin of a fatally wounded soldier or the touch of a nurse's lips to those of a dying man was more important than surgical procedures or medical treatment.

For nurses, comforting touch presented a dilemma. Despite the positive value associated with women's assumed "natural" ability to provide comfort and care, the emotional components of nursing did not always prove useful. In fact, they were often perceived as hindrances to carrying out their duties. Under these drastic circumstances, abandoning traditional "femininity" was recognized as necessary and even encouraged. Writing anonymously in the *Red Cross Herald*, a sister of mercy commented that upon her acceptance into the Red Cross, she and her fellow nurses were told to "forget that you are women, forget that you have personal desires, sorrows or joys." Only then, she maintained, would the nurses be of any significant use.[57] As Farmborough sat clenching the hand of a dying man, her head doctor called to her insistently to leave the hopeless case and attend to those who had greater chances of survival. He had little patience for Farmborough's desire to remain by the dying man's side: "His irate voice sounded: '*Sestra*, we are waiting.' 'Alexander Mikhailovich,' I urged, 'it will be very soon.' 'There is nothing for you to do here,' he replied roughly ... And still more roughly: 'Have the goodness to come *at once*.' His words were final and he turned away."[58] Nurses faced a difficult choice, abandon those beyond the ability of medical science in favor of those who could be treated, or provide solace to those on the brink of death. In essence, they faced a tactile choice, to "harden" themselves against the emotional desire to provide "soft" comfort in the form of their flesh.

A taste of war

The old adage, "an army marches on its stomach" indicates the vitally important role of the gustatory in military conflict. In his chapter for this volume, Steven Jug has related the significance of the sense of taste for soldiers of the Red Army in the Second World War as a defining experience. Food and eating was, however, equally poignant during the First World War. Severe shortages and problems of distribution meant that those at the front, despite being prioritized by the Russian Imperial administration, often suffered from hunger and were fed very substandard food. Soldiers' letters home are full of complaints about food. As one soldier dictated to his nurse in a letter to his wife, "with regard to food, of course, it is bad—so many days we sit in the trenches without anything hot, only some dry crusts and raw cabbage, because it is forbidden to light fires in the trenches. However, this is military life."[59] Frontline nurses shared similar experiences. They too suffered from scarcities of basic necessities and hunger. When they did receive provisions, they were often poor in quality and quantity. Many were exposed to tastes they rarely, if ever, encountered prior to enlistment. Taste therefore further illuminates the nature of war experiences for sisters of mercy and their contrast to peacetime life, while indicating their parallels to male combat experiences. In the adverse circumstances of war, the flavors of simple foods such as potatoes and bread sometimes altered from mundane basics to culinary delights revealing the transformative aspects of wartime nursing.

From their very first inclinations to enlist in medical service during the war, women who desired to become nurses were conscious of the challenges that life at the front would present with regard to taste. When asking her husband for permission to join the Red Cross and train as a nurse, Khristina Semina was rebuffed. Her husband was a military doctor and therefore familiar with the hardships of war. He argued that not only her delicate constitution would be unable to endure exposure to "blood and pieces of human flesh" but also her noble taste buds would never endure the assault on them from the hard, black bread that was the main military fare.[60]

Once at the front, the realities of military rationing, which plagued both medical workers and combat troops, became readily apparent. The "dry crusts," known as *sukharki* were a staple of military life. Florence Farmborough described these vividly: "odd scraps of black bread in various sizes, baked or dried hard, and guaranteed to last for years. They were, indeed, as hard as stones … sometimes, the only way of demolishing them was to soak them in tea or water, until they became a 'sop'."[61] Despite this rather unappetizing description, Farmborough indicated how important these dry crusts were. "There were times," she recalled, "when our *sukharki* meant all in all to us." On one occasion, the unit was overjoyed when they received word that a bakery had been persuaded to supply them with fresh bread. They waited all day, "hungry, angry, tired and wet through, for the weather had no pity on us," but the bread never appeared. They finally were given roughly 36 pounds of bread to feed the entire unit. The bread was given to the rank-and-file (the soldiers who served as orderlies, drivers, and other auxiliary personnel), while the medical staff "had to be content with potatoes." But considering the conditions, Farmborough exclaimed "We were more than content! We boiled some, roasted others in the hot ashes of our fire and, then, under shelter of the overhanging trees … we lay down on the damp earth and dozed."[62]

Moreover, the death and destruction that surrounded them and bombarded their other sensory perceptions with foul odors, terrifying sounds, and horrific sights had to be suppressed in order to allow wartime nurses to eat. British nurse Violetta Thurstan, serving with the Russian Red Cross, wrote about how she and her fellow nurses had to adjust to these sensory assaults, and to eat despite the gruesome conditions:

> About four in the morning there was a little lull and some one [sic] made tea. I wonder what people in England would have thought if they had seen us at that meal. We had it in the stuffy dressing-room where we had been working without a stop for sixteen hours with tightly closed windows, and every smell that can be imagined pervading it, the floor covered with mud, blood and debris of dressings wherever there were not stretchers on which were men who had just been operated upon ... Two dead soldiers lay at our feet—it was not safe just at that moment to take them out and bury them. People would probably ask how we *could* eat under those conditions. I don't know how we could either, but we *did* and were thankful for it, for immediately after another rush began.[63]

Such impressions indicate the ways that taste links to other perceptions. As Priscilla Ferguson argues:

> it is conspicuously dependent upon those senses ... Smell makes taste possible, and touch, or in tasting terms texture, intensifies, and therefore completes, any tasting. Sight and even hearing also enter into the taste experience. If taste rarely impinges on sight or hearing, every cook knows full well how much seeing and hearing have to do with what and how we taste.[64]

The tastes that Russian wartime nurses encountered were also indicators of class and social position, which figured prominently in dictating what they were able to eat. While Farmborough and many others assigned to frontline medical facilities or mobile treatment units ate like soldiers, those with privilege and connections had access to the kinds of food they would have been accustomed to in their peacetime lives. Although paid for their work, sisters of mercy held responsibility for their own upkeep, often purchasing their own food. Despite the fact that many nurses came from comfortable middle- and upper-class backgrounds, some relied on the stipends they received for medical service. When these proved insufficient, or were not distributed as a result of the massive disruptions in financing caused by the war, some sisters went hungry.[65] Those who possessed economic advantage, particularly those who secured assignment to more comfortable medical facilities in the rear, tasted war quite differently. Gustatory sensations reflected the kinds of social stratification that permeated Russian society and continued to dictate experience despite the upheavals of war. Sofia Bocharskaia described dinners of roasted chicken, wine, brandy, coffee, and chocolate.[66] In fact, her memoir of the war reads more like a romantic adventure than an account of the trials of war, where she went on lavish picnics in the countryside and sweet-filled outings with flirty officers. Like most sisters of the nobility, Vanda Stepanova shared meals with the officers of her unit, and often had access to cakes, chocolate, candies, liquors, wine, fruits, and other delicacies in the wartime economy.[67] Chelakova recalled sitting in the well-apportioned private railway car of a high-ranking official of the Russian Red Cross, where they sipped tea and ate cakes and other sweets, and "chatted as if it were a Petersburg social call."[68] The contrast between the tastes enjoyed by the elite in medical service did not go unnoticed by other nurses. Farmborough framed her description of the *sukharki* she and her fellow frontline nurses ate most frequently in class terms. "'Crumbs from the rich man's table,' we called them jokingly and, indeed, they often looked like partly demolished, cast-off scraps."[69] Farmborough further echoed such sentiments when she encountered a group of sisters serving in the city of Minsk. She hesitated to even call them nurses, rather referring to them as "ladies who wore the uniform of Sisters" but with "painted faces and long gold chains hanging down over the Red Cross on their breasts ... befrilled and becurled ..." She could scarcely imagine such women performing the duties of a frontline nurse: "We tried to picture them out there where we had been: passing the long night hours in the open, buffeted by rain and wind; veiled with curtains of thick dust; wearing vermin-infested clothing for days on end; sleeping on benches, floors, under haystacks, in open fields; hunger stricken and thankful beyond measure for dried, black crusts."[70]

Gender and sexuality were equally significant in the food experiences of women in wartime nursing. Nurses were often the subjects of flirtation and sexual advances on the part of male military and medical personnel. Men who desired personal relationships with sisters offered food and drink, particularly sweets and alcoholic beverages, as currency in the coveted exchanges of intimacy. Despite strong admonitions from authorities against this kind of interaction, some sisters of mercy readily accepted attention and gifts of candy, cakes, chocolate, wine, and spirits from male admirers. Others, however, rejected such overtures, instead adhering to the strict codes of conduct for sisters of mercy that prohibited intimate relationships. Although many of her fellow nurses readily accepted such culinary treats from potential suitors, Stepanova admonished them for what she perceived to be "brazen" behavior. She redistributed the sweets or other gifts that flirtatious officers bestowed upon her to the wounded soldiers in her care.[71]

Illusory perceptions

Wartime experiences produced sensations outside of the realm of the generally-acknowledged five senses. Sensory history has, for the most part, focused on analyzing corporeal perceptions. But experiences outside the physical have had equally profound influence on sisters of mercy. Indicative of their traumatic effect, actual sensory experiences are often so powerful that they are sometimes transformed to illusory perceptions. While the actual sights, sounds, smells, and textures of the war and their effects were highly significant to nurses' wartime experiences, some women also experienced hallucinations and other imagined perceptions, further indicating the acute impact of their participation in war.

Hallucinations were not uncommon manifestations of traumas among both nursing and combat personnel. Tatiana Aleksinskaia recalled a soldier in her hospital train who experienced hallucinations as he neared death. "All night long he was haunted by bad dreams," she recalled. "In his delirium he fought the Germans, shouted, leaped from his bed, and hurled himself at his neighbors; the orderlies kept him back: he took them for enemies."[72] Historian Catherine Merridale detailed the ways war trauma affected Russian male soldiers detailing how one specialist treating soldiers noted the psychological impact of technological warfare on soldiers, particularly among the infantry, who were subject to frequent artillery fire. "The symptoms he observed included hallucinations: 'some believe they are still swatting Germans like flies'."[73] Nurses had similar reactions. Zakharova, suffering from a fever brought on by lack of sleep and the onset of pleurisy, described how she felt as if she was viewing everything through the fog of smoke. In what might be described as a psychological coping mechanism to allow her to relate the strange and unfamiliar perceptions she experienced during the war to something reminiscent of her pre-war life, she hallucinated that the patients being brought into her mobile unit were the friends and acquaintances she had made over the last several months while serving as a nurse. But when she asked them how they ended up at her dressing station, instead of their faces, she saw the "strange eyes of the grey figures of soldiers" looking back at her.[74] Even after being evacuated to a rear hospital for treatment, for several weeks she suffered from feverish delusions, Zakharova saw visions of the horrors she had experienced at the front. Images and sounds of "crawling wounded men, blood, distorted sick faces, shots, soul-chilling shots" filled her mind, sometimes even during the day when her fever would subside. In a statement revealing her own consciousness of how similar these experiences were to those of men in combat, she commented that they fostered in her an "increasing, emotional longing for home, like that of soldiers' [war] weariness."[75] Bocharskaia related how one young sister named Lala suffered from "hallucinations of amputated arms and legs that took on a life of their own, and when she slept, they moved about the room."[76]

The psychological impact was so significant for some sisters of mercy that they found themselves unable to cope. The stresses of service combined with the horrors of seeing so many men's bodies destroyed sometimes left women unable to trust their physical senses. A sister of mercy named Shura experienced a nervous breakdown in March 1916, when she became convinced that all of the men in her care had died. Her fellow nurses tried to convince her that the men still lived, making her feel their heartbeats, but to no avail. "Pulses prove nothing," the emotionally shattered young woman said, "everyone dies." When a new round of wounded came in to be prepped for surgery, she tried to prevent the doctor from operating. "Don't, don't, they will die anyway," she pleaded, as "she wrung her hands and wandered about listlessly murmuring of death."[77]

The notion that non-combatants could suffer similar sensory overload and ultimately serious psychological damage was recognized by some even during the war. Military psychiatrist Dr. S. A. Preobrazhenskii insisted on including medical personnel in his study of the psychological illnesses affecting those participating in the war, which he argued deserved equal attention to that of combatants. Preobrazhenskii noted that involvement in medical services was extremely difficult work, which had "significantly negative effects on both the moral and physical constitutions of those engaged therein, and could not be discounted from weakening neuropsychiatric stability." He reported cases of sisters (as well as brothers and other male medical personnel) of mercy suffering from "manic depressive psychosis," "hysteria," "psycho-polyneuritis," and "neurotic constitutions." Some of the nurses, after rest and treatment, were returned to their duties in the theater of war, only to suffer from relapses brought on by the conditions of their service.[78] For some, the trauma was so great that they chose to end their lives. Interestingly, the Red Cross and other organizations providing medical services did not attempt to hide the instances of nurses' suicides. The pages of the various publications of the organizations carrying out medical service during the war report many such cases among wartime nursing personnel.[79] For these sisters of mercy, the sensory experiences of modern warfare proved overwhelming.

Conclusion

The memories of Violetta Thurstan like those of Chelakova related in the opening passage, reveal the strong impression made by multiple sensory perceptions on nurses. Thurstan described the field hospital in which she worked as "more like hell than anything I can imagine. The never-ending processions of groaning men being brought in on those horrible blood-soaked stretchers, suffering unimagined tortures, the filth, the cold, the stench, the hunger, the vermin, and the squalor of it all … was almost enough to make even Satan weep."[80] In this brief passage, Thurstan evokes the sounds of human pain, the sight of blood and dirt, the feelings of cold and hunger, the sensation of insects crawling on the skin, the smell of rotting flesh, taken together to create an experience of "utter hellishness," one that was far from the normative aspects of the lives of civilians who entered wartime service.

By examining both the physical and illusory perceptions, we can better understand the profound impact of the war on the women who served as wartime nurses. They allow us to recognize similarities with male combat experience as well as understanding the gendered aspects of their service. Despite the presence of multiple strange and horrific perceptions, unlike anything they had experienced in their pre-war lives, Russia's wartime nurses had to learn to continue to function effectively and efficiently, and engage in "normal" behaviors despite the distinctly abnormal conditions that surrounded them. The ways that nursing personnel reacted to these strange and often horrific sensual encounters reveal much to us about the impact of war on participants. They demonstrate the extent to which participants were forced to internalize shock and horror to continue to function effectively in the warzone and how they were able to cope with such traumatic kinds of experiences. Despite the initially unnerving effects of many of these sensory perceptions, nurses had to learn to process and absorb them in such a way as to allow them to continue to carry out practical work. The most effective way most found was to dull the impact of sensation, even to the point of numbness. Thus, nurses had to become accustomed to seeing the disastrous effects of modern weapons on human bodies. They had to remain stoic while hearing constant cries of pain from the wounded and dying. They were forced to adjust to the sounds of bombs and shells, to the point where they often no longer registered them as menacing or even heard them at all. They could not allow the smells of decay and death to deter them from their work. They had to retain their composure and overcome their fears and revulsion when they came into physical contact with mutilated bodies, decomposing corpses, and severed limbs. Those who most successfully absorbed these multiple, traumatic sensations continued their work. Those who were not able to suffered from psychoses, which were sometimes debilitating. When coping mechanisms failed, their senses sometimes betrayed them and took on illusory forms such as hallucinations and imagined perceptions and led some to suicide. And even when nurses found ways of managing the dramatic impact of their perceptions, they often held onto them for a long time afterward.

Notes

1   N. Chelakova, "Iz zapisok sestry miloserdiia," *Novoe Russkoe Slovo* (June 14, 1969): 6.
2   Scholarship is somewhat thin on Russian nursing in general. The few works that do address this topic include N. A. Beliakova, *Sestry miloserdiia Rossii* (St. Petersburg: Liki Rossii, 2005); L. A. Karpycheava, "Kto takie *sestry*

miloserdiia? Ot istoricheskoi etimologii k sovremennomu kontekstu," *Pravoslavnyi Letopicets Sankt-Peterburga* 24 (2005): 11–28; A. V. Posternak, *Ocherki po istorii obshchin sestry miloserdiia* (Moscow: Izdatel'stvo Sviato-Dimitrievskoe Uchilishche setry miloserdia, 2001); V. P. Romaniuk, V. A. Lapotnikov, and I. A. Nakatis, *Istoriia sestrinskogo dela v Rossii* (St. Petersburg: SPbGMA, 1998). Those that focus on Russian sisters of mercy in the First World War are even fewer. See Christine Hallett, "Russian Romances: Emotionalism and Spirituality in the Writings of 'Eastern Front' Nurses, 1914–1918," *Nursing History Review* 17 (2009): 102–28; Laurie Stoff, "The 'Myth of the War Experience' and Russian Wartime Nursing in World War I," *Aspasia: The International Yearbook of Central, Eastern, and Southeastern European Women's and Gender History* 6 (2012): 96–116; and Stoff, *Russia's Sisters of Mercy and the Great War: More than Binding Men's Wounds* (Lawrence: University Press of Kansas, 2015).

3   Samuel Hynes, *The Soldiers' Tale: Bearing Witness in Modern War* (New York: Penguin Books, 1997), 67.
4   Ernst Jünger, as quoted in Hynes, *The Soldiers' Tale*, 67.
5   Lidiia Zakharova, *Dnevnik sestry miloserdiia: Na peredovykh pozitsiiakh* (St. Petersburg: Izdatel'stvo biblioteka "Velikoi Voiny," 1915), 51–2.
6   Ibid., 52.
7   Mark M. Smith, "Making Sense of Social History," *Journal of Social History* 37 (1) (2003): 165–86, here 167.
8   Martin Jay, "In the Realm of the Senses: An Introduction," *American Historical Review* 116 (2) (2011): 309.
9   David Howe, "Can These Dry Bones Live? An Anthropological Approach to the History of the Senses," *The Journal of American History* 95 (2) (2008): 442–51.
10 Smith, "Making Sense," 166.
11 Chelakova, "Iz zapisok sestry miloserdiia," 6.
12 Zakharova, *Dnevnik Sestry Miloserdiia*, 20.
13 For a comparison to the Second World War, see Steven Jug's contribution.
14 For a detailed account of the Russian women who served in combat capacities during the war, see Laurie S. Stoff, *They Fought for the Motherland: Russia's Women Soldiers in World War I and the Revolution* (Lawrence: University Press of Kansas, 2006).
15 Rossiskii Gosudarstvennyi Voenno-Istoricheskii Arkhiv (hereafter RGVIA), f. 12651, op. 3, d. 456, l. 71; and Romaniuk, Lapotnikov, and Nakatis, *Istoriia sestrinskogo dela*, 78.
16 Most Russian wartime nurses received six to eight weeks of training before being dispatched into service. This contrasts with the requirement of a full year of training for nurses under normal peacetime conditions.
17 Luigi Russolo, *The Art of Noises*, trans. Barclay Brown (Hillsdale, NY: Pendragon Press, 1989), 49.
18 Sophie Botcharsky and Florida Pier, *The Kinsmen Knew How to Die* (New York: William Morrow & Co., 1931), 7.

19   Chelakova, "Iz zapisok sestry miloserdiia," 4.
20   Ibid.
21   George Alexander Lessen, ed., *War and Revolution: Excerpts from the Letters and Diaries of the Countess Olga Poutiatine* (Tallahassee, FL: The Diplomatic Press, 1971), 31.
22   Steve Goodman, *Sonic Warfare: Sound, Affect, and the Ecology of Fear* (Cambridge, MA: MIT Press, 2009), xvii.
23   Botcharsky and Pier, *The Kinsmen Knew*, 7.
24   Ibid., 33.
25   Florence Farmborough, *With the Armies of the Tsar: A Nurse at the Russian Front in War and Revolution, 1914–1918* (New York: Cooper Square, 2000), 43.
26   Sophia Rosenfeld, "On Being Heard: A Case for Paying Attention to the Historical Ear," *American Historical Review* 116 (2) (2011): 323.
27   Botcharsky and Pier, *The Kinsmen Knew*, 54–5.
28   Russolo, *The Art of Noises*, 50.
29   Ernst Jünger, *Storm of Steel* (New York: Penguin Books, 2004), 8.
30   Zakharova, *Dnevnik sestry miloserdiia*, 11.
31   Farmborough, *With the Armies of the Tsar*, 22.
32   Mary Britnieva, *One Woman's Story* (London: Arthur Barker, 1936), 35.
33   Wilfred Owen, "Dulce et Decorum Est," in *The Oxford Book of War Poetry*, ed. John Stallworthy (Oxford: Oxford University Press, 1988), 189.
34   Britnieva, *One Woman's Story*, 35.
35   Farmborough, *With the Armies of the Tsar*, 42.
36   Khristina D. Semina, *Tragediia russkoi armii: Pervoi velikoi voiny 1914–1918: Zapiski setry miloserdia Kavkazkogo fronta* (New Mexico: Privately published, 1963), 30.
37   Farmborough, *With the Armies of the Tsar*, 220.
38   Botcharsky and Pier, *The Kinsmen Knew*, 9.
39   Ibid., 10.
40   Tolstaia distinctly uses the word "worms" (черви) rather than "maggots" (личники).
41   Aleksandra Tolstaia, *Doch'* (Moscow: Vagrius, 2000), 228.
42   N. Chelakova, "Iz zapisok sestry miloserdiia," *Novoe Russkoe Slovo* (June 18, 1969), 4.
43   Botcharsky and Pier, *The Kinsmen Knew*, 35.
44   Farmborough, *With the Armies of the Tsar*, 233.
45   Santanu Das, "'The Impotence of Sympathy': Touch and Trauma in the Memoirs of the First World War Nurses," *Textual Practice* 19 (2) (2005): 239–62.
46   Zakharova, *Dnevnik sestry miloserdiia*, 54.

47 Ibid., 110, 112.
48 Botcharsky and Pier, *The Kinsmen Knew*, 9.
49 Ibid., 11.
50 Tolstaia, *Doch'*, 231.
51 Das, "'The Impotence of Sympathy'," 239.
52 Jan Plamper, "Fear: Soldiers and Emotion in Russian Military Psychology," *Slavic Review* 68 (2) (2009), 262.
53 Margaret Higonnet, "Authenticity and Art in Trauma Narratives of World War I," *Modernism/Modernity* 9 (1) (2002): 92.
54 Farmborough, *With the Armies of the Tsar*, 130–1.
55 Valentina Kostyleva, "Nashi Amazonki," *Zhenskaia zhizn'* 19 (October 1914): 24.
56 Botcharsky and Pier, *The Kinsmen Knew*, 46–7.
57 "Sestry," *Vestnik Krasnago Kresta* 2 (1915): 598.
58 Farmborough, *With the Armies of the Tsar*, 130–1.
59 Zakharova, *Dnevnik sestry miloserdiia*, 46.
60 Semina, *Tragediia russkoi armii*, 11.
61 Farmborough, *With the Armies of the Tsar*, 148–9.
62 Ibid., 149.
63 Violetta Thurstan, *Field Hospital and Flying Column: Being the Journal of an English Nursing Sister in Belgium and Russia* (London: G. P. Putnam's Sons, 1915), 165–6.
64 Priscilla Parkhurst Ferguson, "The Sense of Taste," *American Historical Review* 116 (2) (2011): 372.
65 Records of the meetings of the Mobilization Department under the Main Administration of the Russian Society of the Red Cross, Journal No. 14, October 6, 1916, RVGIA f. 12651, op. 3, d. 418, l. 102.
66 Botcharsky, *The Kinsmen Knew*, passim.
67 Stepanova, "Zapiskii velikoi voiny," 60–2, 67.
68 Chelakova, "Iz zapisok sestry miloserdiia," 4.
69 Farmborough, *With the Armies of the Tsar*, 149.
70 Ibid., 150.
71 Vanda Kazimirovna Stepanova, "Zapiski velikoi voiny 1914–1918 gg.," unpublished manuscript, Hoover Institution Archives, Collection No. ZZ175, 62, 64, 67.
72 Tatiana Alexinsky, *With the Russian Wounded*, trans. Gilbert Cannan (London: Fisher Unwin, Ltd, 1916), 109.
73 Catherine Merridale, "The Collective Mind: Trauma and Shell-Shock in Twentieth-Century Russia," *Journal of Contemporary History* 35 (1) (2000): 41.
74 Zakharova, *Dnevnik sestry miloserdiia*, 116.

75 Ibid., 150–1.
76 Botcharsky and Pier, *The Kinsmen Knew*, 46.
77 Ibid., 217–8.
78 A. S. Preobrazhenskii, *Materialy k voprosu o dushevnykh zabolevaniiakh voinov i lits, prichastnykh k voennym deistviiam v sovremenoi voine* (Petrograd, 1917) 79–80.
79 *Vestnik Krasnago Kresta*, 1915–6.
80 Violetta Thurstan, *Field Hospital and Flying Column: Being the Journal of an English Nursing Sister in Belgium and Russia* (London: G. P. Putnam's Sons, 1915), 136–7.

CHAPTER SEVEN

The taste of *kumyshka* and the debate over Udmurt culture

Aaron B. Retish

Kumyshka is an alcoholic drink traditionally used in animistic rituals by Finno-Ugrics, especially Udmurts, of Russia's Volga-Kama Region of the northern Urals. This grain-based homebrew captured the public imagination of late imperial and revolutionary Russia. At issue was the sensation, the effect, of *kumyshka* on the body and soul as either a gateway to a higher spiritual plane or an entree to primitive savagery. *Kumyshka*, and the physical sensations it elicited, became a totem for multiple populations in late imperial and early Soviet Russia to debate confession, modernity, national culture, and contagion.

How *kumyshka* tasted, appeared, and affected the drinker were all part of colonial and modernizing discourses flowing through Russia in the late nineteenth and early twentieth centuries. Almost every sensation that *kumyshka* brought—taste, sight, smell, and effect—were contested by state officials and cultural commenters and by Udmurts who used the drink. If sensation, such as the effect of alcohol, is biomedical, descriptions of the experience are culturally and socially constructed. As Pierre Bourdieu noted, social and economic conditions and the systems of dispositions of classes shape taste: "Taste classifies, and it classifies the classifier."[1] Colonial images across the globe have painted portraits of colonial subjects unable to control their desires for alcohol, especially indigenous alcohol, in contrast to the colonial elites who could.[2] It was this sensory primitivism—the hunger of the flesh and immediate sensation from drink—that separated colonial subjects from the colonizers.

Kumyshka also fit into larger debates about proper tastes in a modernizing world. As Alison K. Smith and Anton Masterovoy discuss elsewhere in this volume, taste was a central part of defining national identity in the nineteenth and twentieth centuries. For state officials and cultural commentators, good tasting and healthy food and drink helped raise the culture of the people. For Russian commentators and officials, the putrid taste of *kumyshka* reminded them that this was not a usual or acceptable drink. This contrasted with many Udmurts' feeling that *kumyshka* was an integral and healthy part of their everyday spiritual world. As anthropologist Mary Douglas reminds us, drinks "act as markers of inclusion and exclusion."[3] In this case, the danger of *kumyshka* came in part from how Udmurts used it to keep themselves separate from the unifying Russian nation. *Kumyshka*'s potency came less from its alcoholic content than from what outside commenters feared it could do to its Udmurt and even Russian consumers. As a ritualistic mind-altering drink traditionally made and consumed outside of the state gaze, *kumyshka* essentially represented the antithesis of what the Russian state and the Russian Orthodox Church wanted out of its non-Christian, non-Russian subjects.

Tasting *kumsyhka*

Commentators of rural Russia lamented that all peasants drank too much. But in the ethnically diverse northeastern region of European Russia, they paid special attention to *kumyshka*. Through the major upheavals in the country, *kumyshka* captured the political imagination and became a contentious touchstone for public discussions of larger cultural and social tensions in Russian mass politics. *Kumyshka* became shorthand for Udmurts and all that was wrong with Russia's national minorities. In this way discussions over the sensation of *kumyshka* were also discussions of Russian imperialism and point to how political and cultural elites fashioned non-Russian peoples. Like most cultural signs, *kumyska* was a malleable, evolutionary construction that both elites and Udmurts fought over. The discourse surrounding the effects of *kumyshka* therefore brings to the surface the centrality of ethnicity in understanding the turmoil sweeping the country from the late imperial era through the Civil War.

From the mid-nineteenth century, debates over *kumyshka* began with the preparation of the drink and ended with its after-effects. Writers and commentators paid special attention to how all parts of the process affected the senses of sight, taste, and smell. Udmurts traditionally distilled the beverage at the edge of the village or in the forest because the still was so large. Brass or copper tubing connected the cauldrons in which the cook made the drink. Nineteenth-century ethnographers used a common term to describe the sight of the still: "primitive."[4] They defined the smell of the brewing of *kumyshka* as "burning" and producing "the strongest scent of fusel alcohol."[5] Ethnographers focused less on the taste, distancing themselves from the full experience of, or exposure to, *kumyshka*. When they did describe it, they most often called it sour or repulsive.

There are actually several varieties and tastes of *kumyshka*. The most common recipe calls for distilling grain (usually rye, oats, or barley) and mixing it with a sweetener. Recipes, though, vary by occasion and region. *Lim kumyshka*, for example, is one of its most potent varieties and produces an alcoholic drink of 5 to 20 percent (10 to 40 proof), while *nebyt kumyshka* is designed for children with a nearly non-alcoholic content.[6] In a recent ethnographic survey, Chuvashes of the Volga-Kama region provided various descriptions of what they thought was *kumyshka*. One respondent said, "it is the same as moonshine [*samogon*], but it depends on who is talking" and another said that, "*kumyshka* is a weak moonshine without sugar, using flour, beets, or potatoes instead."[7] Other Finno-Ugric peoples like the Maris and Permiaks made *kumyshka* and used it in their rituals and continue to brew it today to express their national heritage, but popular discourses of the late imperial and revolutionary eras most often linked it to Udmurts. Several writers have confused it with the mildly alcoholic, milk-based drink *kumys* most often associated with Russia's Turkic peoples, especially the Kalmyks, but this is an error based on linguistic similarities of an alcoholic drink made by a non-Russian group.[8] It is this very fluidity in its recipe, definition, and even which people brewed it that helped to make *kumyshka* a vessel for multiple interpretations in discussing empire and the place of non-Russians.[9]

Non-Udmurt writers of the late imperial period struggled to describe *kumyshka* and fell back on its sensory projections. They emphasized its strong smell and especially unpleasant taste. The great Russian lexicographer Vladimir I. Dal' labeled it as a "dark and smelly distilled brew."[10] A contemporaneous encyclopedia on Russia's peoples wrote: "*Kumyshka* is just like vodka only much weaker and made by Votiaks [Udmurts]. It has a strong smoky and fusel alcohol smell and tastes particularly nasty,"[11] while one of the first ethnographers and folklorists of the Udmurts, G. E. Vereshchagin, described it in almost exactly the same terms, as having "a turbid color with unpleasant fusel smell and acidic taste."[12] Taken together, these commentaries describing *kumyshka* as repulsively too sour and essentially undrinkable placed the drink outside the world of cuisine, much as Alison Smith (and Claude Lévi-Strauss) argues for fermentation.

Kumyshka held a special place in Udmurts' spiritual practices and played a symbolic role in their cosmology and creation mythology, especially before state-sponsored conversion to Christianity in the eighteenth century. Udmurts followed a complex attributive worship system of animistic and local spirits and ancestors. In ceremonies often held in local sacred forests or glades they offered agricultural goods such as bulls, cows, stallions, rams, domestic fowl, as well as kasha, cabbage soup, and eggs to the spirits. *Kumyshka* was an intrinsic symbol within every religious service. A cauldron of the drink rested beside the priest when he made his offering, and he consecrated the event by ladling it out onto a ritual coaster and poured into a depression next to a sacred tree.[13] Udmurts also drank the

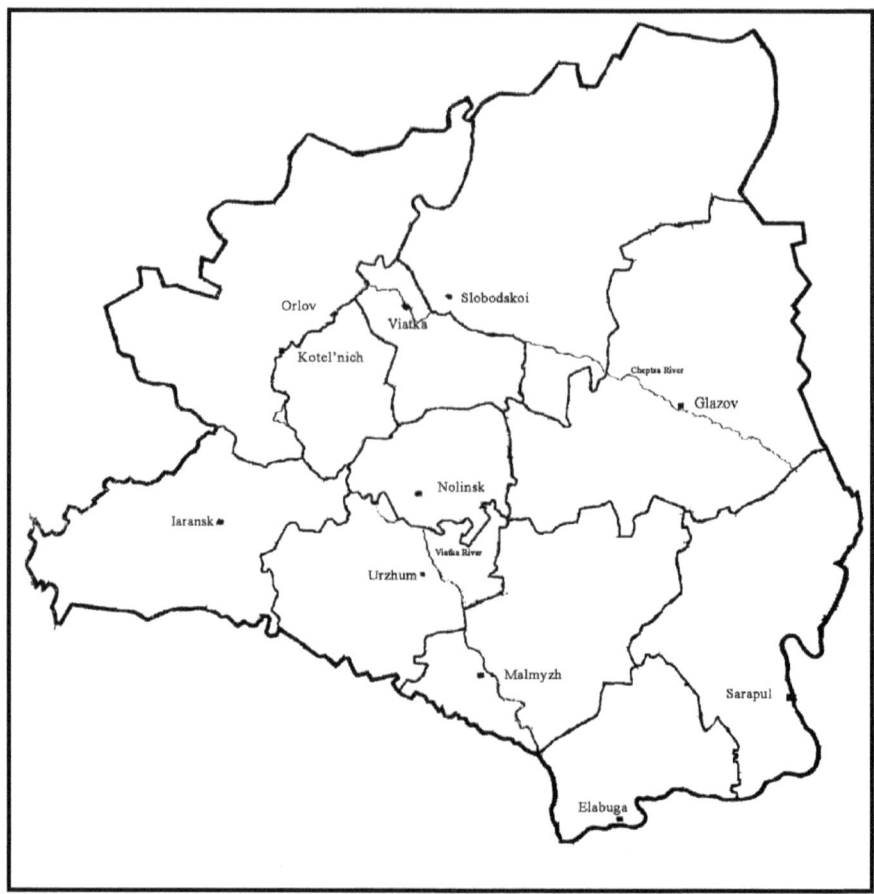

MAP 7.1 *Map of Viatka Province in 1914.*

beverage to mark life cycle events like the birth of a child or a marriage, and *kumyshka* was poured over the deceased during the burial ceremony.[14]

Kumyshka and Udmurt "primitivism" in the pre-war era

Kumyshka became a contested sign in the nineteenth century wrapped up in several overlapping trends of a modernizing nation. The beverage and its effects touched on the governance of a multi-confessional land, growing state control over taxation, the mobilization of ethnography and science in understanding and categorizing peoples of the Russian nation, and fears that cultural backwardness would undermine these modernizing efforts.

The state and outside commentators largely ignored *kumyshka* until the mid-nineteenth century. In 1803, Tsar Alexander I issued a decree (*ukaz*) that upheld the right of Udmurts to brew it for domestic purposes, but prohibited them from selling it so as not to undermine liquor tax farmers. At the same time, Minister of the Interior Viktor P. Kuchebei reminded the governor of Viatka to protect Udmurts from the selfishness and corruption of tax farmers.[15] By the 1830s, though, local enforcement restricted Udmurts from making *kumyshka* stronger than vodka, ostensibly to stop them from selling it and undercutting the liquor market. Church officials and local clergymen supported restrictions of the drink as a spiritual barrier to baptized Udmurts' full conversion to Russian Orthodoxy. As a commodity and a pagan spiritual vessel, *kumyshka* became politicized.

Most Udmurts lived in the area of contested conversions of the Volga-Kama Region.[16] Church officials in the region struggled to convert remaining animist Udmurts to Orthodoxy, to integrate Christian beliefs into Udmurt lifestyles, and especially to prevent spiritual backsliding of the newly baptized. Udmurts continued to make *kumyshka* and use it in spiritual practices. In one case, baptized Udmurts petitioned the state and insisted that they be labeled as so-called new converts "in order not be deprived of the right they have received to brew *kumyshka* for domestic use."[17] Regulating *kumyshka* was one means of controlling spiritual practices. Church officials saw Udmurts who drank the liquor during Christian holidays, especially to excess, as immoral.[18] It also represented an alternative path to achieve a spiritual sensation than sacraments sanctioned by the Church. Church officials worried about the competing spiritual use from *kumyshka*. Tax farmers worried about it as a commodity—as a competitive intoxicant. Yet at the end of the nineteenth century, only 2 percent of Udmurts remained "pagan," that is, neither baptized to Orthodoxy nor Muslim. Many Udmurts practiced some form of syncretism of animism and Orthodox Christianity and brewed *kumyshka*. Some of them also sold it to fellow villagers and Russian and other national minorities nearby. Local merchants who owned the provincial liquor license and concessionaires who sold alcohol put pressure on the state to regulate or ban *kumyshka* because it undercut the liquor market.[19] The government vacillated between prohibiting and tightly regulating brewing until finally, on April 24, 1890, it permanently repealed the Udmurts' right to make *kumyshka*, confiscated stockpiles of the drink, and imposed fines for violations of the law.[20]

As the Church, local state officials, and businessmen expressed concerns about the beverage, local ethnographers and members of the Russian Geographical Society's Ethnographic Division studied Udmurts and their rituals and lifestyles and had much to say about *kumyshka*'s role in non-Russians' cultural level and how it affected the Russian empire and Russian nation.[21] These ethnographers extended and built off previous learned elites' judgment of perceived primitive cultural rituals and tastes of everyday people described by Alison Smith and Matthew Romaniello in

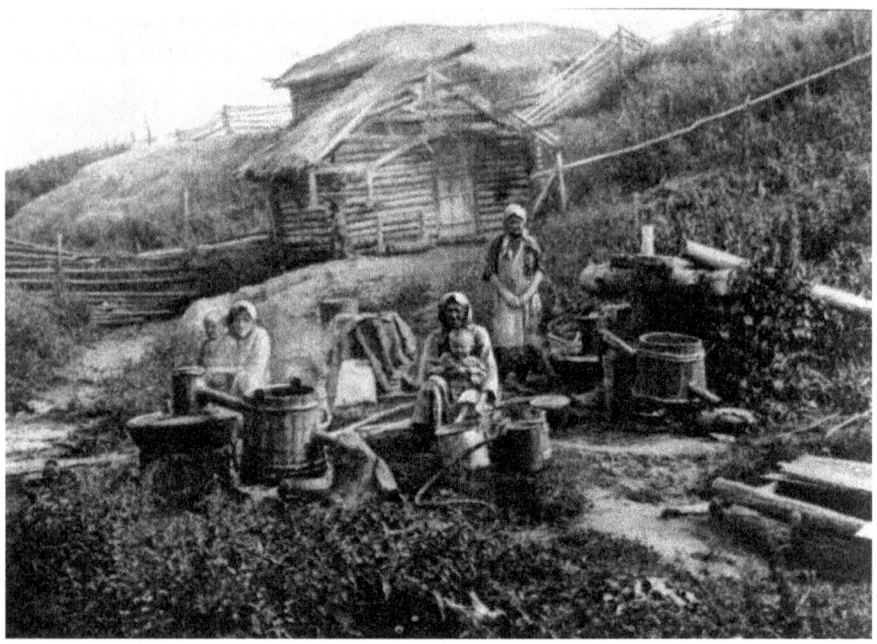

FIGURE 7.2 *"Women and children brewing kumyska," c. 1900. From V. V. Tuganaev, ed.,* Udmurtskaia Respublika entsiklopediia *(Izhevsk: Izdatel'stvo "Udmurtiia," 2000), 43.*

this volume. Nobody did more to express the sensation of consuming the libation than ethnographers of the nineteenth century. Ethnographers acted as food critics or samplers of *kumyshka*—describing and explaining the taste and role of the drink to the state and public.[22] Researchers included the young Alexander Herzen who during his exile to Viatka province penned amateur ethnographic accounts of Udmurts and Maris lamenting their physical inabilities and lack of hygiene or assimilation into the Russian way of life.[23] Later local ethnographers and publications from the capital provided detailed studies of the culture of Udmurts and other non-Russian people of the Volga-Kama region. The Udmurts that emerged in their depictions had hardly been touched by the modernizing world or even Christian missionaries. These were hardly the detached, neutral, ethnographic portrayals of non-Russians of the 1840s and 1850s described by historian Nathaniel Knight.[24] Regional ethnographers in the late nineteenth century characterized Udmurts as meek, unenlightened pagans who lagged behind other local nationalities in culture, physical stamina—in one case referring to them as mice—and sense of hygiene. Studies of Udmurts did paint detailed pictures of national characteristics but, as seen in their colorful description of *kumyshka*, they were also value-laden and linked to larger cultural fears of peasant backwardness and immorality.[25]

Many ethnographers denied the sacred element of *kumyshka*, replacing sanctity with irrational emotions. Its position as a religious icon in Udmurt spirituality is almost wholly absent in ethnographic studies of the time. Instead ethnographers focused on production, look, taste, and Udmurts' emotional attachment to the drink. As a publication at the turn of the twentieth century described it, Udmurts' "love of pleasure is seen in particular in their inexplicable attachment to their *kumyshka*." Many others went out of their way to mention how much Udmurts loved "their *kumyshka*," underscoring that it was a central component to Udmurt culture and that they were addicted to this alcoholic drink.[26] These writings reflected a hierarchy of senses, in which Udmurts could not feel the privileged spiritual sensation but were expected to hunger for more primitive sensations like irrational love.[27] While ethnographic descriptions of non-Russians as primitives did not necessarily have pejorative connotations (in Central Asia, the governor-general Konstantin Petrovich von Kaufman saw Kyrgyz primitivism as a bulwark against an encroaching Islam), ethnographers in the Volga-Kama region certainly portrayed primitivism in negative hues.[28]

In the mid-1890s, Udmurt culture itself stood trial in a case that gripped the national media. Seven Udmurts in southern Viatka were falsely convicted of killing a local peasant and using him in human sacrifice in what would be called the Multan Case. It took three retrials, the intervention of the famous writer Vladimir Korolenko, and a public campaign to bring the Udmurt peasants their eventual acquittal. During the trial, as Robert Geraci has shown, the prosecution relied on ethnographic expertise to show that Udmurts continued to engage in primitive rituals.[29]

By the late nineteenth century, ethnographic descriptions of *kumyshka* increasingly focused on its effects on health and the local medical community hailed the ban of what it saw as a disabling and lethal brew.[30] Criticism from ethnographers continued to focus on the troubling national character of Udmurts as dirty and unhygienic. As one report put it, "*Kumyshka* is brewed through brass tubes which, because of Votiaks' slovenliness, are covered with mud and grass. This is why, in addition to its infamously repugnant taste, it is dangerous to one's health."[31] The Viatka Medical Inspector Sprenzhin, however, shifted the focus from the lacking character of Udmurts to the dangers of brewing. In a detailed chemical analysis of the brewing process, Sprenzhin found that *kumyshka* was essentially just like vodka or beer and, if brewed correctly, could be a high quality alcoholic drink. He sampled three types of the concoction and described the drink in almost the polar opposite of Dal' and ethnographers of the time. He found his *kumyshka* samples to look "milky white," "yellowish," and "clear." Dal' and others described it as looking dark and turgid. Sprenzhin smelled *kumyshka* as "strongly sour" and "burnt." If ethnographers found the drink overpowered the senses—as poisonous and nasty—Sprenzhin's chemical appraisal saw it as just another alcoholic drink. Indeed, even *kumyshka's* potency was contested. Sprenzhin found *kumyshka* to range from 5.71 percent to 6.14 percent alcohol (about the same as porter), significantly lower than the 10 to 20 percent suggested by ethnographers of the time.

Sprenzhin still found *kumyshka* to be harmful because of its impurities such as verdigris from the copper piping, something that ethnographers had seen as stemming from Udmurts' natural propensity toward filth. Sprenzhin contended that verdigris, along with other impurities, damaged hemoglobin, which made it harder for women to bear children. He concluded that even Udmurts came to agree that vodka was healthier and that they "regretted the good old days when they were completely free to make *kumyshka* without any regulations."[32] The conclusion that the decidedly more potent, pure, Russian, state-regulated vodka, was better for Udmurts' health than *kumyshka* is striking, repeating a colonial trope of unhealthy native drinks in favor of healthier, sanitary colonial ones. Sprenzhin ignores Udmurt drinking practices—including allowing women to make and drink *kumyshka*—and focuses instead on undermining the brewing process. The drink was not the problem, but Udmurts' primitivism and distance from state regulations that upheld healthy practices. By regulating Udmurt customary practice, the non-Russian group would not only become healthier and larger with more women being able to bring babies to term but also closer to the dominant, Russian power.

Kumyshka was also tied into educated society and intellectuals' concerns of Russia's peasantry as an isolated and culturally backward people. Fearing social breakdown from a period of rapid industrial modernization, commentators created a rural other that expressed their societal and cultural dreams and anxieties. They saw an idyllic, autarkic village increasingly corrupted by the dangers of a modern world—endemic crime, disease, poverty, and most notably—drunkenness. The primitive peasants needed to be enlightened and tutored to be brought into the modern age, although there were debates if that was even possible.[33] Ethnographers at the turn of the twentieth century reported that Udmurts were slaves to their drink, just as social critics complained that Russian peasants were abusing alcohol. The state had prohibited *kumyshka*, but ethnographic and state reports continued to lament how much drink continued to destroy rural life, undermining social control and customs.[34]

For their part, many Udmurts sharply resisted the restrictions on *kumyshka*, even murdering officials searching for the liquor in Sarapul and Elabuga districts.[35] Udmurt resistance also shows that they equated *kumyshka* with their identity. In 1905, Udmurts in Uzinskaia and Multanskaia townships, Malmyzh district, petitioned the central government to repeal the ban on the grounds of historical rights. They argued that before 1890, Udmurts had always made the beverage and the ban represented a change in their ethnic lifestyle. They also demanded equitable treatment with other non-Russian peoples, citing the recent state acquiescence to Siberian peoples to make their national drink *araka* (an anise-flavored alcoholic beverage).³⁶ The government rejected the petition the following year. In one telling court case, an Udmurt brought up on charges of making *kumyshka* articulated his resistance in terms of religious faith and argued that as an Udmurt he needed the alcohol in order to pray.³⁷ On the eve of war and revolution, despite Church and state efforts, many Udmurts continued to practice their beliefs. Several clergy reports from villages across Udmurt settlements in southern Viatka complained in June 1913 that local Udmurts continued their "pagan" rituals and customs, including brewing and drinking "unhealthy *kumyshka*" and sacrificing livestock to connect to their spirits.³⁸

For state and Church officials, *kumyshka* remained a sign of Udmurts' persistent paganism, cultural and economic insularity, and unhealthy lifestyle. For Udmurts, it was a sign of their cultural heritage. These tensions of empire show the non-Russians straining to maintain a coherent system of spiritual and cultural beliefs in a homogenizing system pushing a uniform nationality. *Kumyshka* went beyond Udmurt-state dynamics during war and revolution, however, when the general prohibition of alcohol combined with larger economic, social, and political pressures, it moved the beverage into a larger discussion of the place of Udmurts in the Russian nation and the state of peasant culture as a whole.

The First World War and the Udmurt corruption

With the First World War, *kumyshka* became a sign that peasants' cultural weaknesses threatened Russia's security in military conflict. During the mobilization for the war in July 1914, Tsar Nicholas II approved a prohibition on the sale of alcohol. Despite reformers' initial hopes that Russia would rid itself of the demon of alcohol and keep its soldiers and peasants sober and ready for war, peasants quickly responded to the prohibition by developing stills or marketing drinks, like *kumyshka*, that they made in the forests or courtyards.³⁹ For public officials and commentators in Russia's Volga-Kama Region, the persistence of alcoholic consumption was cause for concern not only as a potential barrier to the country's victory in the war but also to peasants' (and Russia's) cultural advancement.

In 1915–16, the Duma pushed through a bill to make prohibition permanent. Duma members' efforts enjoyed wide support among the intelligentsia. Representatives of the First Congress of Cooperativists in Viatka passed a resolution that they sent to the tsar himself commending the temporary prohibition and urging him to make it permanent. "For the health of the body and soul of Russia," they demanded that the government step up its efforts to get rid of "alcoholic surrogates" like *kumyshka*.⁴⁰

Ethnographers, state personnel, and clergy had commented on *kumyshka*'s unhealthy role in Udmurt life before the First World War, but the drink took on new strength in popular imagination when Russians feared its detrimental effects on all of society during the war. The discourse on *kumyshka* had followed a rational course with accompanying enlightenment traditions and a modernizing goal. Ritual practice was described in medical language in the late imperial period. The sterilized conversations continued in the First World War.

Reporting to Petrograd on the situation in Viatka during the first month of the war (and prohibition), the governor's office devoted half of its account to the problem of containing *kumyshka*. The report touched on several central cultural constructions of Udmurts as both romantic primitives and backward peoples.[41] The governor's office account drew upon late imperial era ethnographic depictions of Udmurts, calling them "very timid and sober." Drinking *kumyshka*, however, destroyed their calm, childlike nature and reverted them to a violent, untamed people. "Upon imbibing in *kumyshka*," the Governor's office wrote, Udmurts "turned into wild people" and "savages."[42] Local government newspapers during the war also underlined the pernicious effect of *kumyshka* in articles, although they emphasized that it was the hold on alcohol, rather than national character that brought down Udmurts. A typical article stated that Udmurts, "were unable to give up" the drink, wasting "grain, wood, and time" and leading to "many arguments and fights" while drunk.[43] The rise of the illegal liquor trade became a means for the popular press to discuss drawbacks in the government's grain monopoly. It was also a way to admonish peasants for not sacrificing enough grain, while displacing criticism to a marginal group.

Udmurts continued to resist state attempts to prevent the preparation of the beverage. Beyond diverting grain for the sale of the drink, Udmurts overtly protested state laws. In January 1915, policemen arrived in the Udmurt village of Kyrlyt to search for contraband liquor. Their search of huts and storehouses turned up nothing, but a group of seventy armed Udmurts met them on the street. Someone shot and wounded the officer and another peasant struck the village policeman in the head with a shaft. The police wisely fled the village. District police later brought twelve peasants before a military court where they continued to express bitterness toward the police for conducting searches.[44]

Despite the government's fears of the dangers of *kumyshka*, it was in fact its ban that brought a new era of popularity as Russian peasants began to seek it out. *Kumyshka* quickly took on new meaning, moving from ritual drink to popular commodity. In 1913, the Viatka Finance Ministry reported only nineteen cases of the sale of *kumyshka*. In 1914, that number escalated to 184 and in 1915 reached 638 cases.[45] Udmurts had the advantage over their Russian neighbors of already having stills and an established recipe for making moonshine. Certainly, peddling in *kumyshka* was more profitable than selling grain at fixed prices, especially with the growing disparity between prices of agricultural and manufactured goods.[46] In February 1917, the newspaper *Kama* reported that for 36.11 pounds (a *pud*) of flour that Udmurts could sell to the state for two rubles, they could make fifteen bottles of *kumyshka* that sold for three rubles each. After labor and materials, producers made thirty-nine rubles profit.[47] Soldiers, who had already demanded alcohol in riots in August 1914, in particular sought out the beverage. For example, in Vikharovskaia township, Malmyzh district, four soldiers arrived at the home of the village elder in Staryi Kaks and demanded that he stop enforcing the ban on *kumyshka*. They attacked him and the village constable, stole confiscated moonshine and brewing equipment, and yelled, "As it was before, and it will always be, *kumyshka* will be brewed."[48]

Even as Udmurts resisted state pressures against *kumyshka* production, the changing nature of the liquor engendered Udmurt society itself to change. While a very small number of men made the drink for sale before the war, Udmurts still identified *kumyshka* as a cultural icon. During war and revolution, the drink became much more of a central commodity, thereby undercutting the religious symbolism of it. Moreover, *kumyshka* production before the war was also distinctly gendered female as Udmurt women were the ones who traditionally made it four times a year to mark the changing seasons.[49] During wartime, the gender roles changed. Wartime population and economic pressures pushed peasant women to have a larger part in village politics, agriculture, and household economics. As *kumyshka* moved solidly from ritual drink to commercial commodity, however, significantly more men than women appeared in court and administrative reports for brewing and selling it. Newspapers also emphasized that the whole Udmurt household had become involved in making the drink. Government reports during war and revolution paint a uniform picture of men establishing production lines in the back of their hut or in the forest to produce a large quantity of the drink for marketing.[50]

Popular discourse on the destabilizing effects of brewing reached its peak during the period of the Provisional Government following the February 1917 Revolution that overthrew the tsar. New Liberal Constitutional Democratic, local administrative, and Socialist revolutionary newspapers all used *kumyshka* as a sign of the benighted Udmurt nation. *Kumyshka* (as a stand-in for Udmurts) became an enemy of freedom. As the newspaper *Word and Life* reported in March 1917, local "Udmurts interpreted freedom for their own benefit and began a massive brewing of *kumyshka*. Extreme and strict measures must be taken to stop this secret wine brewing."[51] *The Peasant Gazette*, a local administrative newspaper, also described Udmurts as misinterpreting political freedom, writing that, "The brewing of *kumyshka* is an invention of Udmurts, so they are smitten by their skill. The Udmurt says, 'while there is freedom we need to make [*kumyshka*] because there may one day be new laws published and then we will willy-nilly have to give up *kumyshka*.'" The newspaper editorialized, however, that, "The Udmurt loves money a lot and so will obtain it through the easiest method—brewing *kumyshka*. Cooking *kumyshka* does not take much labor and is easy, but is at the same time lucrative."[52] References to Udmurt greed, profiteering, and swindling Russians in a society that was recently gripped by a trial of Udmurt human sacrifice may bring to mind anti-Semitic slurs, but such portrayals of Udmurt cultural failings such as selfishness, greed, and miscomprehension of the political arena, reflect both educated Russia's unease with peasants actively participating in Russia's politics, and popular cultural portrayals of benighted peasants as a whole.[53] But discussions of *kumyshka* went beyond social, or class, tensions. "The Udmurt," the article in *The Peasant Gazette* concluded, "is still not completely enlightened and not completed developed. They see no harm in brewing *kumyshka* and no one reads to the locals about the harm of brewing *kumyshka*."[54]

Township assemblies passed resolutions against *kumyshka* as part of the larger political discourse on freedom and national renewal. The Piniuzhanskaia township provisional committee, Orlov district, Viatka province resolved on March 25, 1917, "for the good of the general welfare of citizens of free Russia, we will engage in a merciless fight against the wicked serpent *kumyshka*" by sending police to every village and electing a township police force to help fight the brewing of *kumyshka*.[55] The popular press widely praised these resolutions. *The Peasant Gazette* published a long article on a township meeting in Sarapul district, Viatka province, which agreed to a "draconian policy in which people convicted of brewing *kumyshka* or storing it will be subject to eviction from the township for the whole duration of the war." The writer noted, however, that such policies exist "only on paper" as *kumyshka* is too prevalent to control.[56]

It was bad enough that democracy was threatened by nationally backward Udmurts and their *kumyshka*, but newspaper writers editorialized that this evil trait was contagious and infecting all of rural Russia—spreading the threat beyond this small nationality. The local newspaper *Kukarsk Life* in August 1917 reported that, "now almost all the villagers of Viatka are making this "boiled mind-dulling drink" and the local intelligentsia do not have the strength to stop it."[57] An article in July stated, "the skill of Udmurts to distill *kumyshka* was adopted perfectly by our peasantry of Troitsksia and Norlianskaia townships. The method of distilling is very easy and the instruments, if you will, are found in every home."[58] The newspaper reiterated two months later that *kumyshka* had invaded Russian regions of Viatka province. "In Nolinsk district, all the population is Russian. Up to the prohibition of the sale of spirits no one made [home brews] and no one was skilled in making beer and *kumyshka*. They learned from the non-Russians living in neighboring districts."[59] The press displayed a growing impotence to stop Udmurt to Russian peasant contagion. As part of educated society's fears that anarchy was taking over Russia, newspaper articles expressed a sense of rampant *kumyshka* by the fall of 1917. In the "Anarchy Reigns" section of *The Peasant Gazette*, the newspaper reported peasants who had resolved not to punish those caught making the brew and to free the policeman from even searching for the illegal substance.⁶⁰

Obviously, local officials were also concerned with *kumyshka*'s effect—to make people drunk. Having prohibited most state-produced spirits three years earlier, *kumyshka* represented an unguarded drink antithetical to controlled alcohol. Drunkenness from *kumyshka* threatened the society and the level of popular culture like other alcoholic beverages, but it now threated the revolution itself. As a prohibited substance produced by a benighted people, drunkenness from *kumyshka* was especially pernicious. Revolutionary committees, however, used the same language as tsarist officials and ethnographers in describing *kumyshka*'s effects. As the members of the Nechinsk township committee of public safety in Sarapul' district noted in its resolution to enact strict measures to destroy the "disease" of *kumyshka* by going after the local *kumyshka* trade, the brewing of *kumyshka* was a "great evil" because "drunkenness leads to one vice after another."⁶¹

National movements emerged from hiding with the political freedom guaranteed by the Provisional Government. National minority intellectuals held several congresses to mobilize popular national sentiment. *Kumyshka* emerged as a central, contentious topic among Udmurts during the meetings. In the short congresses in southern Viatka and Kazan' through the late summer and fall of 1917, representatives comprised mostly of teachers, priests, and educated society discussed the needs of their national groups. While they spoke of political freedoms, cultural enlightenment dominated discussions—the need for schools, language training, and literature so Udmurt peasants could enter society as cultured individuals, aware of their national membership. For the national leaders, *kumyshka* was an unnecessary part of old Finno-Ugric culture. The Udmurt Section of the Congress of Small Peoples of the Volga Region in May 1917 debated the role of *kumyshka* in the revolutionary era. The leadership reiterated the language of ethnographers and state officials. The military doctor T. K. Borisov spoke of a rash of illnesses linked to drinking *kumyshka* and that Udmurts "drink it for weeks on end and during festivals that last as long as two months. The elderly and youth drink it, as do women and children. *Kumyshka* is the misfortune of our people and we need to get rid of it." He followed that Udmurts "did not have interesting books, theater or other forms of entertainment. In order to raise the cultural level of the people, then it is vital to renounce the evil that is *kumyshka*." Other scholars at the conference agreed. For Borisov and others, it was less *kumyshka*'s immediate alcoholic effects and more that it caused problem drinking—that Udmurts were unable to liberate themselves from seeking the immediate pleasure from the drink in order to find the longer-term pleasure of high, acceptable culture. Essentially, Udmurts could not free themselves from their own national cultural and religious practices, much like colonial subjects in Africa and the Americas with palm wine and moonshine or peasants from underclass desires of the flesh, and needed intervention from the state and intellectuals to do so. As I. S. Mikheev reported to fellow delegates, however, Udmurt peasants disagreed. They saw *kumyshka* as "our religious tradition," and an integral part of the sacrificial offering. They argued that when vodka was legal, it was much easier to get than *kumyshka,* which required a lot of "time, labor and risk" to make. The peasants pointed out the problem in the national leaders' argument—that it was not that Udmurts drank spirits, for before the 1914 prohibition they could easily drink vodka, but it was the religious national beverage that somehow uniquely overwhelmed their senses. For what it is worth, recent anthropological studies have shown that community ritual drinking actually brings drinking under control, supporting the peasants' argument.[62] At the 1917 congress, though, the national elite's views won out and they pushed through resolutions against the brewing and consumption of *kumyshka*.[63] They wanted to rid their newly defined national culture of such poison, which fit well into ethnographic studies and the Soviet state that was about to be born.[64]

Kumyshka as class enemy during the civil war

The official struggle against *kumyshka* continued in the Soviet period. In May 1918, the Soviet government nationalized the liquor industry and in December 1919, formally extended the dry laws (although allowing the production of grape wine up to 12 percent).[65] Regional political reports placed strong emphasis on the prevalence of *kumyshka* and the Bolsheviks continued to prosecute those drinking and brewing it.[66] From May to November 1918 in Glazov district (Viatka province) alone, Soviet officials fined 100 people found guilty of brewing or drinking *kumyshka* and put forty of them in jail, while 25 percent of cases heard before the Slobodskoi district Revolutionary Tribunal in fall 1918 involved *kumyshka*.[67]

Definitions and the language surrounding *kumyshka* shifted to match Soviet class perspectives. The Soviet state defined brewers of *kumyshka* as class enemies and ascribed to them the same characteristics as speculators and kulaks, the enemies of the new regime. The state's main concern, though, was *kumyshka*'s drain on grain reserves. It had grounds for its claims. Officials estimated that moonshiners used up nearly 2.35 million pounds (65,000 *puds*) of grain in Elabuga district alone in 1918 and even more in Sarapul' district.[68] In Spring 1918, the First Congress of the Soviets of Peasant Deputies of Viatka district equated those who sell *kumyshka* with grain speculators and businessmen in levying a one-time tax on the well-to-do.[69] When Moscow sent expeditionary forces to Viakta to requisition grain in late summer 1918, soldiers fought against *kumyshka*. In one village, the expeditionary brigade arrested the Soviet head of the village for permitting the brewing of *kumyshka* and confiscated eleven stills and 10,111 pounds (280 *puds*) of grain.[70] In October 1918, during one of the most dire grain crises in Viatka, a member of the All Russian military provisions commission reported from Iaransk district that there was enough grain to feed the population. Speculation hurt the grain supply, but "one of the greatest misfortunes is the brewing of *kumyshka*," which undermined grain requisitions.[71] Instructions for grain requisition brigades in 1919 in the district contained a special multi-tiered clause for punitive measures against peasants found diverting grain for *kumyshka*, calling for the confiscation of all the citizen's grain if the home contained a still. If the peasant made *kumyshka* from his own grain the home would be put on a 10.83 pound (12-*funt*) ration, but if the peasant was found to have made *kumyshka* from distributed grain, then the home would be put on a 5.2 pound (six-*funt*) ration.[72]

In state proclamations and court records, Bolsheviks placed the struggle against *kumyshka* as part of class warfare and the struggle for cultural enlightenment, to create a new Soviet Udmurt.[73] For example, a communist agitator's report portrayed the liquor as a product of rich Udmurt peasants (*kulaks*). In late 1918, G. Prakhov traveled to the mostly Udmurt villages of Belzinskaia township, Glazov district to form so-called committees of poor peasants. While successful in forming two committees, things fell afoul when he discovered *kumyshka*. In a search of homes, he found four bottles of *kumyshka* and labeled the household kulaks. According to the report, the next day poor peasants from the neighboring village ran out to greet him and led him to the kulak homes, which all stored *kumyshka*. The Communist agitator portrayed the liquor as anti-Soviet and as an instrument of kulaks.[74] While possible that peasants with larger grain reserves were more likely to convert excess grain into profitable *kumyshka*, historian Helena Stone has argued that the village poor were in fact more prone to selling moonshine as a means to make ends meet.[75] The Revolutionary Tribunal case in May 1919 against Andrei Berestev for making *kumyshka* is also notable. According to court transcripts, Berestev's daughter stated that he had used the last flour to make a batch of *kumyshka* while his children starved. Berestev had been arrested twice before, was known as a drunk, and had tried to engage in incest with his daughter. The court ruled that this was "an intolerable way of life among free citizens of the Soviet Republic."[76]

The Soviet state tried to balance attacking a central Udmurt cultural sign and winning the Udmurt population's favor. Therefore a 1920 Party-sponsored conference for women in the Udmurt autonomous oblast' came out against *kumyshka* by blaming tsarist oppression for its persistence:

> Udmurt women understand well their suffering under the tsarist regime's Township administrations, prisons, and courts for making *kumyshka*. Tsarist officials got rich, as robber barons, and like beasts they hunted down women for making *kumyshka*. At the same time, they did not

completely prohibit the brewing of *kumyshka* and so Udmurts were killed by *kumyshka*.⁷⁷

Party officials denied Udmurt women ethnic consciousness by transferring agency from women to tsarist officials, who used them for collection of fines and denied them educational access and knowledge of the physical harm of *kumyshka*. In this way, the Party tried to mold the liquor into a gendered-female form of tsarist economic and national exploitation in which Udmurt women became passive observers to their own rituals.

While the Party and state defamed the drink in the courts and press, representatives from the Soviet People's Commissariat of Nationalities, a state division that promoted national minority culture, staged spectacles, plays, and speeches in the Udmurt language to fight it and foster "enlightened" Udmurt culture. Such attempts could backfire. In Buranskaia township in February 1920, People's Commissariat of Nationalities officials gathered a meeting of around sixty Udmurts to answer questions about the Soviet state. At the end of the gathering the chairman proposed a resolution welcoming the Red Army and Soviet power and standing against *kumyshka*. When the resolution went up for a vote, no one would participate or even speak. Finally, one peasant stated, "You must get rid of the wording in the resolution" against *kumyshka*. A cacophony of voices erupted in favor of brewing and the agitators were forced to end the meeting abruptly. Reporting back to his superiors, the agitator blamed his failure on the Udmurts as the village was full of drunkards and lacked revolutionary spirit."⁷⁸

Some Udmurt peasants may have accepted Soviet constructions of *kumyshka* as an anti-Soviet tool of counter-revolution, but most Udmurts continued to resist elite definitions of their ritual drink. The brewing of *kumyshka* represented an ideal means to convert grain that faced requisitioning, a point the Soviet authorities understood in their classification of *kumyshka* production as resistance and economic speculation.⁷⁹ In March 1918, according to the Urzhum district government, local Udmurt peasants were so hostile toward state prosecution of the brewing of *kumyshka* that "there was almost no state power." Udmurts continued to brew it "almost openly" despite local Red Guard attempts to prevent it, including issuing fines for up to 500 rubles.⁸⁰ In February 1919, peasants in Malmyzh district attacked and killed a policeman and attacked several others who caught them drinking *kumyshka* in their hut and moved to confiscate their drinks.⁸¹ That same month, comrade Olenev, a member of the Iarslavskaia township Communist Party cell in Slobodskoi district, served *kumyshka* at a wedding. A Red Army soldier attending the gathering publicly chastised him for making *kumyshka* during such a trying moment of crisis and for disregarding state authority. Olenev became so enraged that he threw himself at the soldier and killed him.⁸²

The Soviet government allowed the sale of distilled liquor only in 1923, but continued its fight against *kumyshka* and other forms of moonshine. Some Udmurts continued to make it for its spiritual and ritualistic properties or as a commodity through the 1920s. Udmurt national culture, though, turned away from the symbol. Soviet nationality policy sought to overcome backward national traits like religion and drink and help national minorities evolve; it was an official policy of overcoming sensory "problems" similar to what Claire Shaw describes for Soviet attitudes toward the deaf community.[83] Officials of the new Udmurt SSSR adopted much of the late imperial ethnographic descriptions of Udmurt culture as backward, including religious practice and drink. The Udmurt national poet and literary father Kuzebai Gerd who did so much to describe the idyllic Udmurt in Soviet Russia did not write of animism and rarely wrote of *kumyshka*. When he did, it was to denounce it as forestalling Udmurts' national progress and keeping them away from consciousness. In the poem "It's Better to Die" (*Med kulo, Es'masa*) Gerd writes, "Udmurts! Dozing all the time, brewing *kumyshka*. Do you want to die in the forests?"[84] These types of stories condemning *kumyshka* also appeared in the Udmurt Republic newspaper *Thunder*.

Conclusion

Discussions of *kumyshka* and Udmurts as a whole in the late imperial and early Soviet eras can only be understood by examining how the drink tasted. Its sensation became an important malleable symbol for various social and political groups to debate the role of non-Russians. In the tsarist era it represented Umdurt national cultural and spiritual backwardness. Udmurts' taste for *kumyshka*, both as a ritual drink and simply as a palatable beverage, excluded them from the Russian nation. For educated Russia in 1917, it was a way to discuss Udmurt and peasant insularity, their fears of popular political participation, and a growing sense of anarchy. Soviet officials saw *kumyshka* as both an enemy of the worker-peasant state and a means to show Soviet frustration over the persistence of grain speculation. The discourse surrounding *kumyshka*, however, also had consistent themes. Ethnographers, media, and government officials portrayed Udmurts as culturally lagging behind Russians and threatening to contaminate the greater society with their primitivism. Discussions on *kumyshka* therefore both paralleled larger conversations of alcohol in the countryside and reveal the often-overlooked underlying conversations of ethnicity and imperialism during the revolutionary era.

The contrast between the positive portrayal of the Russian national drink *kvas* (and to a lesser extent even vodka) and the overwhelmingly negative image among Russian and Udmurt elite commentators of the Udmurt drink *kumyshka* shows how the malleable descriptions of drink reveal cultural tensions of empire and nationality.[85] This extended into the Soviet era. Soviet leaders fostered Udmurt nationality, but tried to extricate *kumyshka* from Udmurt national identity. It was the unhealthy sensations of *kumyshka* that were the problem—drunkenness, laziness, and spiritual transcendence. The Soviet state, like the imperial Russian state, imposed a colonial national discourse that made *kumyshka* a cultural sign of backwardness and the other—dirty, primitive, feminine, and unhealthy. It is only in the post-Soviet Udmurt Republic that national cultural leaders have rediscovered *kumyshka* as a symbol for maintaining and renewing Udmurt ethnic identity, now finally free of the discursive baggage of the late imperial and Soviet eras.[86]

Notes

1. Pierre Bourdieu, *Distinction: A Social Critique of the Judgement of Taste*, trans. Richard Nice (Cambridge, MA: Harvard University Press, 1984), 5–6.
2. See William Taylor, *Drinking, Homicide, and Rebellion in Colonial Mexican Villages* (Stanford, CA: Stanford University Press, 1979); Mónica P. Morales, *Reading Inebriation in Early Colonial Peru* (Burlington, VT: Ashgate, 2012); Emmanuel Kwaku Akyeampong, *Drink, Power and Cultural Change: A Social History of Alcohol in Ghana, c. 1800 to Recent Times* (Oxford: James Currey Publishers, 1997).
3. Mary Douglas, "A Distinctive Anthropological Perspective," in *Constructive Drinking: Perspectives on Drink from Anthropology*, ed. Mary Douglas (New York: Cambridge University Press, 1987), 8.
4. As discussed below, *kumyshka* was not the only Udmurt cultural material that observers described as a manifestation of Udmurt primitivism. They also focused on Udmurt housing and beehives. I discuss this in *Russia's Peasants in Revolution and Civil War: Citizenship, Identity, and the Creation of the Soviet State, 1914–1922* (Cambridge: Cambridge University Press, 2008), 16–18, 34–37.
5. See, for just one example, I. V. Rodionov, *Kumyshka (Ocherk')* (Viatka: Gubernskaia tipografiia, 1900), 7–8. Fusel alcohol, described today as having a hot, sharp, solvent-like, or astringent taste, in this case was probably caused by cooking the drink at a high temperature.
6. E. Ia. Trofimova, "Udmurtskaia traditsionnaia pishcha (uroven' izuchennosti i problemy dal'neishego issledovaniia," in *Voprosy etnosotsiologicheskogo izucheniia sel'skogo naseleniia. Sbornik statei* (Izhevsk: Nauchno-issledovatel'skii institut pri sovete ministrov Udmurtskoi ASSR, 1983), 107; *Kak slozhilas' narodnaia kukhnia udmurtov. Bliuda udmurtskoi kukhni* (Izhevsk: Izdatel'svo Udmurtiia, 1991); I. Mikheev, "Kumyshka. Istoriia kumyshki," in *Izvestiia obshchestva arkheologii, istorii i etnografii pri Kazanskom gosudarstvennom universiteta*, t. 34, no. 1–2 (Kazan, 1928), 154–9; V. E. Vladykin, *Religiozno-mifologicheskaia kartina mira udmurtov*

(Izhevsk: Udmurtiia, 1994), 113. See also G. E. Vereshchagin's works on everyday consumption of *kumyshka*, *Votiaki sarapul'skogo uezda viatskoi gubernii*, rev. ed. (orig. published in 1889) (Izhevsk: Rossiiskaia akademiia nauk ural'skoe otdelenie UIIIaL, 1996).

7   A. V. Chernyk and M. S. Kamenskikh, *Chuvashi v Permskom krae: Ocherki istorii i etnografii* (St. Petersburg: Mamatov, 2014), 115. Chuvash only knew of *kumyshka*. They did not make it themselves.

8   For example, L. V. Belovinskii describes it as a milk-based vodka, although he does say that it can also come from grain. *Entsiklopedicheskii slovar' rossiiskoi zhizni i istorii* (Moscow: OLMA-Press, 2003), 384. The discourse on mare's milk, or *kumys*, though, had much more positive tones. George L. Carrick, a doctor and former secretary of the St. Petersburg Physicians' Society, extolls the medical virtues of the drink, including possibly pulmonary diseases. He describes *kumys* as especially sour (like descriptions of *kumyshka*) and alcoholic, but these tastes are followed by cool sensations felt across the body and the mild alcohol stimulates healthy blood flow. *Koumiss or Fermented Mare's Milk* (Edinburgh: William Blackwood and Sons, 1882), esp. 93–127. See Alison Smith's chapter in this volume for more on the debates over fermentation.

9   For discussion on Russian and Soviet national identity and taste, see Alison Smith's and Anton Mastervoy's chapters in this volume.

10 V. Dal', *Tolkovyi slovar' zhivogo velikorusskago iazyka*, t. 2 (St. Petersburg: Izdatel'stvo tipografiia M. O. Vol'fa, 1881), 182.

11 *Narody Rossii: Etnograficheskie ocherki*, t. I (St. Petersburg: Tipografiia Tovarishchestva 'Obshchestvennaia Pol'za, 1878), 289.

12 G. E. Vereshchagin, *Votiaki Sosnovskago kraiia Zapiski Imperatorskago Russkago Geograficheskago Obshchestva*, Tom XIV, no. 2 (St. Petersburg: Tipografiia Ministerstva Vnutrennykh Del', 1886), 15. Vereshchagin was a clergyman and produced work for the Russian Geographical Society, discussed below.

13 N. I. Shutova, *Dokhristianskie kul'tovye pamiatniki v Udmurtskoi religioznoi traditsii* (Izhevsk: Udmurtskii institute istorii, iazyka i literatury URO RAN, 2001), esp. 266.

14 Vladykin, *Religiozno-mifologicheskaia kartina mira*, 212–13.

15 P. N. Luppov, comp. and ed., *Materialy dlia istorii khristianstva u votiakov v pervoi polovine XIX veka* (Viatka: Gubernskaia tipografiia, 1911), 1–2, 24. Also found in *Vesna narodov: Etnopoliticheskaia istoriia Volgo-Ural'skogo regiona: Sbornik dokumentov*, ed. K. Matsuzatvo (Hokkaido: Slavic Research Center, Hokkaido University, 2002), 154–5.

16 For more on official attempts to convert Udmurts to Russian Orthodox Christianity in the nineteenth century, and popular reaction and resistance to these attempts, see Paul W. Werth, *At the Margins of Orthodoxy: Mission, Governance, and Confessional Politics in Russia's Volga-Kama Region, 1827–1905* (Ithaca, NY: Cornell University Press, 2002); on the Volga-Kama region as a space of multiple contested confessions, see Agnès Nilüfer Kefeli,

Becoming Muslim in Imperial Russia: Conversion, Apostasy, and Literacy (Ithaca, NY: Cornell University Press, 2014).

17 Cited in Paul Werth, "Changing Conceptions of Difference, Assimilation, and Faith in the Volga-Kama Region, 1740–1870," in *Russian Empire: Space, People, Power, 1700–1930*, ed. Jane Burbank et al. (Bloomington: Indiana University Press, 2007), 172.

18 See Werth, *At the Margins*, 97.

19 Mikheev, "Kumyshka," 146. Boris M. Segal, *Russian Drinking: Use and Abuse of Alcohol in Pre-Revolutionary Russia* (New Brunswick, NJ: Rutgers Center of Alcohol Studies, 1987), 115.

20 Decree 6740. *Polnoe sobranie zakonov Rossiiskoi Imperii*, t. 10 (1890) (St. Petersburg, 1881–1913), 307–8; Mikheev, "Kumyshka," 149; G. A. Nikitina, "Rol' galliutsinogenov (kumyshki) v bytu udmurtov (2o-e-nachalo 30-kh godov XX v.)," G. K. Shkliaev, ed., *Ob etnicheskoi psikhologii udmurtov: Sbornik statei* (Izhevsk: NISO URO RAN, 1998), 50–2. I have found no evidence that the temperance movement, which was in its infancy in 1890, pressured the government in this decision.

21 The Russian Geographical Society was established in 1845 to study the Russia Empire's peoples, lands, animals, and places through ethnography, geography, statistics, and the social sciences. See Nathaniel Knight, "Science, Empire, and Nationality: Ethnography in the Russian Geographical Society, 1845–1855," in *Imperial Russia: New Histories for the Empire*, ed. Jane Burbank and David L. Ransel (Bloomington: Indiana University Press, 1998), 108–42.

22 They also provide the vast majority of written sources on *kumyshka*, revealing a tension in finding the "true" sensation of *kumyshka*. See Priscilla Parkhurst Ferguson, "The Sense of Taste," *American Historical Review* 116 (2) (2011): 372.

23 Aleksander Gertsen, *Sobranie sochinenii v tridtsati tomakh*, t. 1 (Moscow: Izdatel'stvo akedemii nauk SSSR, 1954), 371.

24 Knight, "Science, Empire, and Nationality."

25 D. K. Zelenin, *Kama i Viatka: Putevoditel i etnograficheskoe opisanie prikamskago kraiia* (Viatka: Tipografiia Ed. Bergmana, 1904), 74–5. Zelenin repeats the ethnographer N. Blinov's views of the Udmurts.

26 N. Dobrotvirskii, "Permiaki—Bytovoi i etnograficheskii ocherk" *Vestnik Evropy* 18 (3) (March 1883), 250. The chapter discusses Perimaks, but mentions this as a sidenote about Udmurts.

27 Alain Corbin "Cultural History of the Senses," in *Empire of the Senses*, ed. David Howes (Oxford: Berg, 2005), 136–7.

28 Daniel Brower, *Turkestan and the Fate of the Russian Empire* (New York: Routledge, 2003), 42–4.

29 The Multan Case gripped Russia's public imagination at the turn of the twentieth century and continues to enjoy great scholarly interest. The Multan Case has become a cornerstone in shaping the Udmurt national heritage. See Robert P. Geraci, *Window on the East: National and Imperial Identities in Late Tsarist Russia* (Ithaca, NY: Cornell University Press, 2001), Chapter

6; G. V. Korolenko, ed., *Delo multanskikh votiakov, obviniavshikhsia v prinesenii chelovecheskoi zhertvy iazycheskim bogam* (Moscow: Tipografiia russkie vedomosti, 1896); L. S. Shatenshtein, *Multanskoe delo 1892–1896 gg.* (Izhevsk: Udmurtskoe knizhnoe izdatel'stvo, 1960).

30 Seen clearly in V. D. Orlov, "Kumyshka—vodka votiakov," *Vestnik obshchestvennoi gigieny, sudebnoi i prakticheskoi meditsiny*, t. 9, book 2 (1891): 79–93.

31 *Narodyi Rossii*, 289.

32 Sprenzhin's findings originally appeared in *Vestnik obshchestvennoi gigieny, sudebnoi i prakticheskoi meditsiny* and are reproduced in I. V. Rodionov, *Kumyshka (Ocherk)*, 3–7. Quote on 6–7.

33 See for example, Stephen Frank, *Crime, Cultural Conflict and Justice in Rural Russia, 1856–1914* (Berkeley: University of California Press, 1999); Yanni Kotsonis, *Making Peasants Backward: Agricultural Cooperatives and the Agrarian Question in Russia, 1861–1914* (New York: Palgrave Macmillan, 1999).

34 Kate Transchel, *Under the Influence: Working-Class Drinking, Temperance, and Cultural Revolution in Russia, 1895–1932* (Pittsburgh, PA: Pittsburgh University Press, 2006), 39–66.

35 Mikheev, "Kumyshka," 150.

36 Ibid., 151.

37 Ibid., 150–1. Criminal violations of laws regulating *kuymshka* were so common that the state produced a mimeographed document and officials filled in the type of brewing apparatus and name of the instigator. Tsentral'nyi Gosudarstvennyi Arkhiv Udmurtskoi Respubliki (hereafter TsGA UR), f. 94, op. 1, d. 988, ll. 2–2ob, 5, 7–8ob; Gosudarstvennyi Arkhiv Kirovskoi Oblasti (hereafter GAKO), f. 584, op. 5, d. 506, ll. 1–2, d. 556, ll. 1–2, d. 450, ll. 1–3ob.

38 Reports of clergymen of churches in Malmyzh and Sarapul' districts, Viatka province. June 1913. In *Vesna narodov: Etnopoliticheskaia istoriia Volgo-Ural'skogo regiona: Sbornik dokumentov*, ed. K. Matsuzatvo (Hokkaido: Slavic Research Center, Hokkaido University, 2002), 176–8.

39 David Christian, "Prohibition in Russia, 1914–1925," *Australian Slavonic and East European Studies* 9 (2) (1995): 89–118; Patricia Herlihy, *Alcoholic Empire: Vodka and Politics in Late Imperial Russia* (New York: Oxford University Press, 2002).

40 *Pervyi kooperativnyi s'ezd v g. Viatke, 5–12 maiia 1915 g.* (Viatka: Kassa melkago kredita Viatskago gubernskago zemstva, 1915), 22–3.

41 On parallel Russian portrayals of northern peoples see Yuri Slezkine, *Arctic Mirrors: Russia and the Small Peoples of the North* (Ithaca, NY: Cornell University Press, 1994).

42 Rossiiskii Gosudarstvennyi Istoricheskii Arkhiv (hereafter RGIA), f. 1284, op. 194, d. 13. This repeats colonial descriptions of the fallibility of colonized peoples in which their inability to stop the urge to drink transformed them from tranquil benighted people into violent savages. See Taylor, *Drinking,*

Homicide, and Rebellion, 41–5. It also extends criticisms of drinking habits of Russia's peasants.
43 *Krest'ianskaia sel'sko-khoziaistvennaia gazeta*, September 20, 1914, 10–1.
44 *Viatskaia rech'*, "V voennom sude," November 25, 1915, 3.
45 GAKO, f. R-876, op. 2, d. 78, ll. 44–5.
46 Helena Stone makes this argument for moonshine production during the scissors crises in the 1920s, "The Soviet Government and Moonshine, 1917–1929," *Cahiers du Monde russe et soviétique* 27: 3–4 (1986): 374. See also Robert E. Jones, *Bread Upon the Waters: The St. Petersburg Grain Trade and the Russian Economy, 1703–1811* (Pittsburgh, PA: Pittsburgh University Press, 2013) who refers to this pattern in the Imperial period.
47 *Kama*, February 17, 1917. On liquor riots in Viatka province, see Retish, *Peasants and Revolutionary Power*, Chapter 2.
48 GAKO, f. 582, op. 194, d. 3, ll. 2–2ob.
49 RGIA, f. 1284, op. 194, d. 13, l. 3ob. Orlov, "Kumyshka," 85.
50 GAKO, f. R-1322, op. 1a, d. 10, ll. 1–3ob.
51 *Slovo i zhizn'*, March 21, 1917. For the larger context of this debate, see Retish, *Russia's Peasants in Revolution and Civil War*, esp. 103–5.
52 *Krest'ianskaia gazeta*, May 26, 1917, 13.
53 Geraci also remarks that blood libel cases against Jews probably influenced the Multan Case, but does not see any direct connection in the press or academic writings linking Jews and Udmurts. *Window on the East*, 194–5. On zemstvo and intelligentsia misapprehension with peasant political participation see Retish, *Russia's Peasants*, Chapter 3. On educated Russia's negative portrayals of peasants, see Cathy Frierson, *Peasant Icons: Representations of Rural Russia in Late 19th Century Russia* (New York: Oxford University Press, 1993).
54 *Krest'ianskaia gazeta*, May 26, 1917, 13.
55 GAKO, f. 582, op. 194, d. 3, l. 34.
56 *Krest'iansksia gazeta*, May 26, 1917, 9. For reports of other *volost'* resolutions against *kumyshka* see April 18, 1917, 11–2; April 21, 1917, 16; May 2, 1917, 17; *Elabuzhskaia malen'kaia narodnaia gazeta*, "Dlia krest'ian Elabuzhskago uezda," May 30, 1917, 2; and *Narodnoe delo*, "Iz zhizni sovetov krest'ianskikh deputatov postanovlenie," October 15, 1917, 4, on the Third Congress of Viatka Provisional Soviet of Peasant Deputies resolution calling for the end to the brewing of *kumyshka* and other alcoholic drinks.
57 *Kukarskaia zhizn'*, August 27, 1917. I see such fears as akin to educated Russia's fears of urban hooliganism and rural crime in the late Imperial era. Joan Neuberger, *Hooliganism: Crime, Culture, and Power in St. Petersburg, 1900–1914* (Berkeley: University of California Press, 1993); Frank, *Crime, Cultural Conflict*.
58 *Krest'ianskaia gazeta*, July 14, 1917, 20.
59 *Krest'ianskaia gazeta*, September 5, 1917, 13.

60 *Krest'ianskaia gazeta*, November 7, 1917, 9.
61 Protocol of the Nechinsk township committee of public safety, Sarapul' district, April 4, 1917 in *Khristomatiia po istorii Udmurtii Tom 1: Dokumenty i materialy, 1136–1917*, ed. N. K. Korobeinikova (Izhevsk: Komitet po delam arkhivov pri Pravitel'stve UR, 2007), 672.
62 Douglas, "Anthropological Perspective," 6; Corbin, 136–7.
63 "Protocol of the Votiak Section of the Congress of Small Peoples of the Volga Region, Kazan', May 15–22, 1917," in *Khrestomatiia po istorii Udmurtii*, 680–1. See also "The Congress of Udmurt intelligentsia of Glazov district made a similar proclamation, June 13–14, 1917," in which delegates stated that *kumyshka* hurt Udmurts' hygiene, economy, morality, politics, and culture and urged measures to destroy the tradition of making *kumyshka* (686).
64 See N. P. Pavlov, *Samoopredelenie, avtonomiiia: Idei, realii* (Izhevsk: Udmurtiia, 2000), 24–5.
65 Christian, "Prohibition in Russia," 95–6.
66 Rossiiskii Gosudarstvennyi Voennyi Arkhiv, f. 169, op. 1, d. 114, l. 167ob; Gosudarstvennyi Arkhiv Sotsial'no-Politicheskoi Istorii Kirovskoi Oblasti (hereafter GASPI KO), f. 1, op. 1, d. 142.
67 GAKO, f. R-885, op. 1, d. 47, l. 208; f. R-1322, op. 1. d, 24, ll. 115–120ob.
68 E. I. Riabukhin, *V bor'be s kontrrevoliutsiei (Pomoshch' trudiashchikhsia Viatskoi gubernii vostochnomu frontu v 1918–1919 g.g.)* (Kirov: Kirovskoe knizhnoe izdatel'stvo, 1959), 32.
69 GAKO, f. R-879, op. 1. d. 1, l. 2.
70 N. Orlov, *Sistema prodovol'stvennykh zagotovok. K otsenke rabot zagotovitel'nykh ekpeditsii A. G. Skhlikhtera* (Tambov: Otdelenie gosizdatel'stva, 1920), 16–7.
71 Rossiiskii Gosudarstevnnyi Arkhiv Ekonomiki, f. 1943, op. 3, d. 160, l. 542; GAKO, f. R-1062, op. 1, d. 42, l. 63; f. R-3454, op. 1, d. 68, l. 10; f. R-876, op. 1, d. 79, ll. 5,119.
72 GAKO, f. R-746, op. 2, d. 123, l. 36.
73 Soviet discussions of the necessity for cultural transformation of Udmurts, and peasants as a whole, parallel what Claire Shaw describes for the deaf community.
74 GAKO, f. R-876, op. 1, d. 110, ll. 197–198ob.
75 Stone, "The Soviet Government," 368–9.
76 GAKO, f. R-1322, op. 1a, d. 634. Quotation from l. 14.
77 Rossiiskii Gosudarstvennyi Arkhiv Sotsial'no-Politicheskoi Istorii, f. 17, op. 10, d. 176, l. 8.
78 Gosudarstvennyi Arkhiv Rossiiskoi Federatsii, f. 1318, op. 5, d. 27.
79 Nikitina, "Rol' galliutsinogenov (kumyshki)," 55; Stone, "The Soviet Government," 360–1; GASPI KO, f. 1, op. 1 d. 142, l. 118.
80 GAKO, f. R-382, op. 1. d. 13, ll. 263–4.

81 GASPI KO, f. 8, op. 1, d. 45, ll. 13–13ob.
82 GASPI KO, f. 1, op. 1, d. 142, l. 118.
83 Francine Hirsch, *Empire of Nations: Ethnographic Knowledge and the Making of the Soviet Union* (Ithaca, NY: Cornell University Press, 2005), esp. 21–108.
84 From A. V. Kamitova, *Obraznyi mir Kuzebaia Gerda: Original i perevodcheskaia interpretsiia* (Izhevsk: Udmurtskii institut istorii, iazyka i literatury Ural'skogo otdeleniia Rossiiskoi akedemii nauk, 2006), 20.
85 See Alison Smith's discussion of *kvas* in this volume.
86 *Pamiatniki otechestva. Al'manakh Vserossiiskogo obshchestva okhrany pamiatnikov istorii i kul'tury. Polnoe opisanie Rossii. Udmurtiia*, t. 33 (1995): 84–8; *Nezavisimaia gazeta*, (Izhevsk) "Liubimy narodnyi napitok zhitelei Udmurtii variat v kazhdoi derevne," December 15, 2003.

PART THREE
Soviet Russia

CHAPTER EIGHT

Engineering tastes: Food and the senses

Anton Masterovoy

In the early 1930s, in order to overcome the "temporary ... deficit of meat and fish" in the USSR, Soviet newspapers urged food manufacturers to stop being limited by the adherence to "*traditional* raw materials," while agricultural planners were encouraged to abandon their "wheat-barley-rye" psychology that was not appropriate to the "land of the proletarian revolution."[1] Rising salaries for workers and the "joyful ... rise of the village to a higher step in human existence" would lead to the demand for proteins and fats, the journalists argued, but Soviet society was paying too high a price for the "dictatorship of the cooking pot" filled with the usual ingredients.

The solution to Soviet food shortages lay in "changing the traditional menu."[2] *Pravda*, for instance, claimed that scientific experiments "demonstrated the high quality of canned nettles" and pointed out that the bodies of the "millions of squirrels ... hunted annually ... may be canned very well" in response to "worker-consumer" demand.[3] In this chapter, I argue that the Soviet state attempted to adjust consumer taste preferences as a means to deal with food shortages. Soviet government officials, scientists, and food workers believed that taste was simply another factor that they could engineer to better fit the needs of the day. Western, capitalist nations, whether the United States, Britain, or Fascist Italy, also attempted to tinker with the taste preferences of their citizens but had largely abandoned these projects after the Second World War. The Soviet Union pursued this strategy until its collapse in 1991 and, despite its failure, the modern Russian government has not entirely abandoned it. Unknowingly perhaps, Soviet authorities defined national tastes in opposition to the West similarly to the process in the tsarist era observed in Alison Smith's chapter in this volume. Necessity may have influenced the Soviet program, but the campaigns to change taste preferences modified in focus—from the First World War to

1935 when Stalin declared an end to previous asceticism; from 1935 until Stalin's death in 1953, Soviets were told to desire and expect luxurious tastes worthy of a great and prosperous nation; and finally during the late Soviet periods of shortage of 1953–64 and again between 1964 and 1991 Soviets were urged to modify their tastes. The campaigns to change tastes appear surprisingly similar to the advertising campaigns illustrated in Tricia Starks' examination of tobacco marketing, demonstrating one more way in which the Soviet era shared processes with its imperial predecessor.

The origins of the Soviet campaigns to change taste, 1850–1917

The four Soviet campaigns to change tastes had roots both in Russian cultural traditions as well as more recent scientific and political developments. The Russian Orthodox Church maintains a strict calendar of fast days. Leo Tolstoy and Feodor Dostoyevsky, perhaps Russia's most influential writers, shared what Ronald LeBlanc describes as an "almost medieval" belief that "carnality," food and sex, "is something inherently sinful."[4] Russia's nineteenth-century intellectuals, as Alison Smith discusses in her chapter in this volume, used food and taste to define Russian national identity. Their combined appeal both to Western science and Russian culinary traditions as a unique path to modernity would be inherited by Soviet taste reform activists.

The European science of nutrition that was embraced by the Bolsheviks came with its own moral traditions. Taste has been commonly viewed as one of the lower, more animalistic senses, a view that was embraced by nineteenth-century nutritionists.[5] According to scholar of public health and nutrition John Coveney, since Antiquity, eating only for pleasure was morally questionable in Western cultures. After the Enlightenment, the science of nutrition replaced Christianity as the moral force to which every modern diner was to be held accountable.[6] A teacher-student dynasty of German chemists Justus von Liebig, Carl Voit, and Max Rubner from the mid-nineteenth to the mid-twentieth centuries established most of the modern principles of nutrition, the view that food is simply fuel for the "human motor" and that taste, appearance, or tradition have no place in rational nutrition.[7] They in turn influenced American nutritionists such as Wilbur O. Atwater and Harvey Wiley, as well as the Russian-Soviet nutritionists including Emmanuel Pevzner and Mikhail Shaternikov.[8]

The discovery of the chemical composition of food in the nineteenth century led to remarkably similar approaches to solving social problems across the Western world. Now that it was believed that food did not have to be expensive or tasty to satisfy human needs, the demands of the poor for better wages or food aid became immoral whining of the unenlightened, wasteful masses who ignored perfectly good sources of calories and nutrients. During an 1860s famine, Swedish peasants were told to eat mosses and mushrooms, foods that they considered animal fodder, as a replacement for grain. The upper-class reformers openly claimed that the use of recommended surrogates would not just help the peasants but lift the "economic burden of the local tax payers" and "reduce the need for aid… and costly grain imports."[9] In the early twentieth century, highly influential American food reformer Ellen Richards recommended that Americans eat foods that not only fulfilled their nutritional needs but also honestly reflected their class and income. The poor were not to be given tastier foods to avoid stimulating "an artificial appetite" for foods that they could not afford.[10] In late nineteenth-century Russia, Natalia Nordman fed distinguished visitors with her recipes for hay and wild herbs but they were primarily aimed at impoverished Russians. As proof that her hay and vegetable peel soup was good, she pointed out that "her yardman and joiner can eat three bowls apiece."[11] Just like the Scandinavian reformers' efforts of the 1860s, her insistence on feeding the poor with food considered to be cattle feed was not popular.[12]

Unsurprisingly, when faced with such heavy-handed, upper-class attempts to feed them unfamiliar food that the reformers themselves were not expected to eat, the European and American poor rejected the campaigns to rationalize their diets. Even the more democratic approaches stimulated by the very real emergencies of the two world wars were ultimately unsuccessful in forcing Westerners to permanently and radically change their diets. British and American consumers did not follow every bit of the nutritional advice offered to them by the enthusiastic food reformers and "cheated" whenever they could.[13] To their dismay, as soon as the wars were over, nutrition reformers found their efforts marginalized and all the healthy but unattractive wartime foods largely abandoned.[14]

Why then did the Soviet authorities follow in the footsteps of so many failed policies, many of which were specifically designed to marginalize rather than to aid the poor? What makes the Soviet attempts to change consumer taste different from similar attempts in the rest of the Western world? The four attempts to reform Soviet tastes discussed below were the product of the Soviet embrace of scientific reason, communalism, the revolutionary transformation of man, and traditional Russian asceticism. The belief that whatever the policy, all Soviet actions were made on behalf of, rather than against, the workers made the conscious attempts to reform taste a perfectly acceptable tool of the government.

The first campaign, 1917–35

The Soviet government began its first campaign to change tastes because it needed to deal with the effects of almost a decade of war and deprivation. They were not alone in their efforts. The critical situation of the First World War allowed well-known nutritionists to discuss and implement some of their most radical ideas, thanks to the increased toleration for state intervention. Denmark's Mikkel Hindhede convinced the government to slaughter most of the nation's pigs and put the entire country on a diet based on grains, potatoes, vegetables, and dairy.[15] Even in the United States, where consumption limits were essentially voluntary, nutrition specialists such as the chief chemist of the Department of Agriculture, Harvey Wiley, suggested (and practiced) the eating of whales, potato skins, and even dogs and cats, instead of wheat, beef, and pork so that these staples might be sent to the European allies and the US Army.[16]

Russian nutritionists, however, emphasized that a lack of wisdom, rather than a lack of food, was the cause. They argued that irrational prejudices towards the "underutilized or even unknown riches" of unfamiliar foods, allowed Russians to starve "among the colossal stores of food waiting to be developed."[17] In 1919, Soviet food provisioning experts pointed out that the availability of only horse and dog meat in Moscow's markets need not be seen as dire, since only "simple cultural prejudice" prevented consumers from embracing dog eating—a perfectly acceptable practice in ancient Mexico and China.[18] Similarly in 1923, the authors of a book on acceptable food surrogates had little sympathy for hungry people who had to adapt to a rapidly deteriorating food situation. "The starving peasantry, in part through ignorance, narrow-mindedness, and … desperation or apathy" gathered and ate plants of little nutritive value while ignoring those scientifically demonstrated to be nutritious.[19] The same peasants' objections were supposedly the main obstacle to rabbit breeding which could resolve the meat shortages.[20] Relief came with the implementation of the New Economic Policy (1921–8) that allowed the Russian economy to recover and lead to more food being available, not least by allowing the American Relief Administration to offer food aid.[21]

In 1928, Joseph Stalin's turn towards rapid industrialization and collectivization of the peasantry again led to massive food shortages. Stalin envisaged his first Five-Year Plan (1928–32) as a way to rapidly modernize industry and to collectivize peasant landholdings. The violent chaos of collectivization and the sale of food abroad in exchange for machinery and foreign currency instead led to drastic shortages. Though the official system of rationing would be in place from 1930 to 1935, the government downplayed all shortages as purely temporary and the mass famine in southern Russia, Kazakhstan, and the Ukraine that killed millions between 1932 and 1933 was not reflected in the national press.[22] Unlike the early 1920s, a nutritional emergency was occurring in peace time and officials deployed the language of rational nutrition to explain why national improvements meant the deterioration of the individuals' standard of living. Differences emerged in the standard language of nutritionist reforms. While most nutritionists claimed that their ideas were based on natural order, Soviet discourse was dominated by the triumph of science over nature.[23] Any culinary innovations meant to deal with the food shortages were now described as revolutionary reforms, demonstrating not shortages but technological innovations of taste as befitting rational, socialist modernity. As the Soviet press continued to write exposé articles about the starvation of workers under capitalism, it also made the claims that the very same measures used by capitalists to trick workers to accept their impoverishment became progressive when used by Soviets. Writing in 1931, Mikhail Kol'tsov claimed that while the "rations dispensed in … [Soviet] canteens" were something that "German workers could only dream about," Soviets could learn something from the "German professors of starvation cuisine." "Western … technology manages to … extract all nutrients and flavors" out of any ingredient, no matter how "coarse," Kol'tsov wrote, and the Soviet Union needed "chef-engineers" who "have mastered western technology" to do the same.[24]

If Western nutritionists downplayed the unattractive features of replacement foods during times of crisis, the Soviet discourse emphasized them. The disgusting nature of the new food sources which would free Soviets from the "dictatorship of the cooking pot" would demonstrate the ability of Soviet science to transform the sensory experience of consuming the new foods. In 1930, it was claimed that with "rationally organized processing," the "stinking, tough, but cheap and nutritious" dolphin meat could be turned into "sausage and canned meat of good quality and taste."[25] According to the Soviet showpiece magazine, *Our Achievements*, "rational methods of preparation" would allow "shark, dolphin, walrus, seal, [and] beluga whale" to be eaten after being "chemically treated [to] remove their … unpleasant taste and odor." They could then replace the "mollycoddled beluga sturgeon" while "the gannet," a sort of a sea bird, which otherwise "repulsively smells of pond scum" would replace the "traditional grouse."[26]

In the early 1930s, Soviet researchers and press focused their attention on soy as the most potentially malleable and revolutionary new source of protein. The plant was referred to as "the Revolutionary Chinese woman," a "miracle bean" whose discovery in Russia was made possible by the October Revolution. With such credentials, it would undoubtedly bring about "the revolution … in the kitchen."[27] According to Soviet journalists, scientists' reports on soybeans sounded like "young men's confessions of love" in which the head of the State Soy Research Institute called upon Russian peasant farmers to grow more "roast meat and whole milk" by planting the soybean.[28] Contemporary American researchers also looked to soy as a solution for agricultural problems, but planned to use it in animal feed. It took decades for American scientists to remove the "beany, grassy, chalky flavors from soy" to make it palatable to an average American consumer but in the Soviet Union, research into new ingredients was supposed to be applied right away.[29] Tempted by its much touted nutritional equality to meat and milk, soy was said to be ready to resolve the "protein-lipid crisis" in the Soviet Union.[30] Recipe books were published and journalists invited to soy food tastings, where soy hamburgers (*kotlety*), puddings, bread, veal, cheese, deserts, and native Chinese dishes were served.

No amount of enthusiasm could help soy overcome its disagreeable flavor and texture. Even the enthusiastic *Pravda* journalists thought that the hamburger resembled "both cabbage and cream of wheat" simultaneously.[31] The more cautious *Izvestiia* reporter found that soy milk possessed an "aftertaste" that was "fairly disgusting," and that a soy hamburger "was much better than a potato one" but was still "far from meat." He hoped that "man will not live on soy alone."[32] While researchers cautioned against repeating the experiment of Khar'kov canteens that cooked entire meals out of unprocessed soybeans and left many workers disgusted and sick, soy made it into many menus.[33] The senses of the workers of Moscow's Electric Equipment Plant (Elektrozavod) were put to a test as they were consistently fed with sour soy "cheese casseroles" and foreign workers were scared off by the tendency of soy sausage to have a "rainbow-colored" oil slick.[34] Other ersatz foods were also derided by the actual diners. The "admonition[s] from diners" did not stop culinary laboratory specialists from suggesting that the flavor of vegetarian soups could improve with the addition of properly prepared yeast, despite admitting that most canteen cooks would simply stir the uncooked yeast into soups as a condiment while the yeast still possessed a "characteristic, somewhat unpleasant scent" and therefore causing "a series of reactions in the digestive tract."[35]

Along with soy, the rabbit breeding campaign that peaked in 1932 was an attempt to address the protein deficiency in the Soviet diet from a new source and with a different appeal to the palate. As the Soviet government was not willing to discuss the actual reasons for the lack of meat, such as the failure of collectivization and the sale of food abroad in exchange for hard currency, rabbit breeding perplexed foreign observers as an example of the apparent Soviet tendency "to do ordinary things," such as trying to feed its population, "by extraordinary methods."[36] After the mass publication of the decree of the Communist Party that required factories to organize rabbit breeding in the main industrial regions of Russia, the campaign got front cover treatment in most publications including *Ogonek* [*Little Flame*], the Soviet illustrated weekly magazine.[37] Only "ignorance of the useful economic qualities of the rabbit can explain the underdevelopment of rabbit breeding in the Soviet Union," one of the *Ogonek* articles claimed, especially since "in France, Belgium and England rabbit meat is eaten daily in families, restaurants, and cafes."[38] The campaign does not appear to have been taken too seriously, probably because rabbits get sick easily and were difficult to process industrially.[39] The delays in transportation and processing led to most of the rabbit meat becoming unmarketable due to rancid smell and appearance.[40]

The second campaign, 1935–43

After 1935, the official Soviet approach to nutrition and the sensual experience of eating made another rapid turn, radically different from that of most contemporary Western nations. By the middle of the 1930s, collectivized farms could offer a more predictable supply of food for at least some Soviet consumers.[41] The Soviet Union needed to demonstrate the effectiveness of the first Five-Year Plan and that life, according to Stalin's slogan, became "better and more joyous." This was especially important to counterbalance the new European rivals—Nazi Germany and Fascist Italy. These two nations harnessed the language and ideology of nutrition to their goals of autarky and military build up, essentially to "sell the benefits of a diet that would not strain the nation's budget."[42] At the same time they now turned to the solutions that the Soviet Union considered (and would again after the Second World War) for its own food shortages. According to Carol Helstosky, Italian fascists promoted exactly the same foods that were seen by Italian nineteenth-century reformers as the source of national shame and ill health—vegetable stew (*minestra*), polenta, rice (as opposed to pasta), whole-grain bread, and grapes. Fascist magazines recommended rabbit breeding, soy, and peanuts as a way to make up for any nutritional deficiencies, though some patriotic nutritionists argued that Italians needed less fat and protein than other ethnicities anyway.[43] Similarly, Nazi Germany encouraged its housewives to embrace "unused treasures of nature" and reminded its youths that excessive meat consumption led to disease.[44] In order to achieve freedom from imports, Germans also sponsored and then abandoned rabbit breeding campaigns, tried to get consumers to eat more whale and fish, and recommended the use of quark (skim-milk curds) as a protein-rich substitute for both butter *and* meat.[45]

In the United States, the Great Depression and the Second World War prompted concerns about the diet of poor and working-class Americans, leading to the formation of the Committee on Food Habits headed by the anthropologist Margaret Meade. One of the major concerns for the Committee was how to get Americans to eat nutritious but unloved offal. A prominent exiled German psychologist Kurt Lewin used group discussions directed at housewives to break down prejudices against the target foods, suggest ways in which the foods could be best introduced to the rest of the family, and explain why it was necessary to eat something that was not liked. Using techniques which William Graebner called "democratic social engineering," Lewin and the Committee would structure the discussions to have groups of housewives reach the desired conclusions themselves.[46]

The official Soviet policy, by comparison, was now to *increase* Soviet consumer taste for rich and luxurious foods.[47] As the rationing system wound down in 1934, Soviet journalists argued that the heroic Soviet workers "have a right to a luxurious life."[48] Workers at Moscow's major factories were encouraged to compete with each other for the tastiest and most filling lunches, demonstrating the rise of their "culinary culture" with an abundance of attractive meat dishes, since a "dented meat patty is less appetizing."[49] Meanwhile, the traditional peasant reliance on starches was ridiculed and one could be called a "right-wing opportunist" for suggesting that vegetables could replace meat.[50]

The most enthusiastic proponent of progressive tastes was the food minister and a close associate of Stalin, Anastas Mikoyan. "We were used to having only bad foods and that there were few of them" Mikoyan told an audience of Stakhanovite workers in 1935, "but people, ... their appetites ... their demands, ... their tastes are developing and the food industry must move towards the growing tastes and demands of the workers."[51] For Mikoyan, the food industry contributed to the "task of reconstructing man" by working to "awaken new tastes among the populace" and to "actively break down old habits."[52] The people could not be allowed to retain "the old attachments to cabbage soup and porridge."[53] Mikoyan's rhetoric set the tone and as late as 1939, when the Soviet Union began to experience massive shortages due to the wars with Finland and Poland, the main newspaper of the Soviet food industry wrote that the "socialist reconstruction of the people's diet" required food to not only contain enough energy and nutrients but also "be prepared in such a way as to possess a pleasant appearance (color, scent, shape) [and] to arouse pleasant taste sensations."[54]

The Soviets admired the United States as the most prosperous industrialized nation of the 1930s. Mikoyan himself visited the United States in order to learn about and purchase technology in 1936, bringing back flash-frozen vegetables, industrially produced ice cream, and a strong love of hamburgers.[55] The official Soviet cookbook, published in 1939, and rather tellingly called the *Book of Tasty and Healthy Food*, had its pages filled with explicitly American foods: tomato juice, fish filets, whiskey, and convenient breakfast cereals such as "kornfleks" and "greyp-nots."[56] The Soviet popular press was also filled with American food references and advertising including canned corn and ketchup.[57] The realities of the continual food shortages, especially in the countryside where most people still survived on black bread and potatoes, were simply ignored.[58]

Even during the Second World War, officially published culinary texts danced around the real facts of extreme deprivation. The ersatz food solutions were presented as a part of the Soviet pre-war goal of making popular tastes more cultured. A 1944 brochure on wild plant recipes complained that because culinary specialists remained unaware of the high nutritional value of "many of the wild plants that grow on the vast territory of the Soviet Union...wild greens still" had an "extraordinarily unimportant place" in the Soviet diet, unlike Western Europe and the United States. War was only mentioned in passing, while emphasizing that the benefits of wild plants which were "exceptionally important in times of peace take on special meaning now, in time of war."[59] Similarly, *Sweet Dishes without Sugar* (1944) did not mention the war at all.[60] The introduction of the 1945 edition of the *Book of Tasty and Healthy Food* mentions the victorious conclusion of the war, the "tremendous care" of the Party and government in supplying food to the army and the civilians, as well as the "warm response" of the citizens to the calls for economic use of food and for growing and gathering edible plants.[61] It did not, however, explicitly draw the connection between the war and the goal of the book to "give the Soviet housewife a practical guide for food preparation under conditions of the frugal use of a number of foods."[62]

The importance of the campaign of the second-half of the 1930s to instill luxurious tastes should not be underestimated, however illusory it actually was. Even the vast majority of Soviet citizens, who did not have access to the relative abundance of Moscow and Leningrad supermarkets, would have at least *seen* or read of the abundance that Mikoyan spoke about. The Soviet press bombarded its readers with constant images of food in what Sheila Fitzpatrick described as "consumer-goods pornography."[63] Literature of the Stalinist period was said to be permeated by the "delicious scent of dumplings" and its films filled by scenes in which people "ate ... plentifully ... as an entire farm collective."[64]

As a favorite food of the urban working class and an easy way to turn less attractive raw meat into an attractive industrially-processed meat product, sausage was a particularly important feature of these images (see Figure 8.1). Even if the goods were not on the shelves, consumers knew which particular goods *had* to be there. Because sausage formed an important part of the narratives of abundance, it began to be strongly associated with Stalin and his promise of a prosperous life. Mikoyan repeatedly told the anecdote of Stalin reminding him to make plenty of sausage and frankfurters in his speeches.[65] He eagerly pointed out that while Soviet consumers in Moscow and Leningrad could now enjoy frankfurters, long considered to be the "signs of bourgeois abundance and well-being," Germany was running out.[66] A Soviet diarist, concerned about possible arrest was said to add entries of gratitude to Stalin for the sausage that she bought, while another Soviet citizen saw the appearance of even middling quality sausage as a sign of better things ahead.[67] After the end of the Second World War, sausage along with other luxury goods returned to the stores in major cities, though at very high prices.[68] Art critic and memoirist Mikhail German remembered receiving a present of a piece of white bread with a piece of sausage during the war and eating

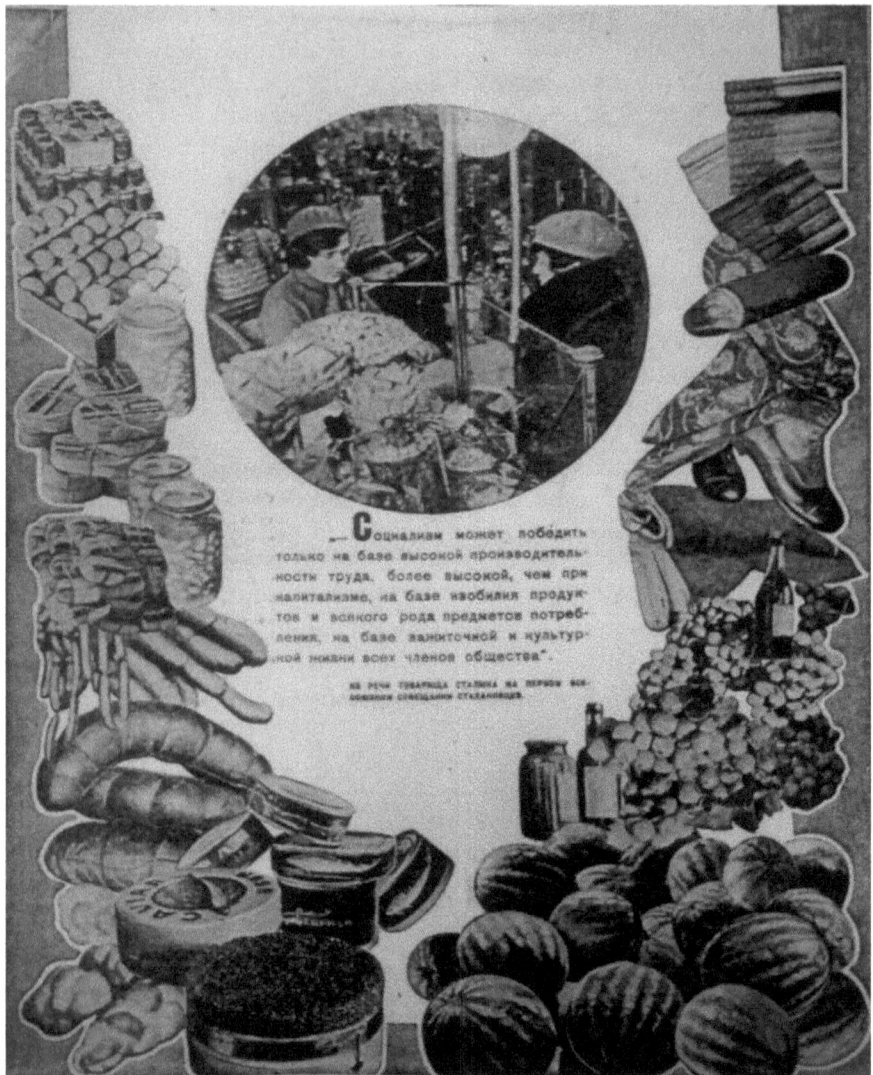

FIGURE 8.1 *A Soviet cornucopia*. Stakhanovets *no. 21–22 (1936): inner rear cover*.

them separately since they were both forgotten luxuries and needed to be savored individually.[69] Returning from wartime evacuation to her room in a communal apartment, a Soviet woman recalled finding a note and a piece of sausage left as a present from her husband and feeling that she "had come home."[70]

The third campaign, 1953–64

After Stalin's death in 1953, Nikita Khrushchev promised not only to return to the true Leninist path to communism but also to "catch up to and overtake" the United States in the consumption of meat and milk.[71] Khrushchev was aware that the Soviet people were expecting better food and more of it. The comparative improvements of the postwar decade in providing more food and housing for Soviet citizens led to what Steven Harris has described as a "crisis of growing expectations."[72] When the production of food could not match the higher expectations of the Soviet consumers, Khrushchev returned to the earlier Soviet legacy and tried to match consumer tastes to what was available.

Khrushchev's goals were essentially to fulfill the promises of the earlier era—to provide more housing and food for Soviet citizens. In multiple letters to the new leader, Soviet citizens wrote that while the people were not starving, one could not "raise a healthy new generation on bread alone."[73] "Our people have lived through a lot," wrote one Muscovite, "and it is time to create normal living conditions for them."[74] His response was rapid but the results were mixed. Starting in 1953, the Virgin Lands campaign plowed up Kazakhstan and Siberia but soon the top soil was blown away by erosion.[75] Khrushchev's promise to "catch and overtake America" in milk and meat production first mentioned in a 1957 speech, ran aground due to lack of proper feed or even proper breeds of livestock. His most notorious program to improve the availability of animal feed by creating an American-style corn belt in the USSR (1955–64) also failed due to significantly different climatic conditions and mismanagement. The overplanting of corn led to a decrease of traditional grains and grass for people and cattle.[76] Raising prices on milk and meat to encourage Soviet collective farms to produce more food was ideologically difficult and led to a massive riot in the southern Russian city of Novocherkassk in 1962.[77]

As food had not materialized as quickly as Khrushchev expected, Soviet state authorities attempted to sweeten the situation by making the food that was available more attractive. Believing in the transformative potential of the Soviet ideal, Khrushchev promoted horse meat not as a substitute for more common meats, but as a demonstration of the gradual abandonment of ethnic, religious, and dietary prejudices that followed the October Revolution. As formerly Muslim Central Asians now ate pork, Khrushchev pointed out, the state could now also ask European Soviets why, so many years after the Revolution, they were still afraid to eat horse.[78] Actual consumer tastes were less susceptible to ideology. When horse sausage appeared in stores, Russian consumers were disgusted, describing it as the "Neigh-brand" (*yego-go*) and threatening to force-feed it to Khrushchev and his ministers.[79] Whale meat sausage was nicknamed *nikitovaia kolbasa*, cleverly combining Khrushchev's first name (Nikita) with *kit*, the Russian word for whale. It left poor college students, the only consumers desperate enough to buy it, with painful memories of how it stank up the hallways of their dormitories when they tried to fry it.[80] Such strange foods led to speculation that the next step would be the use of something even more unpleasantly exotic, with rumors circulating that on his trips to visit Asian and African allies, Khrushchev was actually buying monkey and elephant meat in exchange for warplanes.[81]

Corn was promoted as a major ingredient of all foods including special sausages, *Amber*-brand wine, and most problematically, bread. Though journalists invited to a corn menu tasting tried to claim that adding 10 to 20 percent of corn flour to baked goods could save grain and gave the foods an "appetizing yellowness … as if permeated with an amber sunlight," the actual sale of these breads was unsuccessful.[82] A very poor harvest in 1963 and the growing predominance of corn over other grains led to a shortage of bread. It was a testament to the actual successes of Soviet agriculture that most of the bread consumed was now wheaten white bread, but its shortages led to panic buying and shortages of the dark rye bread as well.[83] Wheat and rye flour was now cut with increasing percentages of the relatively plentiful corn and sometimes even pea meal, which gave loaves an unappetizing green color. The resulting mixed-flour loaf was mockingly dubbed the "Russian Wonder" by Soviet consumers.[84] Khrushchev even claimed that alcohol for industrial and food uses would be henceforth "produced from [natural] gas," of which there was an "unlimited supply."[85] The use of other surrogate materials and the traditional Russian name for cheap vodka (*suchok*, twig) prompted widespread rumors that poor-quality vodka was made of wood or some petroleum-based chemical substance.[86]

Khrushchev's position was especially difficult because he always tied the increased production of grain to the production of meat in his public pronouncements. Corn was supposed to feed animals, not people. "Better foods cannot be created without an abundance of grain," he told an audience in 1954, but the future was bright because "what kind of a Communist society would it be without sausage?"[87] And, according to Khrushchev, corn was "sausage on a stalk."[88] Just as the nineteenth-century Swedish peasants who were told to eat foods that they considered to be animal fodder, Soviet consumers refused to adapt their taste preferences to state needs, and lost trust in their leadership.[89]

The fourth campaign, 1964–91

The campaign to remake Soviet tastes was not abandoned after Khrushchev's removal from power in 1964. Soviet nutritionists and economists joined the call to teach consumers how to eat within the means of the State's ability to feed them. From the pages of newspapers, magazines, and cookbooks,

Soviet consumers heard the call to be rational and modern, to overcome the "psychological barrier" that stood between them and enjoying the food that the state could provide.[90]

Between 1960 and 1991, following the patterns seen in Western Europe over the nineteenth century, the Soviet diet began to improve. Soviets ate about as many calories as Americans and as consumption of meat, dairy, and sugar rose, the role of bread and potatoes fell, while still remaining the primary source of calories.[91] Despite increased meat consumption, proteins mostly came from eggs and dairy.[92] Distribution and quality of food remained extremely uneven, and neither Leonid Brezhnev's nor Mikhail Gorbachev's government managed to provide enough protein to satisfy consumer demand. The Soviet Union became a net importer of grain under Brezhnev but the invasion of Afghanistan in 1979 led to the American grain embargo.[93] While its impact on the Soviet food supply was not great, the embargo did lead the Soviet government, and Mikhail Gorbachev as the Party secretary in charge of agriculture in particular, to look for ways to bolster Soviet food security and to free the country from grain import dependence.[94] The result was the "Food Program of the USSR for the Period up to 1990," which aimed not only to raise the production of food in the country but to also "rationalize" its consumption.[95] Gorbachev's input in the program was crucial since, like Khrushchev, he was a "true believer" in the Soviet cause and embraced the perfectibility of Soviet man.[96] It was his anti-alcohol campaign, after all, that became the hallmark of Gorbachev's first years in power.[97]

The Party, state, and the scientific establishment attempted to adjust Soviet consumer demands to what was available. If the Soviet diet finally approached that of Western Europe or the United States, so did Soviet nutritional advice. In its form, function, and choice of ideal ingredients, it resembled the efforts of Nazi Germany, Fascist Italy, and those of the American Committee on Food Habits. Nutritionists gave the Food Program a scholarly aura, basing it on the "Norms of the Physiological Needs for Food Substances and Energy for Various Population Groups of the USSR."[98] Soviet nutritionists reminded consumers that "obtaining enough complete proteins of animal origin ... [was] a very acute problem in the whole world, including the USSR" and that their efforts were oriented "toward the discovery of new and the maximal utilization of traditional sources of food proteins."[99]

The process began before 1982. Under Brezhnev, meat economy became the watchword of the industry. Meat processing workers were exhorted to increase the "utilization of offal of the second category," as well as previously unusable meat that was somehow "made harmless," all in honor of the next Party Congress or even the 1970 celebration of Lenin's birth centennial.[100] When consumer complaints about sausage quality reached their peak during the late 1980s, beleaguered meat industry workers responded to accusations of theft in the press by explaining that "meat economy" was not their own criminal initiative. From 1969 until 1981 the Soviet Council of Ministers sent out a list of "Measures for the Rational Use of Raw Materials in Meat Processing" and meat processors took pride in reaching meat savings goals—consumer accusations of theft notwithstanding.[101]

Like Nazi nutritionists, Soviet specialists saw skim-milk curds and fish as good meat replacements. In 1964, claiming that they were searching for cheaper, protein-rich substances to benefit all of humanity, Soviet scientists created BELIP—an abbreviation for the rather unappetizing "Proteinic Product of the Nutritional Institute of the Academy of Medical Sciences of the USSR." It combined skim-milk curds, cod fish, and vegetable oil, providing an "especially balanced combination of foodstuffs" which contained the most important nutrients and was also inexpensive. The researchers even published a variety of recipes that promised to transform BELIP into paté or "meatballs" by adding some bread, corn, or oil.[102]

Soviet consumers were again told to get over their conservative tastes and eat more seafood and other "non-traditional" sources of protein. According to the authors of one tome of seafood propaganda, the fear of seafood would soon become "an amusing misunderstanding," just like the one-time European fear of tea and potatoes.[103] In the 1970s, copying a practice from the early 1930s, every Thursday in Soviet public catering establishments was designated as a "fish day" and fish-only supermarkets called "Okean" (the Ocean) were opened.[104] The popular press published articles about progress in cultivating sea scallops and giant Pacific oysters promising vast amounts of "pure meat," "precious protein" that could be eaten raw, imparting a "magnificent taste of oceanic freshness" and nutritionally equivalent to milk.[105] Soviet consumers were also offered nutria rat meat and domesticated moose milk.[106]

The difficulty lay in getting consumers to actually buy these foods voluntarily and not clamor for the traditional meat, sausage, and eggs. Soviet consumers complained about the poorly manufactured "sausages" and "hams" made of pollock with a little pork added or bologna with so much starch filler mixed in that it started to turn blue.[107] The fish and seafood sold in stores were usually of the cheapest kind—hake, pollock, and squid, sometimes only squid tentacles.[108] They were frozen, unprocessed, and visually repulsive, either "crooked frozen corpses" or sawn from a giant block into a "cube ... of fish sold by weight," its "neat geometric shape" containing a head complete with "shining eyes" staring out.[109] Prepared fish that was encountered on fish days was poorly made and often not even properly cleaned.[110] The sausage obsession of an average Soviet consumer was not only influenced by the memories of Stalinism. By the 1970s and 1980s, it was one of the few truly convenient foods for Soviet families where it was expected that all adults would hold a full-time job.[111] On the other hand, cooking offal, such as cow udders, required a lot of preparation to rid it of its unpleasant scent.[112] Soviet taste preferences too would require much work to be adjusted to the state's ability to satisfy them.

A 1986 article in the *Agitator*, an official Communist Party journal for propagandists, neatly explained the policies that guided the Soviet sense-adjustment propaganda from the late 1960s onward. "At the current stage the development of production is incresingly aimed not only to satisfy popular demand," the journal wrote, "but also *to form rational needs, [and] tastes of consumers*."[113] The nutritional needs would be satisfied at "justifiable norms"[114] The population was to be "prepared to use the growing possibilities for rationalizing consumption ... under the conditions of free choice" by the means of "propaganda of the rational norms of consumption and desirable consumer standards" given "the existing objective abilities" of the state economy and to "counteract the negative influences on popular consumer behavior by persons with regressive views, certain groups with a low level of culture, as well as the consumerist notions formed in capitalist nations and not conforming to a socialist way of life."[115]

In a remarkable resemblance to the early twentieth-century food reformers in the United States, the late Soviet discourse on food and taste blamed the consumers for giving in to their taste buds and ignoring the abundance of nutrients available to them. A popular weekly supplement to *Izvestiia* hosted a culinary contest entitled "Jane of All Trades" in 1972. The main part of the competition asked the contestants to submit the most varied menus made out of specific amounts of quark, processed cheese, potatoes, carrots, onions, cabbage, flour, fish filets, and sour cream—the most commonly available ingredients.[116] After the passage of the Food Program in 1982, the efforts to change Soviet tastes began to be more forceful. An economist, Iulia Khodosh, was recruited to connect cheaper and commonly available, if not highly desirable, foods to any topic from saving up for a car to staying thin and beautiful.[117] Though the Soviet Union produced plenty of food, people did not know how to use it wisely, she claimed in the introduction to her book, *The Culture of Consumption* (1984), published as a part of the "Food Program in Action" series.[118] Her 1984 article in *Nedelia*, suggested that Soviet consumers were spend-thrifts, pining after pricy foods when their protein needs could be met with simple and wholesome foods, such as bread and milk. With the money thus saved on food, the article claimed, consumers could buy more interesting goods, perhaps even a car.[119] A later article offered a frugal meal of stewed fish, potatoes, and cabbage as an alternative to pricy delicacies. "You might say: well, what about taste?" Khodosh asked. "Science respects emotions and specifics of individual tastes," but "experience shows that ... taste can be nurtured," the readers were told. Khodosh even claimed to know "many people who ... [never] liked fish or quark/farmers cheese but understood their importance for health and taught themselves to like these foods."[120] A true culture of nutrition, she argued in *Izvestiia*, meant that its bearer thought about how to better use the state resources dedicated to food and not in terms of "meat" but in terms of "protein."[121]

Another tireless promoter of the new tastes was Vladimir Mikhailov, a culinary instructor of the Plekhanov State Institute of Economics. Mikhailov's key argument was that "one should not eat according to taste, but according to science."[122] If the articles of the mid-1930s celebrated the disappearance of the foods of the impoverished Russian peasantry such as offal and *tiuria*, a soup of crumbled bread and water, patriotic Mikhailov mourned them.[123] According to Mikhailov, the Soviet people actually suffered from a "shortage of a culture of nutrition" brought on by the "tradition to eat tastily and a lot that formed in the past decades." "The centuries-old folk experience has been forgotten," Mikhailov complained. "Taste [was] nothing else than a product of the imagination," and regular fasting a sign of a true "culture of nutrition," Mikhailov preached. If people were unable to accept that, they could seek the aid of a psychologist.[124]

Conclusion

As the Soviet state's ability to provide food became increasingly futile, the creativity of the taste reformers rose to new, bewildering heights. The state urged Soviet consumers to adapt the three main senses engaged during meals—sight, taste, and smell—to help deal with a period of economic decline. In 1989, *Eating with an Appetite*, a book published by the recently created Center of Healthy Nutrition of the Main Soviet Economic Research Institute, offered a startling solution for the growing shortages of sausage. Reminding their readers that their "sense of smell was closely tied to the stimulation of the appetite," the authors told a family of three or four to sit around the dinner table, place "a thin slice of sausage on a large dish and surround it with vegetables … look at the sausage and inhale its aroma for 10–15 minutes … relax … close [your] eyes and mentally imagine the taste of the sausage." Once this "psychological preparation" was complete, the diners would eat the vegetables but only gaze at the sausage. After the meal, the sausage slice would be wrapped tightly and returned to the refrigerator, to be reused for up to a month.[125]

Actual Soviet consumers were less impressed by the "innovations" offered to them by the state and the food industry. The semi-vegetarianism offered by the official discourse contradicted its own earlier pronouncements which equated vegetarianism with class oppression, poverty, backwardness, and primitivism.[126] Unlike Western societies of abundance, the perennial Soviet shortages made access to tasty, but also high-fat and high-salt, meat delicacies "stable markers of one's social standing" no matter how "unhealthy" they might have been from a nutritionist's point of view.[127] Vladimir Mikhailov's recipes for grain and leaf mixtures that transparently guided readers only to ingredients that could be grown on their small garden plot or picked in the wild seemed suspect to the *Literary Gazette* as it wondered what was so poetic about "Poetry," Mikhailov's cabbage-core-based gruel.[128] The multi-sensory sausage (non)consumption suggested by *Eating with an Appetite* was met by bewilderment in the more liberal *Komsomol'skaia Pravda*.[129] When *Rabotnitsa*, the most popular Soviet women's magazine published similar recipes, the readers were unhappy. Their author was astonished by the "storm of readers' letters" written in a "suspiciously-ironic" tone which saw in the magazine's "recommendations on how to eat well ... an attempt to justify the empty store shelves, a lack of meat, [and] sugar rationing." It was a pity, she complained, that the times were such that "even a harmless culinary recipe is colored by politics."[130] In 1990 G. I. Bondarev, a prominent Soviet nutritionist, advised the readers of *Komsomol'skaia Pravda* not to panic and to obtain all their "basic nutrients and energy with two loaves of bread and a bottle of milk daily."[131] By 1991, Bondarev was complaining that whenever he lectured on rational nutrition to average consumers, the audience descended into "pure barbarity—you just get started and instantly there are yells 'What are you telling us, just give us meat ... and we'll figure it out ourselves!'"[132]

There was little that was new in the Soviet attempts to get consumers to adapt their senses to the current needs of the state. Most of their ideas and methods have been tried by both authoritarian and democratic governments. But that very familiarity is the key to any attempt to understand the social policies in the Soviet Union and, perhaps, in its present-day successor states. The inadequate farm and food processing equipment and the underdeveloped transportation network and distribution systems were not the only factors holding back Soviet development. Soviet propaganda and nutritional science also held on to ideas current in the mid-twentieth century even as most Soviet citizens were increasingly exposed to images of late twentieth-century European and American abundance.

The tragicomic failure of the last attempt to change Soviet tastes has not entirely dissuaded the modern Russian state from occasionally turning to its arguments as it continues to cling to some of the Soviet technologies of power. As soon as the Russian government announced an embargo on American and European foods in retaliation for Western sanctions in August 2014, the Russian Orthodox Church and pro-government journalists began calls to stop "chasing Western consumer standards," end "food cosmopolitanism," and to remember that "happiness is not found in sausage."[133] How the Russian consumers respond to these familiar exhortations remains to be seen.

Notes

1 L. M. Iol'son, *Soiia: Khimiia, tekhnologiia i primenenie* (Moscow-Leningrad: Snabtekhizdat, 1932), 190; L.B., "Bogateiishie syr'evye rezervy," *Pravda*,

July 23, 1930; V. l. Vasilenko, "Blizhe k soe!," *Krasnaia niva* 32 (1930): 15. Emphasis in the original. All translations are mine, unless otherwise noted.

2   A. Bragin, "Protiv diktatury gorshka i koryta," *Pravda*, April 15, 1930.
3   L.B., "Bogateiishie."
4   Ronald D. LeBlanc, *Slavic Sins of the Flesh: Food, Sex, and Carnal Appetite in Nineteenth-Century Russian Fiction* (Lebanon, NH: University of New Hampshire Press, 2009), 235.
5   For a thorough discussion of the role of taste in the West and elsewhere, see Priscilla Parkhurst Ferguson, "The Senses of Taste," *American Historical Review* 116 (April 2011): 371–84.
6   John Coveney, *Food, Morals and Meaning: The Pleasure and Anxiety of Eating* (New York: Routledge, 2000), 109.
7   Anson Rabinbach, *The Human Motor: Energy, Fatigue, and the Origins of Modernity* (Berkeley: University of California Press, 1992), 124–7.
8   I. Borodulin, B. S. Kaganov, and A. V. Topolianski, "Kanony dietologii i uroki zhizni. Pamiati prof. M. I. Pevznera (1872–1952)," *Voprosy dietologii* 3 (2013): 8; V. A. Shaternikov and L. E. Gorelova, *Mikhail Nikolaevich Shaternikov, 1870–1939* (Moscow: Nauka, 1982), 12. For German influence on American nutritionists, see Harvey Levenstein, *Revolution at the Table: The Transformation of the American Diet* (Berkeley: University of California Press, 2003), 46–8.
9   Ingvar Svanberg and Marie C. Nelson, "Bone Meal Porridge, Lichen Soup, Or Mushroom Bread: Acceptance Or Rejection of Food Propaganda in Northern Sweden in the 1860s," in *Just a Sack of Potatoes? Crisis Esperiences in European Societies, Past and Present*, ed. Antti Häkkinen (Helsinki: Societas Historica Finlandiae, 1992), 134, 142.
10 As quoted in Charlotte Biltekoff, *Eating Right in America: The Cultural Politics of Food and Health* (Durham, NC: Duke University Press, 2013), 42.
11 Darra Goldstein, "Is Hay Only For Horses? Highlights of Russian Vegetarianism at the Turn of the Century," in *Food in Russian History and Culture*, ed. Musya Glantz and Joyce Toomre (Bloomington: Indiana University Press, 1997), 116–7.
12 Ibid., 117.
13 See for instance Ina Zweiniger-Bargielowska, "Fair Shares? The Limits of Food Policy in Britain during the Second World War," in *Food and War in Twentieth Century Europe*, ed. Ina Zweiniger-Bargielowska, Rachel Duffett, and Alain Drouard (Farnham: Ashgate Publishing Ltd, 2011), 132–3 and Derek J. Oddy, *From Plain Fare to Fusion Food: British Diet from the 1890s to the 1990s* (Woodbridge, Suffolk: Boydell Press, 2003), 228–30; and Amy Bentley, *Eating for Victory: Food Rationing and the Politics of Domesticity* (Champaign: University of Illinois Press), 99.
14 Harvey A. Levenstein, *Paradox of Plenty: A Social History of Eating in Modern America* (Berkeley: University of California Press, 2003), 74 and Charlotte Biltekoff, "Critical Nurtition Studies," in *The Oxford Handbook*

of *Food History*, ed. Jeffrey M. Pilcher (New York: Oxford University Press, 2012), 177.

15 For a discussion of Hindhede and Demark, see Svend Skafte Overgaard, "Mikkel Hindhede and the Science and Rhetoric of Food Rationing in Denmark 1917–1918," in *Food and War*, ed. Zweiniger-Bargielowska, Duffett, and Drouard, 201–15.

16 Helen Zoe Veit, *Modern Food, Moral Food: Self-Control, Science, and the Rise of Modern American Eating in the Early Twentieth Century* (Chapel Hill: University of North Carolina Press, 2013), 51–3.

17 L. A. Vasilievskii and L. M. Vasilievskii, *Pishchevye surrogaty* (Petrograd: Nauchno Khimiko-Tekhnicheskoe Izdatel'stvo, 1923), 5.

18 Mauricio Borrero, *Hungry Moscow: Scarcity and Urban Society in the Russian Civil War, 1917–1921* (New York: Peter Lang, 2003), 79.

19 Vasilievskii and Vasilievskii, *Pishchevye*, 40.

20 Ibid., 54.

21 On ARA presence in Russia, see Bertrand M. Patenaude, *The Big Show in Bololand: The American Relief Expedition to Soviet Russia in the Famine of 1921* (Stanford, CA: Stanford University Press, 2002).

22 For in-depth coverage of the famine, see R. W. Davies and Stephen G. Wheatcroft, *The Years of Hunger: Soviet Agriculture, 1931–1933* (Basingstoke: Palgrave Macmillan, 2004) and O. A. Antipova et al., eds., *Golod v SSSR, 1930–1934 gg.* (Moscow: Federal'noe arkhivnoe agentstvo, 2009).

23 Overgaard, "Mikkel Hindhede," 204, 211; Sergei Prozorov, "The Biopolitics of Stalinism: Ideas and Bodies in Soviet Governmentality," paper presented at the IPSA World Congress, Madrid, July 8–12, 2012, 8.

24 Mikhail Kol'tsov, "Sadias' za stol …," in *Izbrannye proizvedeniia v trekh tomakh* (Moscow: Gosudarstvennoe izdatel'stvo khudozhestvennoii literatury, 1957), 1:426.

25 D. S. Shnaider, *Balaklava: Proizvoditel'nye sily, kurort, istoriia* (Simfeeropol': Krymgoizdat, 1930), http://www.krimoved.crimea.ua/balaklava.html (accessed February 26, 2016); "Konservy iz Miasa Del'finov," *Pravda*, August 5, 1930.

26 E. Zagorskaia, "Rastional'noe pitanie. Nauchnyii institute pitaniia," *Nashi dostizheniia* 1 (1931): 94.

27 Vasilenko, *Blizhe*, 14; L. Kassil', "'Bob-transformator ili uzhin s oborotnem'," *Izvestiia*, September 19, 1930.

28 Kassil', "'Bob-transformator'."

29 Christine M. Du Bois, "Social Context and Diet: Changing Soy Production and Consumption in the United States," in *The World of Soy*, ed. Christine M. Du Bois, Chee-Beng Tan, and Sidney W. Mintz (Urbana: University of Illinois Press, 2008), 220.

30 "'Chudo-boby'," *Izvestiia*, June 11, 1930.

31 L. Brontman, "Teliatia iz zemli," *Pravda*, September 20, 1930.

32 Kassil', "'Bob-transformator'."
33 Zagorskaia, "Ratsional'noe pitanie."
34 Szabados Arpad, *Dvadtsat' p'iat' let v SSSR (1922–1947 gg)*, trans. Tatjana Lengyel, http://world.lib.ru/s/sabadosh_a/szabadosmemoirdoc.shtml (accessed October 20, 2013).
35 *Pervaia moskovskaia oblastnaia konferentsiia po obshchestvennomu pitaniiu* (Moscow-Leningrad: Gosudarstvennoe meditsinskoe izdatel'stvo, 1932), 61–2.
36 R. O. G. Urch, *The Rabbit King of Russia* (London: The Right Book Club, 1939), v.
37 For more on the decree (*postanovlenie*) see, for example *Ogonek* 14, May 20, 1932 and *Ogonek* 16, June 10, 1932. For newspaper publications see *Sovetskaia Sibir'*, May 18, 1932 and *Krasnyi sever*, May 18, 1932, and almost any other Soviet newspaper that day.
38 P. Nikitinykh, "Nauchnuiiu bazu krolikovodstvu," *Ogonek* 16, June 10, 1932, 2.
39 Davies and Wheatcroft, *The Years of Hunger*, 305–6, 305 n.23.
40 For receiving unusable rabbit meat see A. Rybkin, "Ratsional'nye metody pererabotki krolikov," *Miasnaiia industriia SSSR* 2 (1937): 41–2 and Rossiiskii gosudarstvennyi arkhiv ekonomiki (RGAE), f.8543, op.1, d.382, l.76.
41 Julie Hessler, *A Social History of Soviet Trade: Trade Policy, Retail Practices, and Consumption, 1917–1953* (Princeton, NJ: Princeton University Press, 2004), 227; and Nikolai M. Dronin and Edward G. Bellinger, *Climate Dependence and Food Problems in Russia, 1900–1990: The Interaction of Climate and Agricultural Policy and Their Effect on Food Problems* (New York: Central European University Press, 2005), 13.
42 Carol F. Helstosky, *Garlic and Oil: Politics and Food in Italy* (Oxford: Berg, 2004), 74.
43 Ibid., 79, 84, 87, 99, 101.
44 Mark B. Cole, "Feeding the Volk: Food, Culture, and the Politics of Nazi Consumption, 1933–1945" (PhD diss., University of Florida, 2011), 163; Robert Proctor, *The Nazi War on Cancer* (Princeton, NJ: Princeton University Press, 2000), 127.
45 Cole, "Feeding the Volk," 149–50, 158, 182.
46 For a discussion of the Committee on Food Habits see Biltekoff, *Eating Right in America*, 54–79 and Brian Wansink, "Changing Eating Habits on the Home Front: Lost Lessons from World War II Research," *Journal of Public Policy & Marketing* 21 (2002): 90–9. For democratic social engineering, see William Graebner, "The Small Group and Democratic Social Engineering, 1900–1950," *Journal of Social Issues* 42 (1986): 137–54.
47 For a detailed discussion on Soviet interest in luxury goods in the late 1930s, see Jukka Gronow, *Caviar with Champagne: Common Luxury and the Ideals of the Good Life in Stalin's Russia* (Oxford: Berg, 2003).
48 Pavel Nilin, "O roskoshnoy zhizni," *Nashi dostizheniia* 6 (1934): 61.

49 *Vkusno i sytno* (Moscow: Profizdat, 1934), 24, 43, 46.
50 E. Mikulina, *Chem vy pitaetes'?* (Moscow: Narpit, 1930), 4; F. Kornushin "Pervenets miasnoi industrii SSSR," *Pishchevaia Promyshlennost'* 1 (1931): 37, 39.
51 Anastas Mikoyan, *Pishchevaia industriia Sovetskogo soiuza* (Moscow: Pishchepromizdat, 1941), 94.
52 Ibid., 186.
53 Ibid., 216.
54 V. Kaganov and B. Sbarskii, "Sotsialishticheskaia perestroika narodnogo pitaniia," *Pishchevaia industriia*, April 2, 1939.
55 Mikoyan described his experience in A. I. Mikoyan, "Dva mesiatsa v SShA," *SShA Ekonomika Politika Ideologiia* 10 (October 1971), 68–77 and A. I. Mikoyan, "Dva mesiatsa v SShA," *SShA Ekonomika Politika Ideologiia* 11 (November 1971): 73–84.
56 *Kniga o vkusnoi i zdorovoi pishche* (Moscow-Leningrad: Pishchepromizdat, 1939), 70, 80, 135, 389–92. For more on the history of the *Book*, see Edward Geist,"Cooking Bolshevik: Anastas Mikoian and the Making of the *Book About Delicious and Healthy Food*," *The Russian Review* 71 (2) (2012): 295–313.
57 Canned corn advertisement. *Ogonek* 8–9 (1936): inner rear cover; ketchup advertisement. *Ogonek* 16 (1936): inner front cover.
58 Jukka Gronow, *Caviar with Champagne*, 121–3.
59 *Bliuda iz dikorastushcheii zeleni* (Moscow: Gostorgizdat, 1944), 3
60 S. Griuner, *Sladkie bliuda bez sakhara* (Moscow: Gostorgizdat, 1944).
61 *Kniga o vkusnoii i zdorovoii pishche* (Moscow: Pishchepromizdat, 1945), 3–4.
62 Ibid., 4.
63 Sheila Fitzpatrick, *Everyday Stalinism: Ordinary Life in Extraordinary Times: Soviet Russia in the 1930s* (New York: Oxford University Press, 1999), 90.
64 V. Pomerantsev, "Ob iskrennosti v literature," *Novyi mir* 12 (1953): 219.
65 Mikoyan, *Pishchevaia industriia*, 134.
66 Ibid.
67 Valentina Bogdan, *Mimikriia v SSSR: Vospominaniia inzhenera 1935–1942 gody Rostov-an-Donu* (Frankfurt-am-Main: Possev, 1982), 132, 13.
68 Mikhail German, *Slozhnoe proshedshee* (St. Petersburg: Iskusstvo-SPB, 2000), 143.
69 Ibid., 95.
70 Cited according to Rebecca Manley, *To the Tashkent Station: Evacuation and Survival in the Soviet Union at War* (Ithaca, NY: Cornell University Press, 2012), 265.
71 N. S. Khrushchev, "Rech' na soveshchanii rabotnikov sel'skogo khoziaistva oblasteii i avtonomnykh respublik severo-zapada RSFSR 22 Maia 1957," in

Stroitel'stvo kommunizma v SSSR i razvitie sel'skogo khoziaistva (Moscow: Gosudarstvennoe izdatel'stvo politicheskoii literatury, 1962), 2: 443–4.

72 Steven E. Harris, *Communism on Tomorrow Street: Mass Housing and Everyday Life after Stalin* (Baltimore, MD: Johns Hopkins University Press, 2013), 9.

73 "Obzor pisem v TsK KPSS, v kotorykh ukazyvaetsia na tiazhelye material'nye uslovia v sviazi s ukhudsheniem snabzheniia prodovol'stvennymi tovarami," *Arkhiv Aleksandra Yakovleva*, 2011, http://www.alexanderyakovlev.org/almanah/inside/almanah-doc/1007441 (accessed November 7, 2014).

74 Ibid.

75 N. S. Khrushchev, *Vremia. Liudi. Vlast'* (Moscow: Moskovskie novosti, 1999), 4: 84.

76 William Taubman, *Khrushchev: The Man and His Era* (New York: W. W. Norton and Co., 2003), 372–4 and Roi A. Medvedev, *Khrushchev, the Years in Power* (New York: W. W. Norton and Co., 1978), 123–8.

77 For the history of the riots in Novocherkassk, see Samuel H. Baron, *Bloody Saturday in the Soviet Union: Novocherkassk, 1962* (Stanford, CA: Stanford University Press, 2001) and I. Mardar', *Khronika neobiavlennogo ubiystva* (Novocherkassk: Press-servis, 1992).

78 N. S. Khrushchev, "Za milliard pudov kazakhstanskogo khleba. Rech' na soveshchanii rabotnikov sel'skogo khoziaistva Kazakhskoii SSR, 28 Iulia 1956 goda," in *Stroitel'stvo*, 2: 256–7.

79 *Kramola: Inakomyslie v SSSR pri Khrushcheve i Brezhneve, 1953–1982 gg.*, ed. V. A. Kozlov and S. V. Mironenko (Moscow: Materik, 2005), 262.

80 Yurii Aksiutin, *Khrushchevskaia "ottepel'" i obshchestvennye nastroeniia v SSSR v 1953–1964gg.* (Moscow: ROSSPEN, 2004), 429.

81 *Kramola*, 145.

82 N. Vorob'ev and V. Zhuravskii, "Sto bliud iz kukuruzy," *Pravda*, September 7, 1961 and V. l. Nakariakov, "Meniu iz sta bliud," *Izvestiia*, September 7, 1961.

83 RGAE, f.195, op.1, d.375, ll.64–65. Of all bread consumed in the USSR in 1963, the share of white bread was 70 to 80 percent.

84 Lit. *Russkoe chudo*. Aksiutin, *Khrushchevskaia "ottepel'*, 426–8; RGAE, f.195, op.1, d.375, l.54; Natal'ia Ermolina, "Kino, kuda zhe katitsa ono?" *Respublika Kareliia*, August 29, 2011, http://rk.karelia.ru/2011/08/kino-kuda-zhe-katitsya-ono (accessed September 28, 2011).

85 N. S. Khrushchev, "Bor'ba KPSS za pod"em sel'skogo khoziaistva," in *Stroitel'stvo*, 4:121.

86 Vladimir G. Treml, *Alcohol in the Soviet Underground Economy*, Berkeley-Duke Occasional Papers on the Second Economy in the USSR no.5 (Durham, NC: Duke University Press, 1985), 9; Vladimir G. Treml, *Alcohol in the USSR: A Statistical Study* (Durham, NC: Duke University Press, 1982), 36–45; and Vladimir Voinovich, *Antisovetskii sovetskii soiuz* (Ann Arbor, MI: Ardis, 1985), 27.

87 N. S. Khrushchev, "Prevratim vse sovkhozy v obraztsovye, vysokodokhodnye khoziaistva," in *Stroitel'stvo*, 1: 154.
88 "Rasskaz ob opyte," *Pravda*, December 10, 1961.
89 Antti Häkkinen, "Introduction," in Häkkinen, ed., *Just a Sack of Potatoes*, 13.
90 L.Trushkina, V. Mikhailov, and N. Mogil'nyi, *Eda s appetitom* (Moscow: Molodaia gvardiia, 1989), 1, 4–5, 27–30, 45; and V. Mikhailov and A. Pal'ko, *Vybiraem zdorov'e!* (Moscow: Molodaia gvardiia, 1985), 149, 152.
91 National Research Council, *Premature Death in the New Independent States* (Washington, DC: The National Academies Press, 1997), 327; US Central Intelligence Agency, *A Comparison of the US and Soviet Economies: Evaluating the Performance of the Soviet System, A Reference Aid* (Office of Soviet Analysis, Directorate of Intelligence, October 1985, Released as Sanitized 1999), www.foia.cia.gov, 62–3 (accessed July 14, 2013).
92 Ibid.
93 Raymond E. Zickel, ed., *Soviet Union: A Country Study* (Washington, DC: Federal Research Division Library of Congress, 1991), 532.
94 On the failure of the grain embargo see Robert L. Paarlberg, "Lessons of the Grain Embargo," *Foreign Affairs* 59 (Fall 1980): 144–62.
95 Mikhail Gorbachev, *Memoirs*, trans. Georges Peronansky and Tatjana Varsavsky (New York: Doubleday, 1995), 116–21 and *Prodovol'stvennaia programma SSSR na period do 1990 goda i mery po ee realizatsii: materialy maǐskogo plenuma TSK KPSS, 1982 goda* (Moscow: Izdatel'stvo Politicheskoii Literatury, 1982).
96 John Gooding, "Perestroika as Revolution from within: An Interpretation," *Russian Review* 51 (1992): 38.
97 On Gorbachev's anti-alcohol campaign see Stephen White, *Russia Goes Dry: Alcohol, State and Society* (Cambridge: Cambridge University Press, 1996) and Mark Lawrence Schrad, *Vodka Politics: Alcohol, Autocracy, and the Secret History of the Russian State* (New York: Oxford University Press, 2014), 256–74.
98 "Nauka o pitanii v realizatsii prodovol'stvennoii programmy SSSR," *Voprosy pitaniia* 2 (1983): 3.
99 Ibid., 3–4.
100 "Polnost'iu isspol'zovat' tsennoe belkovoe syr'e dlia proizvodstva vysokokachestvennykh pishchevykh produktov," *Miasnaia industriia SSSR* 1 (1970): 2 and V. Anufriev, "Uluchshenie ispol'zovaniia subproductov, krovi i drugogo pishchevogo syr'ia, poluchaemogo pri pererabotke skota, i uvelichenie za etot schet resursov miasoproduktov," *Misanaia industriia SSSR* 1 (1970): 7, 8.
101 Letter no.8878 From the State Agro-industrial Committee of the Tajik SSR, Box 48, Folder 110A (Letters from readers to Rubinov on Sausage articles), Anatolii Zakharovich Rubinov Papers, 1968–96, European Division, Library of Congress, Washington, DC.
102 A. A. Pokrovskii, "Biokhemicheskie obosnovaniia razrabotki produktov

povyshennoii biologicheskoii tsennosti," *Voprosy pitaniia* 1 (1964): 16, 14; A. A. Pokrovskii et al., "Belkovyi produkt instituts pitaniia AMN SSSR Belip," *Voprosy pitaniia* 2 (1964): 23–4.

103 Lev Zenkevich et al., *Dary moria* (Moscow: Ekonomika, 1968), 10.

104 Irina Petrosian and David Underwood, *Armenian Food: Fact, Fiction & Folklore*, 2nd ed. (Bloomington, IN: Yerkir, 2006), 115 and Liudmila Pletneva, "Nado li vozrozhdat' 'Okeany'?" *Rybak kamchatki*, March 4, 2009.

105 Arnol'd Pushkar', "Okeanskaia niva," *Nedelia* 15 (1982): 5, 21.

106 V. Tolstov, "Tem, kto vyrastil nutriiu," *Izvestiia*, March 31, 1982 and A. Sabirov, "Zachem losiu byt' domshnim," *Izvestiia*, July 14, 1983.

107 Letter no. 10096 from Voronezh and Letter no. 16768 from Perm', Box 48 Folder 110A (Letters from readers to Rubinov on Sausage articles), Rubinov Papers; Nigel Wade, "Russians Shun Ersatz," *Daily Telegraph*, November 14, 1984.

108 Vetkin, *Dnevnik perestroiiki. Bloknot, Proza.ru*, https://www.proza.ru/2014/12/06/1658 (accessed February 26, 2016).

109 Alkesandr Savel'ev "Ot lodki do glotki: rybnomu dniu—80 let," *ProdMag*, http://prodmagazin.ru/2012/09/11/ot-lodki-do-glotki-ryibnomu-dnyu-80-let (accessed August 11, 2014), and "Kukhonnye taiiny: Russkaia eda v Izraile," *Ekho Moskvy*, http://echo.msk.ru/programs/cook-secret/46723 (accessed August 11, 2014).

110 Boris Denisov, "26 Oktiabria 1976 v SSSR poiavilsia rybnyii den'," *Vecherniaia Moskva*, March 23, 2010.

111 Jonathan Steele, "Women: Shop talk on the Streets of Moscow," *The Guardian*, December 13, 1990.

112 See for instance the article and subsequent discussion "Gotovim vymia," *4vkusa.ru*, http://4vkusa.ru/мясные-блюда/14988/готовим-вымя (accessed July 28, 2014).

113 G. Sarkisiants, "Mnogo li cheloveku nado?" *Agitator* 5 (1986), 25. Italics are mine.

114 Ibid., 26.

115 Ibid., 27.

116 "Masteritsa na vse ruki," *Nedelia* 4 (1972), 10.

117 On staying thin and attractive see Iu. Khodosh, "Vasha vesovaia kategoriia," *Sovetskaia kul'tura*, November 22, 1983.

118 Iu. R. Khodosh, *Kul'tura potrebleniia* (Moscow: Izdatel'stvo politicheskoii literatury, 1984), 7.

119 Iuliya Khodosh, "Kak nayti lishnii rubl'," *Nedelia* 5 (1984): 14.

120 Iu. Khodosh, "Ekonomit' li na ede?" *Rabotnitsa* 8 (1985): 1–2 of the supplement.

121 Iu. Khodosh, "Kukhnia, stol, i miliony ili iz chego slagaetsia kul'tura pitaniia," *Izvestiia*, August 30, 1985.

122 Mikhailov and Pal'ko, *Vybiraem zdorov'e!*, rear cover.
123 K. Komarov, "Ushedshee ...," *Obshchestvennoe pitanie* 1 (November 1935), 9.
124 T. Iurkova, "Kak dolzhen pitat'sia satirik?" *Literaturnaia gazeta*, May 13, 1987.
125 Trushkina, Mikahilov, Mogil'nyi, *Eda s appetitom*, 15–6.
126 Ronald LeBlanc, "Vegetarianism in Russia: The Tolstoy(an) Legacy," *The Carl Beck Papers in Russian and East European Studies* 1507 (2001): 24.
127 Natalia Lebina, "Plius destalinizatsiia vseii yedy... (Vkusovye prioretity epokhi khruschevskikh reform: opyt istoriko-antropologicheskogo analiza)," *Teoriia Mody* 21 (Fall 2011): 234.
128 Ilia Foniakov, "Poeziia i kocheryzhka," *Literaturnaia gazeta*, June 5, 1985.
129 P. Tolstoy, "Nu i nu. Dyshite glubzhe: Pakhnet kolbasoy," *Komsomol'skaya Pravda*, August 3, 1990.
130 L. Petrova, "Chto na vashem stole?" *Rabotnitsa* 5 (1990): 21.
131 "K voprosu o vkusnoii i zdorovoii pishche," *Komsomol'skaia pravda*, December 15, 1990.
132 A. Bystrov, "Ispytanie pitaniem," *Pravitel'stvennyi vestnik* 42 (1991): 6.
133 "V RPTs odobriaiut ogranichenie importa, meniaiushchee standarty potrebleniia," *Ria Novosti*, 2014, http://ria.ru/religion/20140807/1019176169.html (accessed August 9, 2014); "Budem zdorovy: Povedenie v zharu," *Ekho Moskvy*, http://www.echo.msk.ru/programs/zdor/1373202-echo (accessed August 9, 2014); Ul'iana Skoiibeda, "Ne v kolbase schast'e," *KP.ru*, http://www.kp.ru/daily/26266/3144781 (accessed August 9, 2014).

CHAPTER NINE

Deafness and the politics of hearing

Claire Shaw

In 1983, the linguist, teacher, and child of deaf parents Iosif Florianovich Geil'man published a brochure about the Leningrad Rehabilitational Center, a vocational school for young deaf adults founded in 1965. The brochure outlined the Center's activities, noting the diverse opportunities open to deaf-Soviet citizens, but it also raised questions about the very nature of deafness. Geil'man remarked that:

> We live in a world of surprisingly diverse sounds. A mother's lullaby, the school bell, the rhythmic drone of the machine or the frightening sound of an alarm bell, the radio transmission and the musical symphony, the rustle of pages and the peal of thunder, the voice of a loved one, a friend, a mentor, a comrade… all these are the companions of our everyday lives, without which life, of course, seems unimaginable. In actual fact, speech, music, and natural sounds, which carry long-lasting and active information, play a significantly important role in the formation of a person's identity, in his creative activity.[1]

For Geil'man, the significance of sound—and of the related phenomenon of hearing and speech—lay in its relationship to the construction and experience of human selfhood. "Hearing ability," as he termed it, allowed individuals to "orientate themselves in space, master spoken language, communicate with those around them, work productively and enjoy their relaxation."[2] This eliding of hearing and speech is not uncommon; as historian Mark M. Smith has argued, histories of hearing have tended to privilege "orality and linguistic sounds over aural, paralinguistic, and non-vocable sounds—the sounds of the mundane and everyday originating outside of the mouth."[3] For Geil'man's deaf students, however, their lack of access to sound represented a "complex problem" that had far-reaching consequences for their lives and identities, and required significant effort and intervention, both technological and educational, to overcome.

At first glance, Geil'man's words are strikingly reminiscent of Western discourses of language, hearing, and deafness that had developed since the Enlightenment, when thinkers began to trace the "interrelations between language, mind and human civilization."[4] Whilst early Enlightenment discourses had explicitly included deaf citizens in their debates on language and the self, and made room for visual and gestural signs as part of their understanding of this linguistic paradigm of humanity (such as the Abbé de L'Épée's famous attempts to "civilize" his deaf students through the use of a "methodical" sign language in the 1760s), the following centuries saw the emergence of a clear sensory hierarchy of language in deaf education. As oral speech came to be understood as superior to the gestured word—the "privilege of man, the sole and certain vehicle of thought, the gift of God"—educators attempted to return deaf individuals' humanity by helping them to master the spoken word, regardless of its difficulty.[5] Following the Milan Congress of 1880, sign language was banned in deaf education throughout Europe and the United States.[6] This dominance of "oralism" (and the oppositional framing of contemporary Deaf identity as rooted in the linguistic community of sign language users) has come to define the struggles and tensions of Western deaf history.[7]

Against this Western historical backdrop, the significance given to oral speech in Geil'man's brochure is perhaps unsurprising; the early education of the deaf in tsarist Russia was driven by German educators, proponents of the "oral method," and Soviet language politics were intimately bound up with Marxism and the rationalist legacies of the European Enlightenment.[8] Yet Geil'man's brochure reveals nuances within the Soviet understanding of hearing and selfhood that complicate this straightforward picture of the valorization of oral speech. Indeed, his explicit focus on sound and the "problem" of deafness belied the strong deaf identity that had developed in Soviet Russia since the Bolshevik Revolution. United within the institutional frameworks of the All-Russian Society of the Deaf (*Vserossiiskoe obshchestvo glukhikh*, VOG), a deaf-run state organization founded in 1926, Soviet deaf people had asserted their identity as equal citizens, working alongside the hearing in all branches of industry and the creative arts.[9] Even as they framed themselves as equal, Soviet deaf citizens celebrated their social and cultural distinctiveness, defined through their visual understanding of the world and celebrated in the widespread use of sign language.[10] This other, visual model of deaf identity is also present, albeit implicitly, in Geil'man's brochure, through references to the widespread use of sign-language interpreting and photographs of happy, confident deaf groups engaging in art and social activities. By advocating this alternative model of sensory perception, deaf people thus called into question the significance of hearing in the construction of Soviet individual and collective selfhood, and challenged the paradigms of sense and self that had emerged in Europe (and beyond) in the preceding centuries.

This chapter will explore the Soviet implications of sound and its lack by examining issues of hearing and speech in the Soviet deaf community. As such, it will engage with the growing scholarly interest in sound and speech as a fundamental and contested part of Soviet constructions of identity, a "sonic turn" that seeks to ground discussions of abstract "subjectivity" in the concrete experience of hearing.[11] Soviet identity, as Stephen Lovell argues, was contingent on the development of a "new orality," through which Soviet citizens could frame themselves as integral members of the new Soviet society.[12] At the same time, however, cultural experiences of silence have been seen to open up pockets of alternative sensory experience in the early Soviet period. As Emma Widdis has shown, experiments with silence and visual formalism in early Soviet film represented a "challenge to speech" that posited new, non-verbal forms of communication.[13] A focus on deafness represents a productive addition to these debates; examining deaf identity and sign-language culture further complicates this binary opposition between "speaking Bolshevik" and "feeling Soviet." Looking at a group of people who, through a quirk of fate, were physically unable to engage with this Soviet culture of sound allows us to test the boundaries of these bigger visions of Soviet identity, and consider the impact of hearing loss on the structures of Soviet selfhood.

This chapter thus seeks to interrogate the complex linkages between sound, speech, and bigger conceptions of identity and selfhood in the Soviet context by looking at the history of the deaf community over the course of the Soviet era, and exploring the tensions which the historical experience of deaf people exposes within the contested narratives of Soviet orality.[14] By focusing on how influential Soviet theorists understood the "tragedy" of deafness, it will explore how Soviet ideology conceptualized sound and speech as fundamental to human experience and development. Yet it will also consider how the deaf community engaged with and challenged such theories, shaping themselves as exemplary Soviet people, and carving out pockets of silent "sovietness" amidst the sound and fury of oral culture. Government attempts to foster a uniform identity amongst its citizens—the figure of the "New Soviet Person"—through social control and state policy represented a type of top-down sensory "biopolitics," traced elsewhere in this volume by Anton Masterovoy. By contrast, the deaf community's bottom-up attempts to redefine Soviet selfhood in line with their own sensory capacities, challenged and complicated established notions of what it meant to be deaf, and to be "Soviet."

The paradoxes of revolutionary hearing

Discussions of hearing, and its lack, began surprisingly early after the Bolshevik Revolution of 1917, in the context of broader discussions on the body and health as matters of "survival, duty and political change."[15] The first congress on disability and child development was held in the midst of Civil War in 1919.[16] In 1924, Lev Semenovich Vygotskii, the "father" of Soviet special education, published a set of scholarly papers in which he set out his understanding of what hearing signified in the new, socialist context.[17] Vygotskii understood hearing not in strict medical terms, but as a social phenomenon, drawing on the ideas of Karl Marx, the behavioral psychologists Vladimir Bekhterev and Ivan Pavlov, and the widespread debates about man and society that characterized the Soviet 1920s. The early Soviet Union was a society with a transformative mission, to turn the "dark" and "backward" peasant masses into "new people"; rational, collectivist individuals who would build and ultimately inhabit the socialist society of tomorrow.[18] Such individuals would be forged primarily through social interaction: as Marx had suggested, "it is not the consciousness of men that determines their existence, but, on the contrary, their social existence that determines their consciousness."[19] Hearing and speech, therefore, were not simply communicative tools, but key to the development of the mind: as Vygotskii put it, "speech is not simply a tool of communication, but a tool of thought; our consciousness develops, for the most part, with the help of speech and emerges from our social sphere."[20]

In this light, hearing loss had significant consequences. Vygotskii saw deaf people's lack of hearing and, by extension, speech, as a direct challenge to Marx's understanding of the individual as shaped by communication. By perceiving and analyzing the world around him, the "normal" child could orientate himself towards his surroundings and develop self-understanding through interaction with his peers. By contrast, deafness, according to Vygotskii "turns out to be the most tragic of disabilities, because it isolates a person from all interaction with people. It deprives him of speech; it cuts him off from social experience."[21] The gravity of deafness, it seems, could not be overstated. In Vygotskii's eyes, a deaf person would have to master lip-reading and oral speech in order to become "Soviet" and gain agency and independence in society. Sign language would not suffice: although Vygotskii recognized sign as "the natural language of deaf-mutes" and said that it would be wrong to ban it entirely (a statement which appears particularly radical after the Milan Congress of 1880), he also dismissed it as "a poor and limited language" which condemned deaf people to life in a narrow social sphere and did not allow for the development of abstract or conceptual thought.[22] Oral speech, however, had the potential to be transformative: he argued that "to teach a deaf-mute to speak means not only to give him the opportunity to communicate with others, but to develop in him consciousness, thought, and self-consciousness."[23]

From Vygotskii's perspective, therefore, the line between sound, speech, and sovietness was easily drawn. Yet the notion of the articulate, communal subject was not the only model of selfhood present in the early Soviet ideological landscape. Early Soviet society also valorized the notion of the independent worker, liberated from capitalist oppression by the Revolution, and overcoming personal obstacles through the will and the transformative power of labor.[24] This vision proved significant for the deaf community. Before 1917, the lives of deaf individuals had been particularly limited; according to Russian Imperial law, the deaf were equated with the insane, deprived of all legal rights, and kept under permanent guardianship. They could apply for the status of "legally competent" and have their guardianship revoked, but only by means of an examination which assessed their written and oral language skills, as well as their logic and reasoning. In a country where hardly any deaf people were educated and the majority of hearing people were illiterate, for most deaf people this obstacle remained insurmountable.

After the Revolution, however, the category of "legal competence" was replaced by that of "labor competence" as a marker of inclusion within the Soviet body politic. This shift in category proved transformative for deaf people. As Vygotskii himself admitted, deafness was not in itself an obstacle to labor: "as a labor apparatus, as a human machine, the body of a deaf-mute barely differs from the body of a normal person and, consequently, a deaf person retains all the fullness of physical possibilities, bodily development, the acquisition of skills and labor abilities."[25] As such, deafness was both the "most tragic" of disabilities, and the "happiest" of disabilities, as deaf people's lack of hearing did not impact on their ability to become workers. In the aftermath of 1917, therefore, and this reconceptualization of "capability," most of the legal restrictions on deaf people were simply swept away. Deaf people gained the right to work, to vote, and to stand for election to local Soviets: the first deaf deputy, Evgenii Zhuromskii, was elected in Petersburg in 1918.[26] In 1926, VOG, the deaf-run government organization which would oversee all aspects of deaf people's lives until the collapse of the Soviet Union, was finally established. With its network of grassroots deaf clubs, industrial training workshops, and deaf educational and cultural spaces, VOG provided the foundation of a lively, institutionalized form of "deaf space" that shaped Soviet deaf people's lives.[27]

Within this push towards labor and independence, conceptions of hearing and speech inevitably became more nuanced. As deaf people entered the factories and proved themselves competent laborers, they began to actively question the ideological predominance of hearing and oral speech. In 1921, for example, in the build-up to the creation of the national deaf society, deaf representatives met with state educators to debate the issue of speech in schools. The deaf delegation pointed out that the oral method of education took six to seven years, and yet the deaf masses wanted to enter the factories immediately: "We have the power to work and to lead. According to the constitution all workers must work, with the exception of prisoners; deaf-mutes can work too, and they want to help their brothers."[28] Learning to speak took far too long, given the pressing need to start building the new Soviet industrial infrastructure; far better, they argued, to learn literacy and labor skills immediately and to use sign language where necessary as a practical tool of instruction. Indeed, in the context of early factory culture, deafness was often viewed as a positive attribute, with deaf workers able to communicate easily over the din of machinery and, by taking jobs in the "noisy shops" of the factory, to protect the ears of hearing workers from noise-induced hearing damage.[29] In light of this, as delegation leader Savel'ev asserted, the insistence on oral speech represented a "fundamental difference of opinion" with hearing government workers.[30]

The early Soviet period thus saw a tension between two separate but interrelated paradigms of Soviet identity: on the one hand the independent worker (a vision dependent on notions of the body and the plastic gesture) and on the other the articulate, speaking subject.[31] This tension manifested itself in rather confused attitudes to speech and sign language on the ground. In the workplace, which saw a massive influx of deaf industrial workers both before and during Stalin's first Five-Year Plan, sign language was increasingly relied upon—and indeed promoted by the state—as a tool to facilitate deaf labor. Deaf industrial brigades were served by a sign-language instructor-interpreter, provided by the deaf society and funded by the state, who used sign language as a tool of training and day-to-day communication. In fact, it could be argued that urbanization and the Stalinist industrial revolution were the primary driving forces in the development of a Soviet sign language and Soviet deaf community. Most deaf people at the start of the 1920s did not sign, but were required to learn basic sign language to enter the factory: as one deaf worker pointed out, "if a person comes from the countryside, it is necessary to teach him sign language first, so that he knows city sign."[32] As such, the Soviet state was in many ways facilitating the creation of a Soviet sign language. This sign language was initially localized and dialect-driven, but thanks to the developing social networks put into place by VOG activists, both within and outside Soviet Russia, deaf citizens from across the USSR were increasingly able to understand each other.[33] At the same time, however, Soviet educational and psychological theory continued to stress the paucity of sign language, and its unsuitability as a language of culture and communication, with the Soviet education system banning sign in the classroom for most of the Soviet era.[34] Tellingly, however, both the Soviet state and the deaf community itself continued to employ the term "deaf-mute," accepting the essential nature of deaf people's silence even in the face of educational intervention.

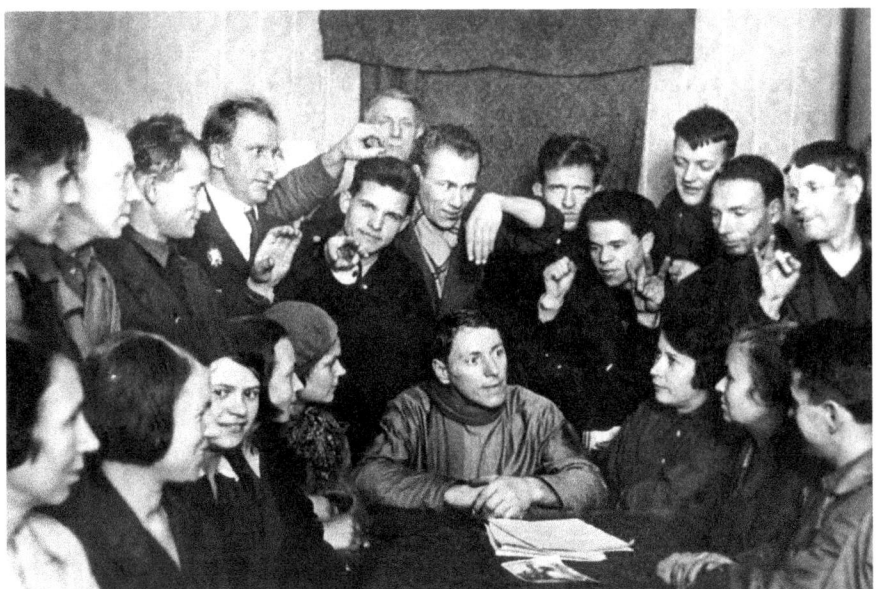

FIGURE 9.1 *A meeting of deaf workers of the "Paris Commune" factory with the Stakhanovite Smetanin in 1935. The men are fingerspelling his name. Courtesy of Viktor Palennyi of the All-Russian Society of the Deaf.*

From the outset, therefore, Soviet attitudes to speech and sign language were complicated. In a society such as the USSR, complicated attitudes inevitably had ideological implications. It soon became clear that the ambiguous position of sign language could lead to it being viewed as politically suspect. In 1929, Anatolii Lunacharskii, the first Commissar of Enlightenment, gave a speech to the Second All-Russian Congress of Deaf-Mutes. This speech was remembered by the deaf activists present as positive and utopian in its attitude to deafness, but, to a contemporary reader, it seems deeply ambivalent towards signing and the deaf.[35] Lunacharskii used deafness as a metaphor for selfishness and egotism, cardinal sins in a socialist society: "in this business, in our fight against muteness, I see a sort of sign, a symbol of our general battle against human unresponsiveness. ... He who thinks only of himself is deaf. He who does not unite in a single thought and action with his brother people is deaf."[36] Like Vygotskii, whom he quoted at length, Lunacharskii agreed that teaching oral speech to the deaf would allow them to overcome their isolation and re-enter the Soviet community. His use of language was telling; learning to speak, he argued, would allow the deaf to become "*like* living people"—only ever "fellow travelers" on the road towards communism.[37]

It is important to note that no matter the ideological complications, Soviet state officials never suggested that deaf people should be excluded from society. The practical and symbolic integration of deaf people into the Soviet collective of laboring people was seen as an achievable goal; a goal that would prove the Soviet Union's status as the world's most progressive and most humane society. In this respect, deafness was no more of a problem than peasant "backwardness," a practical obstacle that could be "overcome" through hard work and education. Strikingly, the insistence on viewing deafness as a social, rather than a medical, problem meant that eugenicist theories were never applied to deafness in the Soviet context, in stark contrast to policies of treatment, sterilization, and euthanasia enacted across the "Eugenic Atlantic" to minimize the incidence of genetic deafness.[38] Marriage between deaf people was never banned in the USSR, and memoirs have shown that deaf intermarriage was common throughout the Soviet period, with hearing children of such marriages often integrated into the deaf community as sign-language interpreters.[39] There were occasional moments where suspicions about deaf people came to a head, such as during the great purge of 1937, when a group of deaf society activists in Leningrad were arrested and sentenced for being German spies. Whilst this case was driven by existing contacts between the Leningrad Oblast branch of VOG and a group of deaf German refugees, the ambiguity and seeming secretiveness of the plastic gesture served to exacerbate the perception of the deaf as "other."[40] There was never a moment, however, when the deaf were the target of state repression simply for being deaf (as they were in Nazi Germany).[41]

Yet the very idea that deafness had to be "overcome," and that speech had to be "mastered" in order for deaf people to become Soviet did have an inevitable impact on how they were seen by the state and by wider society. There were often suggestions that deaf people were inherently "backward"—that like women or peasants they had considerably further to go to join the "first ranks" of the Soviet proletariat—and it was very easy for that thinking to slip over into a belief that deaf people, particularly signing deaf people, might not be able to "overcome" at all. Stalin himself would underline this interpretation in 1951, when on the pages of *Pravda* he dismissed "deaf-mutes, having no language" as "abnormal people." For Stalin, spoken language was an indicator of progress, and its lack inevitably marginalized deaf people within society.[42] Whilst sign language could be tolerated as a tool of labor, it would never, he implied, be an acceptable language of communication for a conscious, Soviet citizen.

Rethinking sign language

Stalin's intervention in sign-language politics framed sign—and, by extension, the visual—as a poor and imperfect substitute for hearing and speech. It would be tempting, therefore, to see the widespread use of sign language within the Soviet deaf community as evidence of resistance to an overbearing state. An exploration of the use of sign language and its symbolic meanings, however, reveals the deaf community's attempt to reconceptualize sign as a language of Soviet expression, borrowing the language of logocentrism and "culturedness" to remake the visual as inherently Soviet. As early as the 1920s, the use of sign as a marker of sovietness was implicit in articles within the deaf press, with young deaf people portrayed "carrying out lively debates amongst themselves" and singing "The Internationale" in sign language.[43] In 1936, the Saratov newspaper *Young Stalinist* published an article about one Petr Spiridonov, a young deaf man from the Volga region who found success as a Stakhanovite safe-maker.[44] Through a sign-language interpreter, Spiridonov described his successes and the benefits he enjoyed as a leading industrial worker. At the end of the interview, "the Brigadier-Stakhanovite, with special expressiveness, signed the phrase: 'Life has become better, life has become more joyous.' Having made sure that we understood him, he headed for his brigade in the depths of the workshop, from where the clatter and clang of metal could be heard."[45] By "signing Bolshevik" in this way, Spiridonov and his interviewer underlined the expressiveness and ideological orthodoxy of sign.

It was after the Second World War, however, that sign language and the visual finally came into their own, as both a means of expression and marker of sovietness. The Thaw era, in particular, became known as the "golden age" of the Soviet deaf community, with the development of new forms of artistic creativity allowing the deaf to posit a new sensory model of being.[46] New deaf institutions, such as the VOG Studio of Fine and Applied Arts in Leningrad, and the Theatre of Sign and Gesture (TMZh) in Moscow, showcased the silent, visual creativity of the deaf community.[47] Following an exhibition of deaf fine art in 1958, for example, the reviewer V. Sungarin commented that "here there is much that is typical and characteristic of the work of those people who live through the visual perception of the world. This is above all the prevalence of cheerful, life-affirming tones. Our artists do not love gloom."[48] Through the TMZh, in particular, the expressive ability of sign as a silent, visual medium, and its capability of transmitting high artistic content was underlined. The notion of the eloquence of silence was central to these debates: deaf theater practitioners referenced Greek mime and contemporary mime experiments on the Soviet stage, as well as a visit to the USSR by Marcel Marceau in 1959, to demonstrate the solid cultural foundations of this new, sign-language-based art form. They contrasted speech and sign, with sign itself often portrayed as the richer and more cultured language; one article praised the theater for the "great labor of their transformation of words into gesture ... which unexpectedly proved to be stronger, more effective and more voluminous than speech."[49] Notions of art and silence, therefore, represented a new framework of selfhood for the deaf community, positing visual, affective performance as an alternative to spoken language and rationality.

The significance of silent theater was also seen to lie in its derivation from the everyday communicative experiences of deaf people: "Our mime must not and cannot be a cold copy of classical art. It grows out of life itself, as a distinctive art of the masses."[50] As such, it framed itself within the debates on democracy and grassroots activity that characterized the Khrushchev era. Yet sign also derived much legitimacy from the growing power of the deaf community. In the aftermath of the Second World War, during which deaf laborers had played a vital role in evacuating Soviet armaments factories behind the Urals and keeping them running throughout the turbulent war years, the leadership of VOG had begun a fundamental restructuring and strengthening of all services for deaf people. This included the re-establishment of a vast network of deaf clubs and trade union organizations; deaf recruitment in heavy and skilled industry and agriculture, further education in night schools, workers faculties, and technical universities, deaf theaters, deaf housing, and even investment in new technologies such as hearing aids and movie subtitling. As part of this restructuring, the society overhauled its system of deaf-run industrial workshops: so successfully, in fact, that from 1954 the organization was making enough money to refuse all further financial support from the state, and from the early 1960s, it was able to give money *to* the state to build and equip deaf schools. In the context of this burgeoning, institutionalized deaf community—which served as proof, deaf activists argued, of the inherent capabilities of deaf people—it became increasingly possible for the deaf to mount a spirited defense of sign language and visual selfhood against Stalin's charges.

The 1950s and 1960s saw a reconceptualization of sign language, from a tool born of "bitter necessity," as it had been referred to in the 1930s, to a language of high culture and capability. Sign language had been a lived reality and a unifying factor for the deaf since 1917; it now needed to become a marker of sovietness. In many ways, this reconceptualization was simply a matter of sign basking in the reflected glory of deaf people's successes. Propaganda pamphlets produced by the deaf society detailed the heights to which Soviet deaf individuals had risen.[51] The majority of deaf people worked in skilled industry and agriculture, with many winning coveted state medals for production. There were deaf engineers, designers, skilled metalworkers, chemists, sculptors, historians, lecturers, doctors, and physicists.[52] A deaf engineer, Sergei Usachev, worked in the team that sent the world's first artificial satellite, Sputnik I, into space in 1957.[53] The vast majority of these workers used sign language in their everyday working practice, relying on the services of an instructor-interpreter to communicate with their co-workers. The link was thus made between the high achievements of deaf people and their use—and celebration—of sign.

Alongside this burgeoning sense of deaf cultural power, the postwar period saw the framing of sign language in explicitly linguistic terms. Much of this shift was driven by the work of Iosif Geil'man, who published the first dictionary of sign language in 1957: a watershed moment in the re-evaluation of sign. In his introduction, he underlined that sign language was both a "means of communication" and a "tool of the embodiment of thought," thus aligning sign with other, spoken languages.[54] The deaf society's monthly magazine, *Life of the Deaf* was regularly given over to polemical debates on sign-vs-speech, with readers increasingly writing in to argue that sign language was "vitally necessary" and should be recognized as a language in its own right.[55] This explicit alignment of sign and speech was problematic, however, as it continued to define the sensory value of sign in reference to the dominant logocentric framework of Soviet selfhood and to posit sign as in some way an inferior variant of speech. For many, the importance of oral speech to Soviet society made this celebration of sign language dangerous: as one letter writer pointed out, "sign language holds deaf people back, discouraging them, as with a Chinese wall, from real knowledge of language."[56]

To combat this reading of sign language as inferior, deaf activists and scholars employed certain mediating practices in order to make sign language more ideologically acceptable. One of these was the concept of "cultured sign language," which began to appear in discussions of sign language in the mid-1950s. Cultured sign was seen as a progressive corrective to the "crude, distorted forms of sign" that were frequently used by deaf people in everyday conversation. In contrast to the "rude, vulgar ... ugly gestures" that characterized much colloquial sign-language conversation, cultured sign was articulate, rich in vocabulary, and graceful and controlled in its movements.[57] As literary scholar Catriona Kelly has pointed out, the notion of "cultured speech" was much discussed in the late 1950s and early 1960s, as sociolinguists began to formulate the links between the fostering of an abstract Soviet "consciousness" and the normative rules of linguistic etiquette.[58] The use of this term indicated that many deaf people, particularly VOG activists, sought to rework and reformulate the language in order to transform both the behavior and thought processes of its users. At the same time, the use of the term "cultured" referenced discourses that had permeated Soviet social norms from the Stalin era, showing an ambition amongst deaf people to write themselves into the narratives of Soviet high culture.

A pamphlet produced by VOG in 1958 explained the distinction between "cultured" sign and its inferior opposite "simple" or "natural sign."[59] As the author Dmitriev explained, "simple sign" referred to colloquial sign language that had developed organically and not been influenced in any way by a knowledge of spoken Russian. This language, Dmitriev pointed out, was "the most primitive and imperfect means of communication, peculiar to those deaf-mutes who either have not mastered spoken language (of whom, by the way, there are few), or master language to an insufficient level (of whom there are quite many)."[60] In an echo of Stalin's condemnation, "simple" sign language was seen to be incapable of transmitting "abstract concepts ... with the exception of the simplest concepts such as 'good,' 'bad,' 'easy,' 'hard'." By contrast, the author stated:

> in order to raise the educational level of deaf-mutes, simple sign is slowly giving way to a more perfect sign language—cultured, or literal, sign, which is based on spoken language. Whilst this sign language does not yet represent the grammatical forms and syntactical levels of speech, it is significantly richer than simple sign, and with its help it is possible to represent the majority of abstract concepts. Therefore cultured sign more-or-less successfully replaces oral speech, especially when it is combined with lip reading and fingerspelling.[61]

By using the term "cultured sign" Soviet deaf people were able to bridge the rhetorical gap between condemnations of sign by Soviet ideologues, and its everyday use, and even celebration, by the deaf. Whilst "simple" or "natural" sign language might still be considered "backward," the promise of cultured sign allowed deaf people to reclaim sign as a Soviet language and recast the visual as a complex and nuanced means of communication.

Beyond the rhetorical promise of cultured sign, the reality of this impulse to manipulate sign to conform to the patterns of spoken Russian was deeply problematic, often undermining the communicative value of the language itself. In the utopian vein of the early 1960s, attempts were made to develop new forms of sign on the stage of the TMZh, where the hearing-dominated audience and the tradition of using announcers to dub the sign language of its actors, created a particularly fertile arena for linguistic experimentation. According to its founders, the TMZh was always intended to become "a school of correct, precise, and colorful language."[62] In practice, however, the use of cultured sign appealed to the aesthetic values of hearing, rather than deaf audiences, producing performances that were profoundly alienating. Footage of "cultured" sign on stage can be seen in Mikhail Bogin's 1965 film *The Two*, which features a scene from the theater's production of *Romeo and Juliet* starring the real life deaf actors Marta Grakhova and Valerii Liubimov. The film clearly shows the attempts to align the spoken language of the "announcers" with the sign of the actors, the reliance on "voicing" and fingerspelling, and the attempts to limit the scope of the signs and give them a controlled, graceful flow. The film, and other performances by the TMZh, was a big hit with hearing audiences; for the deaf, however, the "calque" language seen on the stage was often incomprehensible.[63] Far from positing a new model of sensory selfhood that celebrated the silent and the visual, discussions of sign language in the late Soviet era had the result of reinforcing logocentrism and orality (even within the very structures of sign itself) as the predominant path to sovietness.

It is very difficult to establish whether "cultured sign" ever became a lived reality beyond the pages of VOG pamphlets or the stage of the TMZh. Equally, the attempts to discredit "simple" sign appear to have had little impact on the widespread use of sign within the deaf community, with the further institutionalization of sign-language interpretation in the 1960s absolving deaf people of the need to speak in the vast majority of their interactions with the hearing world, from the workplace, to the courts, and the doctor's surgery.[64] As the mother of a deaf child complained in 1961, her daughter had learned to speak at school, but following graduation "she attempts to avoid speech" and "has even started to get angry at me for not speaking to her in sign."[65] Yet the attempts by the deaf community to frame sign language and the visual as an alternative model of Soviet communication practice revealed complex ideological and practical tensions. VOG promoted sign language as a language of culture and high art, whilst at the same time bemoaning the vulgarity of its colloquial forms. They promoted sign language on the stage, but they overlaid it with dubbed speech, and pushed it increasingly to conform to the vocabulary and patterns of spoken Russian, in order to appeal to hearing audiences, with the result that, by the 1970s, the deaf community were increasingly complaining that the plays were incomprehensible and that the theater "does not serve us."[66] The inability of the deaf community to find an ideological vocabulary for sign language that could explain its worth in its own terms ultimately undermined its position in Soviet deaf culture.

Technology and the return of hearingness

Whilst the ideological meaning of sign remained contested in the Thaw era, the practical usefulness of sign for the deaf community, and their need to rely on visual forms of culture and propaganda, was never called into question. In the context of the "scientific-technological revolution" of the Brezhnev era, however, the essential nature of hearing loss again became open to debate. In 1973, the magazine *Life of the Deaf* published an article praising the new hearing aids that had been introduced in the USSR. As a result of these aids, the author Gushev pointed out, scientists had proved that many of those children whom they had assumed were profoundly deaf had some residual hearing that could be amplified. For those conducting these experiments, this discovery had changed the very meaning of deafness. Far from dividing the world into the deaf and the hearing, scientists now claimed that "between deafness and hearing loss there is no clear line. The boundary is in many ways relative."[67] Through technology, the "miraculous world of sounds" could be made accessible to the deaf, too, challenging the assumption that "if you are deaf, you can't hear. That's the rule."[68]

In many ways, hearing aids represent an awkward footnote to Soviet deaf history. The first aids were introduced in the 1930s, but thanks to the vagaries of the command-distribution system, it remained very difficult to acquire and fit a suitable aid or to supply it with batteries on a regular basis: an instruction pamphlet from 1940 explained how to modify torch batteries for use with hearing aids.[69] In 1953, free access to hearing aids was guaranteed to all Soviet citizens by the Ministry of Social Welfare, yet attempts to develop Soviet mass-produced hearing aids were continually thwarted by the supply of materials. Moves by VOG to establish its own hearing aid laboratory were similarly unsuccessful.[70] In the 1970s, imported hearing aids from Yugoslavia and from the Danish firm Oticon improved matters considerably.[71] Yet for ordinary Soviet deaf citizens, hearing aids never became an object of everyday use. According to a survey conducted by the Moscow branch of VOG in 1978, only two of the ninety late-deafened and deaf individuals who completed the questionnaire, and six of the sixty hard-of-hearing respondents, regularly used a hearing aid.[72]

For such a peripheral technology, the hearing aid had significant theoretical and ideological implications. In the 1950s and 1960s, the promise of free hearing aids for every Soviet citizen regardless of their level of income was used as a key weapon in the deaf Cold War; foreign visitors to the USSR were often offered hearing aids during their visit, and aids would be sent abroad to needy comrades in China and India.[73] In the 1970s, the rhetorical value of hearing aids lay in their ability to transform deafness from a biological reality into a temporary state requiring technological intervention. No longer did deafness represent an obstacle to be overcome through education and individual willpower, or a challenge to reconfigure the sensory experience of the world. Instead, deaf people were recast as temporarily or partially "non-hearing" open to the intervention of specialists who had the technological ability to cure their sensory lack.

The introduction of hearing aid technology thus had far-reaching consequences for the understanding of deafness, speech, and Soviet identity. Deafness had emerged in the Thaw era as a visual and cultural identity; with the advent of hearing aids, deaf people were again viewed as passive objects of specialist intervention in the hope of returning them to the "norm" of speech and hearing.[74] In 1965, Geil'man opened the Leningrad Rehabilitational Center (LVTs), a vocational college for deaf citizens of the RSFSR, tasked with the "cure, education and professional training and retraining" of deaf people through which "defect will be overcome in practice, and a [deaf] person will receive a 'start in life'."[75] By 1983, the year of Geil'man's celebratory brochure on the LVTs, this overcoming of deafness "in practice" had come to signify the mastery of spoken language, which would, in Geil'man's words, represent "the 'golden key' [which] opens the way to knowledge, to abstract thought, to active work."[76] This, for Geil'man, represented a stark departure from his earlier celebration of sign as a complex and valuable form of communication. Indeed, the LVTs recast sign as a stepping stone to speech: "It is expedient for organizations of the deaf society to attract qualified interpreters to work in their speech and language surgeries. They serve as social workers in collectives of non-hearing people, carrying out their noble mission."[77]

For many deaf people, this promise of the return of hearing and speech represented a positive step. Deaf publications in the early 1980s continued to refer to deafness as a "tragedy" that deprived an individual of the ability to communicate with those around them and lead fulfilled lives.[78] Education, medicine, and technology promised to mitigate this tragedy and remake deaf people as "full citizens of the state." This was certainly not an easy or straightforward process; as Geil'man pointed out, graduates of the LVTs had traveled a "difficult, long path for many years" in order to gain speech ability and remake themselves as "citizens."[79] Yet, rhetorically at least, the power of science to return deaf people to "hearingness" allowed them to resolve the tensions implicit in the Soviet discourse of sign language between the ambiguity of the visual and the ideological clarity of spoken and written language.[80]

The rejection of sign and the reassertion of hearing and speech as the standard model of Soviet selfhood could not help but raise questions about the identity of deaf citizens who communicated in sign language. One of the dominant cultural models through which such questions were explored in the early 1980s was that of Rudyard Kipling's *The Jungle Book*, particularly its hero Mowgli, the little boy who was raised by wolves and thus remained unexposed to human language. A publication on deafness from 1984 challenged the "fantastic" narrative of Mowgli's return to speech and civilization after his lupine childhood:

> Unfortunately, we must consider [Mowgli] to be a beautiful fantasy. In all those cases known to science in which it has been possible to return children who have grown up amongst animals to human society, the mastery of a few words was only possible for those who were no older than five years. For children aged nine to ten it was not only speech that was inaccessible. It was even hard for them to learn to stop walking on all fours.[81]

This dismissal of the "uncultured" behavior of wild children echoed those of two centuries earlier in France, when the feral child Victor, the "Wild Boy of Aveyron," was discovered in the woods outside Paris and taken in by specialists at the National Institute of Deaf-Mutes, who attempted unsuccessfully to return him to society by teaching him language and reason.[82] The Enlightenment overtones of such narratives were clear; only by mastering oral speech and hearing-like behavior could an individual be considered a fully-fledged member of society: "a person's intellect is directly linked to speech, to vocabulary, to their ability to think literally and abstractly."[83] Whilst neither Mowgli nor Victor were deaf, the implication of their narratives was clear: without speech, an individual would always remain beyond the bounds of society.

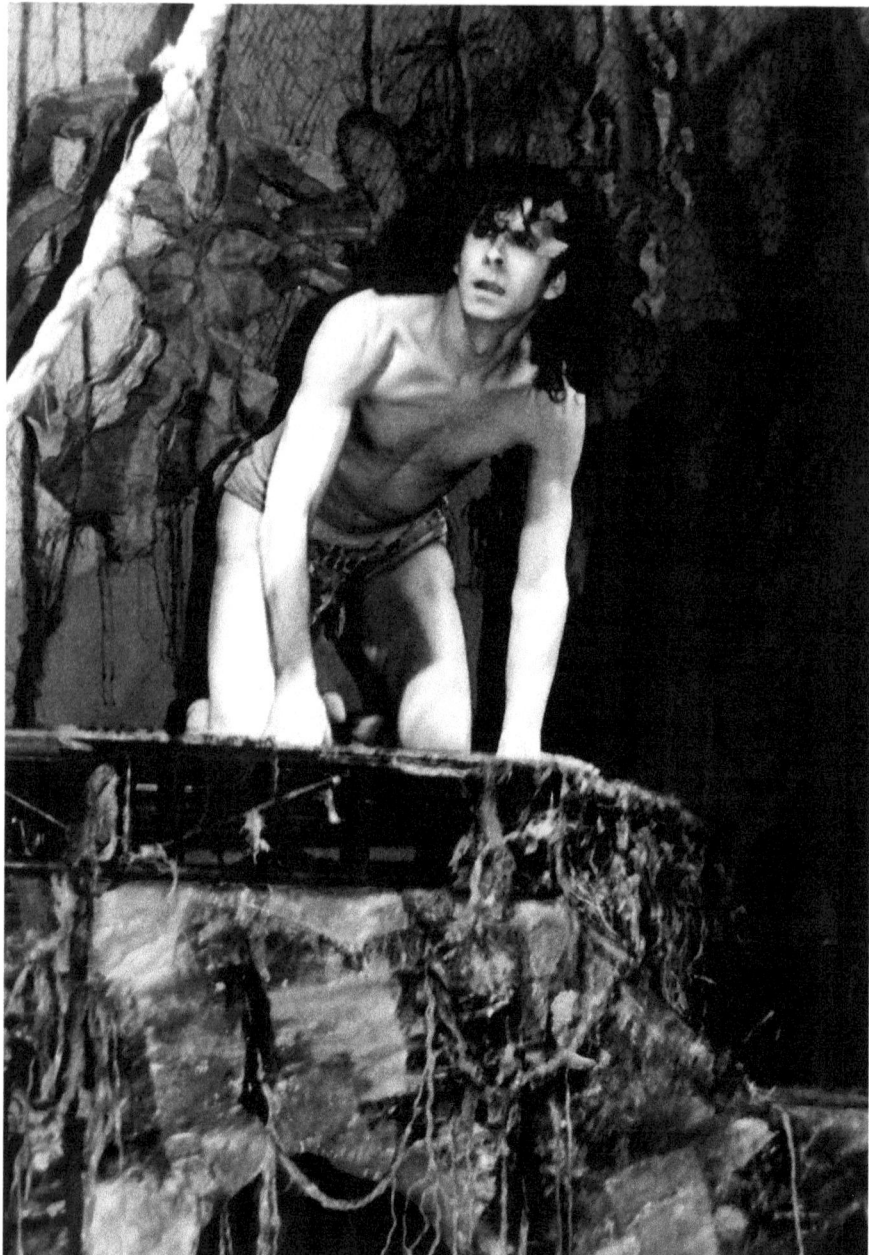

FIGURE 9.2 *Actor M. Muzafarov in the role of Mowgli. Theatre of Sign and Gesture, Moscow, 1982. Courtesy of Viktor Palennyi of the All-Russian Society of the Deaf.*

Within the deaf community, however, the ambiguities of this logocentric model of selfhood continued to be exposed. The sign-language play *Mowgli*, based on Kipling's book, was premiered by the TMZh in 1982, going on to break all records for audience attendance.[84] The deaf actor Mudaris Zagirovich Muzafarov portrayed Mowgli, through sign language and mime, as childlike, playful, yet also fiercely moral, defending the animals of the jungle from the forces of evil. Reviews of the play noted the narrative arc, which traces Mowgli's transformation from a "tiny, silly human" to the "apotheosis of a rational, thinking person, a person who protects the weak and upholds the good."[85] The notion of the visual as offering an alternative path to sovietness continued to surface in discussions of the TMZh; as the hearing director A. V. Mekke confirmed in 1989: "In a sphere where the visual perception of the world and the visual method of communication is predominant, the theater offers the most varied possibilities for moral and ethical perfecting of a personality, experience of the surrounding world, education, or even simply entertainment, without which the life of any person could barely be considered full."[86] Such discussions continued to underline the creative potential of sign-language performance, particularly in the creation of characters who are "strong, courageous personalities, capable of overcoming all difficulties that are caused by their physical ailment; personalities who have learned to live in this world that is difficult, but full of life."[87] The artistic and everyday use of sign was far from curtailed in this period; indeed, many linguists continued to advocate for the use of sign language in the classroom, and its practical significance for the lives of ordinary deaf citizens remained constant.

The implication that a lack of speech was a step away from savagery was telling, however, particularly in relation to how deafness was viewed both by wider society and by the deaf community itself. Mowgli represented an overt portrayal of a silent, signing "savage" on the stage, albeit one whose moral values conformed to Soviet codes. Other performances by the theater underlined the confusion and ideological ambiguity engendered by lack of speech and a reliance on the visual. As Anastasia Kayiatos has pointed out in her analysis of the "speechless pantomime" *Enchanted Island* premiered by the TMZh in 1972, the experience of silent, affective performance on the stage, with its elements of queer and drag, called forth confused and angry responses from Soviet hearing audiences: "What is it? What's it about? What's the use?"[88] Performances by the TMZh showed that the plasticity of the body and the ambiguity of the visual had no place in a society that was moving towards, as Aleksei Yurchak puts it, a "hegemony of form" under late socialism. The silence of deaf performers thus recast them as marginal within Soviet society: in Kayiatos's words, "socialism's silent others: the queer and the deaf, the unspeakable and the unspeaking, respectively."[89]

Mowgli and the silent actors of *Enchanted Island* represented the very few identifiably "different" characters to be portrayed on the stage of the TMZh, where dubbed performances of the "classics" of Shakespeare and

Ostrovskii continued to predominate. As Mekke pointed out, there were very few recognizably "deaf" stories portrayed by the theater, as "many deaf people consider the fate of hearing people to be an unachievable ideal, and therefore by experiencing the fate of a hearing person in the theater, a deaf person can in a sense come nearer to it. For non-hearing people are often ashamed of their deafness and consider that their life should not be the subject of theatrical art."[90] Reviewers of the TMZh often noted the "skill" with which deaf actors feigned hearingness on the stage, responding to auditory signals or dancing rhythmically to music.[91] The notion that hearing represented the "norm" of Soviet selfhood thus had the result of recasting deafness, and the celebration of the visual and silent sensory, as its anti-Soviet other. It is perhaps not surprising that mainstream cultural and social understandings of deafness continued to equate the deaf with the insane, a throwback to the oppressive tsarist laws that the Soviet deaf community had fought so hard to overcome. Similarly, the ideological and cultural ambiguities surrounding sign language explain the fact, noted by Anna Komarova and Michael Pursglove, that "Russian has no established terms for 'deaf culture,' 'deaf awareness,' 'deaf identity,' 'deaf pride,' or 'deaf heritage'."[92] The notion that deaf people could take pride in the visual framing of their own self-identity could not compete with the dominant cultural figure of the Soviet speaking (and hearing) subject.

Conclusion

The history of the deaf community reveals tensions and complexities in how sensory perception was understood, in both practical and ideological terms, during the Soviet era. It was all very well to point out, as Viktor Krainin did in 1984, that "over 98% of information about the outside world is carried by sight, and only about 2% by hearing."[93] In the Soviet sensory hierarchy, hearing and speech, with their ability to foster communication, orientate the self in their surroundings, and facilitate the learning of written language, were placed definitively above the visual. Whilst the context of theoretical discussions shifted, from the utopian social welfare debates of the 1920s, through Stalin's linguistic interventions of the 1950s, to the growth of "surdo-technology" in the 1970s, the fundamental enlightenment belief in language and speech as fundamental to the rational Soviet mind remained consistent. A lack of hearing thus remained an obstacle to the ideological existence of Soviet deaf subjects.

Yet the continued presence of sign-language culture within the deaf community, despite its problematic ideological status, hinted at the existence of experiences and selves beyond the standardized, logocentric Soviet person. These pockets of visual culture, which were consistently facilitated by the Soviet state, suggest that whilst logocentrism remained ideologically dominant, visual perception also had its place in the Soviet sensory imaginary. The Thaw, in particular, with its fostering of alternative forms of culture and communication, laid the groundwork for the flourishing of silent theater and the rediscovery of deafness. Yet the use of sign both predated and outlived the cultural moment of the Thaw, and the value of the visual in the creation of the Soviet self remained a consistent point of discussion. This consistency was in many ways pragmatic; the practical value of visual communication and the flourishing of silent cultural forms for the deaf community ensured their continued use throughout the Soviet era. Beyond this, however, Soviet deaf individuals sought to reframe the visual in Soviet terms to legitimize their place in Soviet society. Their efforts proved partial, problematic, and frequently borrowed the language of logocentrism to validate deaf culture in linguistic terms. Yet these ideological rewritings of sensory experience demonstrated the limitations of a model of selfhood posited on speech and hearing to the exclusion of other realms of perception.

The link between language and selfhood was never unproblematic for Soviet deaf citizens, therefore, in a way that has resonances for Soviet society as a whole. For many deaf people, sign language was a path to sovietness—a means to become workers, to overcome backwardness, and to gain independence and agency—and in the 1950s and 1960s, this hybrid deaf-Soviet identity became prominent. Visual experiences of the world, which formed the sensory foundation of Soviet deaf people's individual and collective self-understanding, were unpacked and explored, particularly in the 1950s, in an attempt to posit an alternative model to the Soviet-speaking subject. Yet the ideological ambiguities of sign, and the privileging of the voice and the ear in Soviet culture, mean that for many deaf people, sign and the visual were not unequivocally positive. In this respect, the experience of the deaf community showed how "marginal" identity coexisted and interacted with dominant Soviet practices of shaping and forming the self. Sign language in the Soviet Union was at the same time a lived reality, a marker of sovietness, and a threat to it. This ideological Gordian knot was finally cut in the mid-1970s by the advent of technological innovations, which suddenly—on paper, at least—made "hearingness" accessible to almost all deaf citizens. In the aftermath of this seismic shift, discussion of sign was significantly limited, and people like Geil'man could claim, in a brochure aimed at deaf people, that "sound is what makes us human." The history of the signing deaf community thus betrays the complexities inherent in Soviet understandings of sound, speech, and identity, and problematizes the relationship of imperfect individuals to the Soviet "project."

Notes

1. I. F. Geil'man, *Leningradskii vosstanovitel'nyi tsentr VOG* (Leningrad: Leningradskii vosstanovitel'nyi tsentr VOG, 1983), 3.
2. Ibid.
3. Mark M. Smith, *Sensing the Past: Seeing, Hearing, Smelling, Tasting, and Touching in History* (Berkeley: University of California Press, 2007), 41.
4. Avi Lifschitz, *Language and Enlightenment: The Berlin Debates of the Eighteenth Century* (Oxford: Oxford University Press, 2012), 1. See also Matthew Lauzon, *Signs of Light: French and British Theories of Linguistic Communication, 1648–1789* (Ithaca, NY: Cornell University Press, 2010). Geil'man's words are also indebted to a contemporaneous British publication, which suggested that as deaf people "live within a world of sound but are not fully part of that world," they can best be categorized as "outsiders in a hearing world." Paul C. Higgins, *Outsiders in a Hearing World: A Sociology of Deafness* (Beverly Hills, CA: Sage, 1980), 22.
5. Augusto Zucchi, cited in Harlan Lane, *When the Mind Hears: A History of the Deaf* (New York: Random House, 1984), 392.
6. On de l'Épée, see Sophia Rosenfeld, "The Political Uses of Sign Language: The Case of the French Revolution," *Sign Language Studies* 6 (1) (Fall 2005). Rosenfeld traces a slightly different hierarchy of the senses in the hearing world, in which "the empiricism of the eye" was valued more highly than "the ostensibly more subjective, more spiritual, and, ultimately, more primal ear." Sophia Rosenfeld, "On Being Heard: A Case for Paying Attention to the Historical Ear," *American Historical Review* 116 (April 2011): 321.
7. On language and the Deaf community, see Carol Padden and Tom Humphries, *Deaf in America: Stories from a Culture* (Cambridge, MA: Harvard University Press, 1988).
8. On late-imperial deaf education, see Howard G. Williams, "Founders of Deaf Education in Russia," in *Deaf History Unveiled: Interpretations from the New Scholarship*, ed. John Vickrey Van Cleve (Washington, D.C.: Gallaudet University Press, 1993), 224–36. On Marxism and Enlightenment rationalism, see David L. Hoffmann, *Stalinist Values: The Cultural Norms of Soviet Modernity, 1917–1941* (Ithaca, NY: Cornell University Press, 2003).
9. On the creation and development of VOG, see Claire Shaw, "Deaf in the USSR: 'Defect' and the New Soviet Person" (PhD diss., University of London, 2011).
10. On the social and cultural history of the deaf community in the late Soviet era, see V. A. Palennyi, *Istoriia Vserossiskogo obshchestva glukhikh: Tom I, II i III* (hereafter *Istoriia*) (Moscow: Vserossiiskogo obshchestvo glukhikh, 2007, 2010, 2011); Susan Burch, "Transcending Revolutions: the Tsars, the Soviets and Deaf Culture," *Journal of Social History* 34 (2) (2000): 393–9; Anastasia Kayiatos, "Sooner Speaking than Silent, Sooner Silent than Mute: Soviet Deaf Theatre and Pantomime after Stalin," *Theatre Survey* 51 (1) (2010): 5–31; Claire Shaw, "'Speaking in the Language of Art': Soviet Deaf

Theatre and the Politics of Identity during Khrushchev's Thaw," *Slavonic and East European Review* 91 (4) (2013): 759–86.

11 See, for example, Lilya Kaganovsky and Masha Salazkina, eds., *Sound, Speech, Music in Soviet and Post-Soviet Cinema* (Bloomington: Indiana University Press, 2014).

12 Stephen Lovell, "Broadcasting Bolshevik: The Radio Voice of Soviet Culture," *Journal of Contemporary History* 38 (1) (January 2013): 78–97, here 81. See also Lovell, "How Russia Learned to Listen: Radio and the Making of Soviet Culture," *Kritika: Explorations in Russian and Eurasian History* 12 (3) (2011): 591–615; Michael Gorham, *Speaking in Soviet Tongues: Language Culture and the Politics of Voice in Revolutionary Russia* (Dekalb: Northern Illinois University Press, 2003).

13 Emma Widdis, "Making Sense without Speech: The Use of Silence in Early Soviet Sound Film," in *Sound, Speech, Music,* ed. Kaganovsky and Salazkina, 100–18, here 101.

14 In this respect, the history of the deaf supports Jochen Hellbeck's contention that Soviet identity politics were "not repressive, but productive." Jochen Hellbeck, "Working, Struggling, Becoming: Stalin-Era Autobiographical Texts," *Russian Review* 60 (3) (2001): 340–59, here 341. See also Jochen Hellbeck, *Revolution on My Mind: Writing a Diary under Stalin* (Cambridge, MA: Harvard University Press, 2006), 13. At the same time, this history of Soviet sensory politics also engages with recent scholarship on deaf identity, which considers how deaf communities shape their identity in dialogue with the norms of hearing society. See, for example, Karen Nakamura, *Deaf in Japan: Signing and the Politics of Identity* (Ithaca, NY: Cornell University Press, 2006); Christopher Krentz, *Writing Deafness: The Hearing Line in Nineteenth-Century American Literature* (Berkeley: University of California Press, 2007).

15 Tricia Starks, *The Body Soviet: Propaganda, Hygiene, and the Revolutionary State* (Madison: University of Wisconsin Press, 2008), 4.

16 Irina Sandomirskaja, "Skin to Skin: Language in the Soviet Education of Deaf–Blind Children, the 1920s and 1930s," *Studies in East European Thought* 60 (4) (2008): 321–37.

17 L. S. Vygotskii, ed., *Voprosy vospitaniia slepykh, glukhonemykh i umstvenno-otstalykh detei: sbornik statei i materialov* (Moscow: Izdanie otdela sotsial'no-pravovoi okhrany nesovershennoletnikh Glavsotsvosa Narkomprosa RSFSR, 1924).

18 See, for example, Hoffmann, *Peasant Metropolis*, 158–69.

19 Karl Marx, *A Contribution to the Critique of Political Economy* (Chicago: University of Chicago Press, 1994), 11.

20 L. S. Vygotskii, "K psikhologii i pedagogike detskoi defektivnosti," in *Voprosy vospitaniia slepykh, glukhonemykh i umstvenno-otstalykh detei*, ed. L. S. Vygotskii, 5–30, here 23.

21 Ibid.

22 Ibid.

23 Ibid., 24.
24 On the figure of the worker, see Katerina Clark, *The Soviet Novel: History as Ritual* (Bloomington: Indiana University Press, 2000), 10.
25 Vygotskii, "K psikhologii i pedagogike detskoi defektivnosti," 21.
26 Palennyi, *Istoriia, Tom I*, 30.
27 For more on the concept of "deaf space" in the Soviet context, see Claire Shaw, "'We Have No Need to Lock Ourselves Away': Space, Marginality, and the Negotiation of Deaf Identity in Late Soviet Moscow," *Slavic Review* 74 (1) (Spring 2015): 57–78.
28 Gosudarstvennyi arkhiv Rossiiskoi federatsii (GARF), f. A–511, op. 1, d. 5, l. 19.
29 See A. F. Raikh, "Glukhonemykh—v shumnye tsekha," *Zhizn' glukhonemykh* 14 (1934): 23. Hearing loss was considered a particular danger during Stalin's first Five Year Plan. Lewis Siegelbaum, "Industrial Accidents and Their Prevention in the Interwar Period," in *The Disabled in the Soviet Union: Past and Present, Theory and Practice*, ed. William O. McCagg and Lewis Siegelbaum (Pittsburgh, PA: University of Pittsburgh Press, 1989), 85–117, here 99.
30 GARF, f. A-511, op. 1, d. 5, l. 19.
31 On the plastic gesture, see Oksana Bulgakova, *Fabrika zhestov* (Moscow: Novoe literaturnoe obozrenie, 2005).
32 GARF, f. A-511, op. 1, d. 45, l. 27.
33 For example, some of the founding members of VOG traveled to neighboring Soviet republics in the 1930s to establish local deaf organizations, taking their traditions of signing with them; see Agrippina Kalugina, "Zhizn' v tishine," in *Vspolokhi tishiny*, ed. V. A. Palennyi and I. B. Pichugin (Moscow: Vserossiiskoe obshchestvo glukhikh, 2005), 5–102, here 76. See also *Za zhestovoi iazyk! Sbornik statei*, ed. A. A. Komarova and V. A. Palennyi (Moscow: Vserossiiskoe obshchestvo glukhikh, 2014).
34 On the early history of Soviet deaf education, see A. I. D'iachkov, *Sistemy obucheniia glukhikh detei* (Moscow: Akademiia pedagogicheskikh nauk, 1961).
35 For a positive deaf account of Lunacharskii's speech, Kalugina, "Zhizn' v tishine," 65.
36 GARF, f. A-511, op. 1, d.13, l. 42.
37 Ibid.
38 On the "Eugenic Atlantic", see Sharon L. Snyder and David T. Mitchell, *Cultural Locations of Disability* (Chicago: University of Chicago Press, 2006), 100–32. The reluctance of Soviet scientists to engage with eugenicist policies of sterilization is discussed in Daniel Beer, *Renovating Russia: The Human Sciences and the Fate of Liberal Modernity, 1880–1930* (Ithaca, NY: Cornell University Press, 2008), 123–4.
39 See, for example, Mikhail Shorin, "Vzorvannaia tishina," in *Vspolokhi tishiny*, 121–86, here 131.

40 For details of the "Deaf-Mute Affair," see D. L. Ginzburgskii, "Pomniu tragicheskii 1937–I," and A. I. Razumov and I. P. Gruzdev, "Delo leningradskogo obshchestva glukhonemykh," in *Leningradskii martirolog 1937–1938, Tom 4*, ed. A. Ia. Razumov (St. Petersburg: Rossiiskaia natsional'naia biblioteka, 1999).

41 On the repression of deaf people in Nazi Germany, see Horst Biesold, *Crying Hands: Eugenics and Deaf People in Nazi Germany*, trans. William Sayers (Washington, DC: Gallaudet University Press, 1999).

42 I. V. Stalin, "Tovarishcham D. Belkinu i S. Fureru," *Pravda*, August 2, 1950, 2.

43 S. Usachev, "Zhizn' komsomola: 4-ia godovshchina Saratovskoi iacheiki RLKSM," *Zhizn' glukhonemykh*, October 1, 1925, 2.

44 GARF, f. A-511, op. 1, d. 34, l. 72 ob.

45 Ibid.

46 See A. Slavina and V. Kuksin, "Tak kakaia u nas biografiia?" *V edinom stroiu* 7 (1996): 4–5. Within Deaf studies literature, the utopian notion of a deaf "golden age" is defined as "literacy and pride in all things deaf," commonly associated with the period of history before sign language was sidelined in favor of oralist education. Paddy Ladd, *Understanding Deaf Culture: In Search of Deafhood* (Clevedon: Multilingual Matters, 2003), 394.

47 The Theatre Studio was founded in 1957 and officially registered with the state as a professional theater in 1963. The Studio of Fine and Applied Arts was created in 1960. GARF, f. A-511, op. 1, d. 887, l. 14. For more on Soviet deaf theater, see Shaw, "Speaking in the Language of Art"; V. P. Skripov, *Vernost stsene nam sily davala… Teatr mimiki i zhezta—50 let tvorchestva* (Moscow: Vserossiiskoe obshchestvo glukhikh, 2012).

48 V. Sungarin, "Prazdnik iarkikh krasok," *Zhizn' glukhikh* 6 (1958): 19.

49 T. Smolenskaia, "Ia uchus' na volshebnika," *Zhizn' glukhikh* 10 (1964): 15.

50 T. Nevskaia, "Kak stat' volshebnikom," *Zhizn' glukhikh* 1 (1962): 19.

51 See, for example, E. Vartan'ian and I. Gitlits, *Of Those Who Cannot Hear* (Moscow: Vneshtorgizdat, 1963); V. G. Dmitriev, *Glukhie i glukhonemye v Sovetskom Soiuze* (Moscow: Sovetskaia Rossiia, 1958); F. E. Fishkovaia, ed., *Vystavka izobrazitel'nogo tvorchestva chlenov vserossiiskogo obshchestva glukhonemykh: zhivopis', skul'ptura, grafika, prikladnoe iskusstvo* (Moscow: Sovetskii khudozhnik, 1958).

52 Palennyi, *Istoriia. Tom III*, 163.

53 Sergei Usachev, "Stupeni," in *Vspolokhi tishiny*, ed. Palennyi and Puchugin, 187–213, here 211.

54 I. F. Geil'man, *Ruchnaia azbuka i rechevye zhesty glukhonemykh* (Moscow: Vsesoiuznoe kooperativnoe izdatel'stvo, 1957), 9.

55 A. Shishkov, "Ia golosuiu 'za'," *Zhizn' glukhikh* 12 (1961): 16.

56 V. Cherkizova, "Dat' zelenuiu ulitsu," *Zhizn' glukhikh* 12 (1961): 16.

57 Letter by E. Sidorov, *Zhizn' glukhikh* 3 (1967): 20.

58 Catriona Kelly, *Refining Russia: Advice Literature, Polite Culture and Gender from Catherine to Yeltsin* (Oxford: Oxford University Press, 2001), 334.
59 Dmitriev, *Glukhie i glukhonemye*, 10.
60 Ibid.
61 Ibid.
62 *Otchet tsentral'nogo pravleniia VOGa za 1963–66 gody*, Private VOG collection, 29.
63 *Dvoe* was a huge success, both domestically and internationally; it won the Fipresci Prize at the 1965 Moscow International Film Festival. On the use of a "calque" language on the stage of the TMZh, see A. V. Mekke, *Teatr glukhikh i dlia glukhikh* (Leningrad: Leningradskii vosstanovitel'nyi tsentr VOG, 1989), 12.
64 A. S. Korotkov, *50 let Vserossiiskomu obshchestvu glukhikh* (Leningrad: Leningradskii vosstanovitel'nyi tsentr VOG, 1976), 43.
65 T. Sevost'ianova, "Ne mimika li vinovata?," *Zhizn' glukhikh* 12 (1961): 16.
66 TsGA Moskvy, f. 3089, op. 1, d. 132, l. 8.
67 S. Gushev, "Uvidet', uslyshat', poniat'…," *V edinom stroiu* 6 (1973): 10–11, here 10.
68 Ibid., 11.
69 Nauchno-Issledovatel'skaia Surdo-Akusticheskaia Laboratoriia NKSO RSFSR, *Instruktsiia dlia pol'zovaniia slukhovym apparatom tipa 'SA-39' i 'Liliput'* (Moscow: n.p., 1940).
70 GARF, f. A-511, op. 1, d. 480, l. 71. See Minsobes Order No. 586, December 10, 1953.
71 See E. P. Kuz'micheva, "Ispol'zovanie razlichnykh tipov slukhovykh apparatov v obuchenii glukhikh uchashchikhsia," *Defektolotiia* 3 (1976): 44–57, here 45. For an overview of the new types of hearing aid technology and the issue of residual hearing in the 1970s, see also V. D. Laptev, "O tekhnicheskom osnashchenii zaniatii po formirovaniiu proiznosheniia i razvitiu ostatochnogo slukha u glukhikh i slaboslyshashchikh detei," *Defektologiia* 2 (1976): 69–75.
72 TsGA Moskvy, f. 3010, op. 1, d. 642, l. 9.
73 Anon., "Sen'ora Polia o sebe," *Zhizn' glukhikh* 20 (9) (1967): 24. GARF, f. A-511, op. 1, d. 490, l. 3.
74 A regular publication of the 1960s and 1970s was "Speech and Hearing in Norm and Pathology": Geil'man, *Leningradskii vosstanovitel'nyi tsentr VOG*, 11.
75 I. F. Geil'man, "Leningradskii vosstanovitel'nyi—est'!", *Zhizn' glukhikh* 1 (1966): 12.
76 Geil'man, *Leningradskii vosstanovitel'nyi tsentr VOG*, 13.
77 Ibid., 17.
78 V. Krainin and Z. Krainina, *Chelovek ne slyshit* (Moscow: Znanie, 1984), 8.
79 Geil'man, *Leningradskii vosstanovitel'nyi tsentr VOG*, 28.

80 On the tension between gesture and speech, see Kayiatos, "Sooner Speaking Than Silent," 5–7.
81 Krainin and Krainina, *Chelovek ne slyshit*, 16.
82 On Victor's case, see Harlan Lane, *The Wild Boy of Aveyron* (Cambridge, MA: Harvard University Press, 1976).
83 Krainin and Krainina, *Chelovek ne slyshit*, 32. As Londa Schiebinger points out, European scientists in the eighteenth century argued that humans could be distinguished from the apes by their capacity for speech. Londa Schiebinger, *Nature's Body: Gender in the Making of Modern Science* (New Brunswick, NJ: Rutgers University Press, 1993), 82.
84 Skripov, *Vernost stsene nam sily davala …*, 63.
85 T. Sergeeva, "Zdravstvui, Maugli! Novyi spektakl," *V edinom stroiu* (1983), 4, 28.
86 Mekke, *Teatr glukhikh i dlia glukhikh*, 3.
87 Ibid., 7.
88 Anastasia Kayiatos, "Silent Plasticity: Reenchanting Soviet Stagnation," *Women's Studies Quarterly* 40 (3–4) (2012): 105–25, here 107.
89 Ibid., 108.
90 Mekke, *Teatr glukhikh i dlia glukhikh*, 7.
91 See, for example, Dmitrii Brudnyi, "Mimika i Zhest," *Teatr* 11 (1971), 37–43, here 43.
92 Michael Pursglove and Anna Komarova, "The Changing World of the Russian Deaf Community," in *Many Ways to Be Deaf: International Variation in Deaf Communities*, ed. Leila Monaghan, Constanze Schmaling, Karen Nakamura, and Graham H. Turner (Washington, DC: Gallaudet University Press, 2003), 249–59, here 254.
93 Krainin and Krainina, *Chelovek ne slyshit*, 8.

CHAPTER TEN

Sensing danger: The Red Army during the Second World War

Steven G. Jug

On a quiet night in November of 1944 at the front on the Polish side of the Narev River, a squad of Soviet soldiers sat in a dugout without doors:

> So Valery Semykin gave us a hint about how we could illuminate our shelters. He gave us a whole roll of German phone cable that had rubber coating and tar-covered insulation. We hung the wire from the ceiling, so that one end would be a bit higher than the other, and ignited its upper part. Fire gradually consumed the rubber insulation and went on down the wire. One had to pull the upper part of the wire, at the right time, further from the roll. It did not produce much light, but produced a lot of stench and soot. In the morning, when we left the dug-outs, we looked like demons from hell. It took a lot of effort to wash off the awful soot mask with snow and soap.[1]

Mundane yet complex sensory experiences contributed to the distinctiveness of frontline service for Red Army fighters. For a soldier such as Pyl'tsyn, who had been at the front for a year, a peaceful night in a dugout proved memorable. Only at the front did one have to generate enough light to be able to see the writing on the page, but not so much as to provide a target for enemy mortars. The burning of telephone wire provided a new foul odor that stood out from various ammunition explosions, burned fuels, and types of decaying organic matter. Likewise, it was in the context of rare bathing opportunities that a "demon" soot mask actually necessitated a cold, hard scrubbing.

This chapter examines the interaction and mutual constitution of individual and official-cultural interpretations of the sensory experience of Red Army soldiers during the Second World War as a distinct but significant facet of Russian sensory history in the Soviet period. Drawing from scholarship on the senses, embodiment, and subjectivity, I analyze Red Army soldiers' and propagandists' engagement with the new sights, sounds, feelings, tastes, and smells that set war apart. By considering both popular and official discussions of how it felt to be in the Red Army, I adapt intellectual historian Martin Jay's comparative approach, which considers the senses to be "more than the sources of knowledge, orientation, and meaning, [because] they serve as well as the avenues of pleasure and pain, whose thresholds may well vary on both the individual and the cultural level."[2] I likewise draw from the approach of sensory historian Mark M. Smith, which aims to "understand the senses as communicators of knowledge and, especially, as expressions of power and identity."[3] Smith emphasizes how war produces novel and extreme sensory experiences: "War is hell on them; the violence of it engraves sensory memory in ways other experiences cannot approach, memory so powerful it can be relived, over and over again."[4]

Descriptions of sensory experiences appear almost exclusively in retrospective materials like memoirs and published oral history interviews, while troops' wartime writings—whether letters, journals, or petitions—typically focus on relationships, goals, and achievements beyond the war.[5] Drawing from literary scholar William Cohen's claims about "the body as a sensory interface between the interior and the world" and that "autobiography, by its nature, describes the internal experience of the self, and ... embodied selfhood," I treat memoirs as a medium for fighting men to interpret their sensory experiences as part of a reflection on an embodied notion of the soldierly self.[6] Soviet soldiers had grown up with a journal culture that encouraged reflection on their experiences as they strove to affiliate themselves with collective struggles, and many veterans wrote postwar memoirs with related objectives in mind.[7] Russian Civil War historian Sean Guillory argues that "it is, after all, ultimately the body that serves as the depository for experience and, by extension, for the veterans' very senses of self."[8] In the next generation of Russian combatants' sensory experiences and their significance, I find the evolution of embodied subjectivities, which distinguishes the Russian sensory experience of the war from that of both enemy and allied combatants.

Simon Creak, a historian of Southeast Asia, has argued, "physical or embodied practice reinforces national consciousness and, through it, state power by solidifying it through everyday experience."[9] As anthropologist Ana María Alonso has demonstrated, the basis of modern state rhetoric about mobilization and national sacrifice rests on "the fusion of the ideological and the sensory, the bodily and the normative, the emotional and the instrumental."[10] The Soviet pre-war foundation for physical and sensory training rested with the Stakhanovite movement in labor, militarized youth athletics, and the celebration of quasi-military national exploits, all of which appeared in slightly adapted form in wartime propaganda.[11] I argue, however, that official rhetoric about the senses and embodied practices of national sacrifice failed to resonate with Red Army soldiers. The Soviet fusion, in Alonso's formulation, privileged the ideological over the sensory, which resulted in disembodied heroic figures that bore little resemblance to real fighting men and the extreme sensory experiences they encountered.[12] Scholarship on Soviet wartime propaganda primarily focuses on how the truthfulness of official rhetoric, or lack of it, affected soldiers' reception of heroic ideals and norms of frontline conduct.[13] In examining the sensory, I relegate degrees of honesty in official rhetoric to secondary importance, and instead scrutinize how accurately propaganda depicted the sensory experiences of combat as a means of assessing its influence on soldiers.

The intensity of wartime sensory experience varied, as did the combinations of senses that distinguished participants' perceptions. I engage the senses not as five isolated categories but based on how they contributed to the embodied subjectivity of Red Army fighters.[14] As troops struggled to interpret and cope with the feel of battle, they encountered official rhetoric that seemed to make their war experiences less comprehensible. I proceed from the least to most distinct sensory expression of embodiment in the Red Army, and consequently from most to least present in the disembodied depictions in soldier-specific propaganda: beginning to fight, engaging the enemy, mastering combat skills, building comradely contacts, and gendering the battlefront. By highlighting the incongruity between soldiers' most intense sensory memories and the disembodied heroes of official rhetoric, this chapter clarifies the distinctly Russian depiction of sensory experiences in war.

Beginning to fight

Germany's invasion of the Soviet Union in June of 1941 shattered Soviet citizens' relative isolation from the war in Europe. Soldiers who entered the Red Army typically endured hardship as they deployed, uncertainty about how to recognize battle, and the shock of combat in a three-phase initiation to the status of frontline combatants. While total war challenged the civilian's senses through deprivation, uncertainty, and danger, Red Army soldiers' perception of war played out with higher stakes because those challenges affected how well troops resisted the enemy. Tasked with more than just survival, fighting men responded to their sensory experiences in order to prepare their minds and bodies for the battles to come.

Smell confronted soldiers early on in their transition from entry to the ranks to participation in battle. As Mark M. Smith noted in his history of the senses in the American Civil War, "Unlike the eye and the mouth… the nose 'cannot close the gates'. Smells are transgressive, punching their way inside, the only real defense being not to breathe at all."[15] One of the earliest such transgressive smells was that of other soldiers in close quarters, as a cavalryman recalled:

Some men were sitting, some were sleeping under the table and benches, some were lying on the stove, some were dozing off on their feet, leaning against the neighboring man. The air was so thick that if someone opened the door, he was almost knocked down by the warm smell of sweat, old foot rags, and bodies that had not been washed for a long time.[16]

When troops first confronted, and then learned to tolerate, the smell of their comrades' frontline exertions (even sleeping through it) they began a passive initiation into the sensory life of soldiers. Closer to the front, Red Army men confronted another transgressive odor: "the temperature rose to 25–27 C ... if a man gets killed, his corpse is already reeking within two hours. Such a stench, and they'd bring up a meal—you couldn't force down any food, so we drank water."[17] The shock of rank odors could overpower other bodily sensations, like hunger, but provided soldiers with clues about the extremes of war before they encountered danger or violence directly. While possible experiences for civilians in wartime, the two central smells of war—others and death—were not outliers for troops, but instead provided a link between the core sensory experiences and bodily practices of soldiering: relying on comrades and killing the enemy.

Once at the front, most soldiers had a keen appreciation of how unprepared they were to make sense of the new sights and sounds that awaited them in their first battle. On his first patrol, Joseph Piliushin, a sniper, noted how "the mysterious silence of the woods was unsettling, and our ears pricked up at any soft rustle. Everything around me seemed unusual; even the starry sky seemed to be suspended just about the tips of the pine trees."[18] Knowing they were at war, soldiers struggled to see and hear their surroundings differently, not unlike the experience of nurses that Laurie Stoff examines in this volume, who could mistake bullet sounds for the buzzing of bees. Many remained tied to civilian frames of reference, as artillerist Petr Mikhin described how "some artillery fire could be heard in the distance to the left and right. It sounded like an approaching thunderstorm, though there wasn't a single cloud in the sky. ... These sounds produced more alarm in our young hearts."[19] New sensations or misperceptions could produce significant emotional responses, as another artillerist remembered: "that night I fell asleep in my foxhole without eating dinner. I don't know what woke me up, but when I saw several unknown men standing over me, I was gripped with terror."[20] Efforts to immediately perceive the first sight or sound of battle and limited trust of one's own senses plagued new arrivals at the front. A pilot recalled first encountering combat veterans after the war had begun: "Crowds of men from the rear who had not tried frontline life who were craving real and not official word of the war listened attentively to the stories of their experiences, full of dramatic tension. The accounts weighed heavily and oppressively upon our souls."[21] Reference to the "soul" reflected a common feeling that troops' first exposure to battle would do more than test their senses, as the veterans seemed to be different from recruits by virtue of what they had endured in battle. The new link between the senses and soldiers' very survival suggested that the experience of combat would change their identity.

The sensory experiences that Russian soldiers eventually encountered in war were often completely new. A loader in a self-propelled artillery unit struggled to explain the scene of his first battle: "Bullets were whistling and armour-piercing rounds swept past us with a howl. From some unknown direction, an aircraft appeared and started to bomb—friendly or enemy, I don't know. I was trying to run, but my legs were wobbly and the ground was shaking. I fell down several times. I looked back—it wasn't a battle, but a scene from hell!"[22] Even after disengaging, troops felt strong sensations for having faced death and survived: "It was dark and quiet in the woods ... but we couldn't yet recover our breath, our hearts were still pounding in our throats, and the sounds of screaming wounded, smashing metal, submachine-gun bursts and grenade explosions still rang in our ears."[23] After surviving, many troops considered the meaning, as much as the feelings of war: "Before the attack, each of us was silently asking if he would be able to kill. Now there was a reply: I can if I have to. At the start of the war, hardening people to killing was a reconstruction of the whole human mentality."[24] The reconstruction process for soldiers began with their first battle, and continued in life and combat in the months to come. The sensory experiences of war changed troops' fighting ability and began the development of an embodied sense of self that challenged their pre-war, civilian subjectivities.

The outbreak of war seemed quite different in the pages of *Krasnaia Zvezda* (*Red Star*), the official newspaper of the Red Army. The vast majority of its content originated from generals' and political officers' reports, as well as the observations of headquarters-dwelling newspaper correspondents.[25] Even the most intrepid correspondents could not report firsthand experience of battle. Vasily Grossman served as one of a handful of war correspondents who was already a respected Soviet writer before the war. Grossman's interview style and candid writing distinguished his articles, not his personal experience of battle. At the front by August of 1941, he interviewed soldiers and generals, learning details, and making notes that "it was remarkably interesting when Netsevich [commander of the aviation regiment] told us all about the first night of the war, about the terrible, swift retreat."[26] Like soldiers at the front awaiting their first battle, he encountered new sensations from a distance: "A cemetery. Fighting is going on below in the valley, the village is burned out. Twelve German bombers are diving over to the left. The cemetery is quiet, [but] chickens are cackling in the smoking village." He also experienced the aftermath of battle: "Morning. We went to the field hospital to see Utkin, whose fingers had been torn off by shrapnel. ... There were bloodstained rags, scraps of flesh, moans, subdued howling, hundreds of dismal, suffering eyes."[27] Even as a more reckless correspondent than most, Grossman lacked sufficient proximity to battle, and had to rely on secondhand accounts and rear-area observations. The war coverage that appeared in *Krasnaia Zvezda* as a result of his and more removed writers' efforts could only succeed in providing disembodied accounts of combat.

The process by which soldiers reached the front and their first battle exposed them to progressively more distinct wartime sensory experiences, from which the process of embodied identity formation began. Proximity to combat, without actual exposure, brought partial change and induced anxiety and fear, but the sights, sounds, and smells of distant or past fighting required no direct response. Virtually all *Krasnaia Zvezda* correspondents' sensory experience of war failed to surpass the non-combat but frontline level of soldier recruits, remaining limited to the effects of war, rather than the experience of it. Many soldiers' introduction to battle overwhelmed their perception. The shock effect of intense new sights, sounds, and feelings persisted after the first battle ended and manifested itself bodily: through balance, heart rate, breathing, salivation, and hearing. The conditions that threatened fighting men's physical survival prepared their bodies for the hardship to come and challenged them to embrace violence.

Engaging the enemy

Once they entered combat, violence became the central aspect of Red Army troops' war experience: they inflicted it and suffered from it. While their senses registered the danger, pain, and horror, Red Army fighters' hatred reflected the broader impact of violence. Similarly, the ease with which soldiers did harm, especially through sight, constituted an embodied experience that transcended self-defense or the need to follow orders. The sensory experiences surrounding violence and the enemy aroused powerful emotional responses that reflected significant changes to the Soviet servicemen involved. Propaganda accounts of violence contained gruesome detail when presenting German atrocities against Soviet civilians, but rarely evoked the brutality of battle, even that exacted on the hated enemy.

Red Army troops faced the constant threat of attack, but the sensory experience of violence combined specific weapons and their impact. An artillerist, Nikolai Shishkin, recalled the complex, or perhaps confusing, combination of sights and sounds that accompanied a bombardment: "At the end of the fight I had only six shells left; the ammunition bearer Ozerov had been wounded, the gun had been knocked out of alignment, and we were bleeding from the nose and ears. These metal beams, with which we had covered our earth and timber emplacement, rang so loudly that we were completely deafened."[28] Troops had to endure the consequences of enemy violence on themselves and their comrades to continue fighting effectively, but the struggle could be more emotional than physical. Seriously wounded soldiers were removed from action, but suffering comrades had to be overcome; as an artilleryman explained: "The Germans encircled our wounded in some kind of depression in the ground, about a hundred meters from us. We could not get through to their rescue. The wounded cried out to us for a long time: 'fight through to us, brothers!' … That cry has been haunting me my whole life."[29] Hearing wounded comrades could thus prove more traumatic than seeing them, and effectively dealing with the sensations and emotions of suffering and loss required a different response to sounds of human suffering.

While weaponry usually removed the immediate, personal experience, soldiers exhibited combatant subjectivity when calmly recounting the violence of comrades. An artillerist recalled the reaction of the infantry guarding his battery during an artillery barrage:

> A command to the battery followed, and a shell swept away the fleeing Fritzes. The soldiers kicked up an ever louder row, and now each man was trying to point out to me the group of fleeing Germans to shell next. The joy of revenge quickly restored their energy, freed them from the fear that they had experienced in the [German] attacks, and softened their sorrow over the comrades they had lost in the fighting. Watching the enemy die in front of them was like balm to their rattled nerves.[30]

The sight and sound of enemy death constituted a powerful sensory experience:

> The flame-throwers destroyed almost the entire column. There was almost no machine-gun fire from our side, but the heart-rending screaming and yelling of burning Nazis rang in our ears for a long time. I guess it is no wonder that the screams of those burning enemy soldiers cheered up our extremely exhausted men, so strong was our hatred of the enemy.[31]

Killing induced bodily responses involving adrenaline and endorphins that energized and then calmed fighters and linked the senses to feelings of hatred, joy, exhilaration, and vengefulness. The sights and sounds of dying enemy soldiers, even when the victims of a comrade's fire, bolstered the mental and physical resolve of Red Army troops, who had embraced vengeance. Fighting men who not only killed enemy soldiers but also celebrated killing, no longer possessed civilian subjectivity.

The transition from a civilian to soldierly subjectivity was an embodied process of responding to frontline sensations, accepting risks, and managing stress. To maintain long-term combat effectiveness, soldiers first had to survive, and that meant embracing the sensations of frontline combat. A self-propelled gun commander, Boris Nazarov, described the challenge of such a course: "When I came out of one battle, I dropped by a house ... in a mirror I saw an unfamiliar man and reached for my Walther [pistol]. He did the same ... only then did I recognize myself in the reflection, and I was just about to fire."[32] Both his readiness to shoot anything that moved as well as his literal inability to recognize himself were indicative of the change to Nazarov's sense of self. Pilot Vasily Reshetnikov believed he could perceive when a fighting man could no longer endure the violence he heard, felt, and witnessed: "A strong and sturdy, swarthy man with the build of a boxer, iron muscles, and a stubborn character, he was a fine, brave flyer who had lasted longer than the rest of Tokunov's group. Now he appeared to be without spirit, broken, deprived of his former enviable dashing appearance and self-confidence."[33] Through a sort of hermeneutics of the fighting spirit, troops trusted their visual senses to assess character, and believed that emotional states and changes in mentality manifested bodily. Such an assessment of comrades reflected Reshetnikov's own change from civilian to military affiliations and values, so that he sought out men as combat capable as himself, and pitied, if not avoided, others who were unable to endure violent experiences and keep up with frontline norms. Both Nazarov and Reshetnikov developed an embodied, soldierly subjectivity in response to their new violent reality.

In heroic propaganda, the significance of violence and the sensory shared a different relationship. Articles in *Krasnaia Zvezda* conveyed the violent experiences of war, but usually reserved details of violence for enemy atrocities. In one such article, a soldier recounted entering a recently occupied village: "the Germans had tied Russian children to trees and used them for target practice. The children were already dead, and their mothers were crying, trying to tear them down."[34] Even this example relies more on the overall scene than details of what the soldier saw and heard. Depictions of battle violence often emphasized details linked to, but not actually of a violent act, such as an artillery spotter's decision to order the bombardment of his own trench: "The Germans were ten steps from him. Suddenly, the thunder of explosions shook the air. The ground around him trembled. The shells exploded in a dense pattern around the position of Bragonin and his comrade infantrymen. However, the earth of the motherland protected them from death"[35] Despite the visual, auditory, and even tactile details about the bombardment, no mention of the harm coming to either the Red Army troops or the enemy appears. Instead, a romantic *deus ex machina* saves the Red Army hero—the Soviet soil. As a result, he becomes a disembodied figure, fearlessly calling in orders but lacking a body to inhale smoke or dust, shield from debris, suffer injury, or be wounded. The article reflects Soviet propaganda's consistent omission of violent details and impacts on bodies in coverage of even close-quarters fire and battle. This may have stemmed, in part, from correspondents' lack of combat experience.

To understand why propaganda lacked the violent details that shaped soldiers' experiences and memories, the role of Soviet ideology deserves mention. The disembodied depiction of Red Army heroes in danger reflected concerns over morale, but the lack of violent ends for the enemy, whose atrocities received consistent attention, exposed ideological goals. In early 1942, military political workers, and then *Krasnaia Zvezda*, began to promote Stakhanovism in the Red Army, thereby applying the 1930s production movement to the killing of enemy soldiers.[36] Echoing Stakhanovite narratives, a *Krasnaia Zvezda* report praised a unit because "in one day of fighting, it destroyed more than 300 fascists," before breaking down the number of enemy dead discovered in individual villages to emphasize this quantitative success.[37] Disembodied heroes produced kill counts in dozens of articles that year, but discussions of how the bloody competition looked or sounded received virtually no attention. With such figures, close combat violence faded from exploit descriptions, and even skill warranted little attention, since the proper ideological priming would yield extraordinary results. In this regard, the 1930s approach to mobilization remained key, as *Krasnaia Zvezda* explained, "the order of Comrade Stalin, requiring soldiers to destroy the German occupiers as snipers do, inspired ardent [affirmative] responses among the defenders of Sevastopol."[38] Stalin's word could turn every fighter into a sniper, for whom killing became a precise but routine task, and one that took place away from the immediate proximity of typical battle sensations.

The role of the enemy as a hated purveyor of violence proved the strongest link between soldiers' and propagandists' depictions of frontline fighting. Red Army troops focused far more, however, on the violence that shaped so many of their sensory experiences at the front. The pain and danger that afflicted Red Army men reflected a view of their bodies and themselves in terms of national sacrifice and service to a mission or comrades. A reduced sensitivity to violence developed among veteran troops, though limits remained, and could bind them together or exclude those unable to cope. Soldiers' hatred of the enemy and wish to do him harm reflected further development of an embodied and militarized subjectivity, as they not only endured violence, but pursued and celebrated the sight or sound of it. Such an interpretation of the sensory dimension of wartime violence distinguished Soviet Russia from those of its main allies, the United States and Great Britain. In British newspaper propaganda, the enemy appeared as an overly-militarized but professional soldier: focused only on war and combat, always in the company of other soldiers, quick to show dominance and aggression, and utterly devoid of civilian relationships or interests. In contrast, British soldiers appeared as typical citizens above all: husbands and fathers who retained their civilian personas and morality in wartime through humor, camaraderie, and reserved emotions.[39] The prevailing American view of the German enemy was essentially that of an honorable foe, although a clear competitor in physical power.[40] In both cases, much more limited experiences of German soldiers in battle and occupation likely produced a more restrained presentation of the German enemy, just as violent encounters and atrocities appeared as a consistent feature in Soviet views.

Mastering combat skills

After learning to survive the extremes of the front, skill mastery served as the next level of sensory adaptation to war and embodied development of a soldierly subjectivity. Although training typically preceded frontline combat, it rarely prepared recruits to master the weapons they would actually use, let alone mimic the sensory reality of battle conditions. Only combat allowed bodily practice to create successful fighters, while propaganda emphasized disembodied exploits and ideologically-driven heroes.

Red Army training became a hurried and inconsistent process after the 1941 German invasion. Sharpening the senses figured as a goal, as one artillerist recalled:

> I dug a hole and sat down in it. He disappeared for a moment, and then a burst of submachine-gun fire struck around the hole where I was sitting. He shouted. "Where am I? Stick your head up, I won't fire." "And how should I know," I replied. "Listen again." That's how you teach someone who doesn't yet know how to determine the source of incoming fire![41]

Training the senses to distinguish weapon sounds and their direction provided crucial aid in combat, however good a recruit's hearing might be in civilian life. Such training was rare, and others, like coordinating sight with distance estimates and equipment use or the bodily practice of aim, received little attention. Another artillerist, Moisei Dorman, trained with drills and tactical lectures, explained:

> At the front we had to learn much all over again. We had little gunnery practice... We fired at wooden mock-ups of tanks that were towed by a long cable only twice. We saw German tanks only in illustrations ... An understanding of the combat situation, the dynamics of combat, as well as a "sense of terrain" comes only through real combat experience.[42]

While critical of the lack of live-fire training, the assessment suggests that skills cannot be truly developed outside combat. The larger sensory experience of battle, as Dorman knew, complicated skills like aiming with its attendant needs for assessing the terrain, deciding which target posed the greatest threat, and filtering out extraneous sights, sounds, and feelings.

Skills comprised part of the embodied experience of combat and contributed to the development of a soldierly subjectivity that practice alone could not produce. The first sniper assignment of an infantryman, Mansur Abdulin, illustrates the contrast between training and combat:

> My rifle is in excellent condition—I can hit a tin can from 100m. Suddenly I'm hot. The target is getting larger as it approaches. Germans. … But what's going on? I can't seem to get the slit, the sight, and the target in line: if I line-up the target and the sight, I lose the slit! If I find the slit, I lose the sight! I'm sweating. It fills my eyes. The gun is shaking in my hands.[43]

Although he would demonstrate medal-worthy aim after missing his first shot, Abdulin's experience of actual combat prompted bodily responses—sweat, nervousness, and shaking—absent from training. Experienced simultaneously, they disrupted the familiar practice of marksmanship centered on sight. Troops in close combat faced different bodily limits on their skills: "When I crawled out again and took a look in the sight, the side of the gun barrel was no longer visible. A black aperture was gazing directly at me. I placed the crosshairs of the gun sight on this aperture—and fired. Then—I blacked out."[44] Artillerist Vasily Ulianov demonstrated his skill but suffered the bodily impact of the resulting shockwave. Whether too nervous to aim or rendered unconscious by the result, the bodies of Red Army fighters limited both their sense-guided skills and their dedication to inflict harm. Having one's body in mortal danger changed the sensory experience in ways which training could scarcely simulate.

Mastery of combat skills fit awkwardly with the presentation of Red Army propaganda heroes who distinguished themselves with extraordinary feats. Skills and sensory perception typically appeared separately in *Krasnaia Zvezda* articles. When propaganda presented superior sight or touch, they seemed as something willed or bestowed as much as shaped by training and experience. Soldiers' hands appeared as a noteworthy subject in *Krasnaia Zvezda*, as a captain narrated the exploits of his deputy: "I knew that senior sergeant Leonov was an excellent shot, he had a keen eye and a firm hand."[45] Hardness, a reflection of touch and a quality, emphasized both the steadiness of aiming weapons as well as psychological determination to wield them. Occasionally, soldiers' masterful touch appeared in contrast to that of the enemy as in coverage of Stalingrad: "And when all his rounds were gone, Farafonov managed to snatch a machine gun from the hands of a German, and he again began to shoot enemy soldiers."[46] The article sent the message that a Red Army fighter would not give up due to a lack of ammunition, and his hands would break the enemy's weaker grip. Overall, such articles emphasized an abundance of strength more than special dexterity, but reinforced the ideal of disembodied soldiers overcoming challenges with determination and firmness.

Similarly, articles about skill emphasized determination. The article "We will become masters of our domain," was representative of several waves of Stalin-inspired coverage in *Krasnaia Zvezda* underscoring "the order of the great leader about fighters' need to perfectly learn their weapons and become masters of their domain." As the title suggests, the soldiers of the Southern Front who heard the order replied in the affirmative, and "feeling that the [next] day was special ... our riflemen, snipers, machine-gunners, and mortar men struck the enemy with exceptional power."[47] Stalin's inspiration produced an immediate improvement in fighting ability, but lacked an embodied exercise of skill to exemplify the change. Much as with Stakhanovism and violence, propagandists' depiction of war skipped to the increased casualties they wished to promote, and omitted the specific skills required.

Building comradely contacts

In his treatment of homosocial relationships in the Russian Civil War as foundational for both the Red Army and Soviet political culture at large, literary scholar Eliot Borenstein explains how "comradeship seeks to break down the wall of the self," and "is implicitly collective," so that "suffering and danger cannot create friendship, but they make all the difference in comradeship."[48] While shared danger, battle performance, and the conversations that punctuated them provided the foundation for camaraderie, touch, and to a lesser extent sight and taste, distinguished the embodied experience of comradeship among fighting men reflecting new affiliations that transcended the needs of combat.

In battle, troops consistently experienced different aspects of comradeship through touch. In some cases, touch represented comrades' familiarity, established tactics for combat success, and unit-specific means of communicating: "I stood with my shoulders at the level of the tank commander's boots, so he pressed me on the left or on the right shoulder, [and] I turned the tank respectively to the left or to the right, [when he] hit my head—[it meant] stop."[49] Despite the superficially harsh mode of touch, the tanker's kicks reflected a level of mutual dependence rare in the civilian world and emerged from shared experience to overcome the noise that might lead to a fatal misunderstanding. Soldiers frequently felt the helpful touch of a comrade in better position on the battlefield, or with a better grasp of the situation: "The mortar battery commander, a senior lieutenant who I knew from his time in the reserve, spotted my senseless face, grabbed me by the belt around my sheepskin coat, and yanked me down into a trench. Not far away, enemy shells and mortar rounds began to explode."[50] Such contact was again sudden and violent, but involved risking one's life to provide life-saving care to a fellow soldier in need. In the frontline context, a jolting move could display comradeship between men who had the slimmest of connections to one another by any other standard.

Embodied sensory experiences also reinforced comradeship in collective or unit-sized contexts. In near-starvation conditions, hunger drove troops to think about consuming anything plausibly edible: "I remember somewhere we unloaded cattle skin in a group of about ten men. And then I saw the guys gather. Skin with streaks of meat. We gnawed that skin. ... Like dogs ... I was scared. I tried it—unpalatable. But I began to gnaw. It was incredible."[51] The collective act meant that the wretched taste was not borne alone, but instead served as a shared hardship that might reassure squeamish comrades and unify the hungry group. In other cases, certain sights prompted an emotional response and directly reinforced solidarity. A lieutenant who volunteered for the front explained the power of fighters' responses to the torture and killing of comrades: "Yesterday I buried eight men (corpses) of our tortured soldiers and commanders ... Such are the actions of the enemy ... Every comrade who saw this with his own eyes or whom we told about it has vowed to take revenge."[52] Viewing enemy atrocities could provide an immediate and shared additional motivation to men in a unit, which distinguished them from fellow fighters driven by individual or national reasons to fight. Seeing other fighters, like oneself, enduring hardship or grief, rather than showing fear, might also buoy the spirits and preserve the discipline of troops who would otherwise waver.

Soldiers' experience of the death of a comrade involved more than immediate visual recognition of the deceased. Instead, the rituals that surrounded comrades' deaths provided an elaborate sensory experience that centered on the body of the fallen. The burial of a comrade followed a relatively consistent pattern and involved all of his fellows:

> If there were time, we dressed the body in clean underwear and uniform. We would wrap deceased tankers in a piece of tank tarpaulin, and infantry soldiers, as a rule, in their own greatcoats. We lined the bottom of the grave with pine boughs or straw or whatever was available. We carefully lowered the body into the excavated grave, being attentive always to inter from west to east [head west, feet east]. We did not use caskets. Accompanied by a volley of rifle fire or main-gun salvos, we threw the dirt in on top of our comrade and then we installed a simple pyramid with a star. Right there, at the fresh grave, we drank our daily ration of a hundred grams of vodka, in memory of the fallen. And then we returned to battle.[53]

Touch figured prominently in many stages of the burial process, and a physical connection with the deceased's body served as a key means of showing respect. The process of dressing, wrapping, and lowering a dead comrade involved considerable physical contact with his body and likely more touch than fighting men would have shared while living. Essentially interrupting the war to prepare the deceased for burial by hand, Red Army soldiers further expressed, by touching a non-family member so much, an embodied soldierly subjectivity anchored by affiliation with a group of men who would still be considered at most acquaintances in the civilian world.

Propaganda depictions of comradeship rang hollow when dealing with life-saving touch in battle and the burial of comrades. Coverage of medics was rare and somewhat problematic, given the standard downplaying of wounds as a short- or medium-term problem at the front. When they received mention, touch scarcely factored into the coverage: "Medic Khachatyrian was himself wounded by an enemy bullet, but did not quit his post. He carried from the field of battle twenty-one wounded men together with their weapons."[54] Both the medic and his patients appeared in disembodied form, so that neither the careful touch of first aid provision nor the wounded men's feelings of pain received mention. Similarly, the burial took place without a body as a point of contact for their comrades: "The coffin was lowered into the grave. An artillery salute sounded. Close to the [burial] mound men tossed pine and willow branches into a pile."[55] The depiction of a frontline funeral service in *Krasnaia Zvezda* was just as passive: "Soldiers stood by a white pyramid, crowned with a Red Army star and a wreath. On it was written: 'Platoon Commander Senior Sergeant Grebennikov …'"[56] Neither article described an actual body, but instead allowed a coffin or a tombstone to serve as substitute. All three articles ignored the sensory experiences and corporeal realities of life and death at the front, and in so doing showed none of the comradely care that motivated young men to fight.

Gendering the battlefront

The frontline and combatant presence of women in the Red Army, especially after 1942, proved to be a distinguishing feature of the Soviet war effort.[57] Despite the sacrifices and successful combat performance of Soviet women, their male counterparts largely focused on the visual experience of women's presence at the front. Women were present in headquarters and medical sectors of Red Army units from the early months of the war, but jealous officers typically limited their proximity to the forward line and their contact with rank and file troops.[58] New opportunities for soldiers to see women later in the war further solidified a frontline experience rooted in, and gendered as, brotherhood. Frontline propaganda likewise paid little attention to women's accomplishments, and it largely ignored women's bodily potential and visual appeal by highlighting traditional, female, wartime contributions. The sight of women, proximity of their bodies, and resultant heterosexual desire linked male comrades and bolstered the gendered facet of Red Army troops' embodied understanding of self.

After troops' sustained isolation from women, the mere sight of a feminine form could elicit both a bodily response and serious reflection about what that sight meant. The young artillerist who likened artillery to thunder years earlier, recalled the occasion of seeing a woman again in 1945: "I was now no longer looking at the newspaper, but more covering myself with it, as I looked at the shapely backside of the young woman ... I was accustomed to seeing only the filthy padded pants of combat soldiers, and now the sight of bare female calves seemed like a dream."[59] His dream involved both the image of a woman's body, but also the contrast of such a sight with the scenes of war. In his work on embodiment, Cohen has asserted "the non-alignment between body and subject suggests that the body has the capacity to unmake the human."[60] The shock of seeing a woman again reminded Mikhin that he had spent the past few years in a homosocial environment looking at men, which changed his sense of self, just as the normalization of sights of death and destruction had. In the absence of women, heterosexual desire had been absent. An erection confirmed the sight of a woman as a novel sensory experience. Mikhin's reaction reflected a greater shift among Red Army fighters, who responded to the influx of women after a long absence by contrasting the frontline as masculine to a complementary "femininity."[61]

In her work on the "gaze," feminist film theorist Laura Mulvey claims "in a world ordered by sexual imbalance, pleasure in looking has been split between active/male and passive/female. The determining male gaze projects its fantasy onto the female figure, which is styled accordingly."[62] Mansur Abdulin, a mortar crew leader by then, thus recalled comrades' reaction to meeting nurses:

> The men are staring at the women around them. Some soldiers have not seen a female face for a couple of years! The women begin with soaping the heads of the wounded, so they would not be looking at them with those begging, eager eyes. But through the acrid, smelly suds the men are still admiring the female figures. The women again splash their faces with soapy water: "Don't you look!" But the soldier jerks his head, throws off the suds and keeps on staring.[63]

The wounded soldiers not only focused on the nurses' potential as sexual objects, despite the improbability of such an outcome, but also ignored their professional role in caring for the wounded. The fantasy view of female nurses underscored how troops had adapted to the absence of women at the front. For men who expected to see sacrifice and hardship with and through their male comrades, the presence of women in a clean and safe context seemed to promise new possibilities. Of course, a few images of female sacrifice circulated widely at the front and shaped wartime culture, such as the image of hero-martyr Zoia Kosmodemianskaia's naked corpse, as Adrienne Harris examines in a later chapter. Unlike the tortured partisan, young, healthy nurses revealed no signs of sacrifice or hardship, reinforcing the masculine dimension of troops' embodied subjectivity, in which heterosexual desire served no purpose, and homosocial comradeship eased the deadly realities of frontline life.

The pages of *Krasnaia Zvezda* lacked any mention of how women's entry into the ranks or physical presence at the front would require a period of adjustment, let alone any suggestions for soldiers hoping to cope with what they saw. The closest any article came to addressing soldiers' interest in seeing women, let alone their sexualized bodies, was an article about a pen pal program. The article contended that fighting men were interested in seeing women's letters arrive in the field post, concluding with the assessment that "such correspondence warms the souls of the frontline soldier, [and] brightens his harsh life on the front line."[64] The article thus reflected an incorporeal view of both soldiers and the women whom they might like to meet. While the article upheld the notion of masculine and feminine roles and spaces in the war effort, it had no real bearing on men's responsiveness to the visual or their isolation from women as an embodied experience.

Frontline propaganda considered men's bodily needs and engaged the gendered, sensory experience only through taste. As a kind of mid-war promise to soldiers, *Krasnaia Zvezda* articles explained: "It is not enough just to provide the cooking of hearty and delicious food, she must also promptly prepare and promptly deliver it to fighters."[65] To this end, soldiers could count on young women who had volunteered for training in the "Central courses of cooks of the Main quartermaster administration of the Red Army… in conditions approaching those of the front," which began operating in December of 1942. In those courses, the article explained, "Young women learned not only culinary arts, but also military affairs. Theoretical work in classes on the organization of nutrition in the Red Army and practical work in kitchens contributed to the training of qualified military cooks."[66] The need for young, female cooks to train in front-like conditions and engage in practical work preserved the distinction between masculine front and feminine rear roles. The articles thus presented taste as male soldiers' concern but female cooks' specialty, and an important way for young women to help meet one of the bodily needs of soldiers. Despite a shared conception of gendered contributions to the war effort, frontline propaganda remained out of touch with soldiers' sensory experiences or bodily needs as conditions changed in the late war period. *Krasnaia Zvezda* suggested that troops apparently avoided the experiments, improvisations, and rogue canteens that Anton Masterovoy's chapter highlights among food supply developments in the prewar Soviet Union. Given that Red Army troops had shown no concern for the particular ability of women to improve their experience of taste at the front, propaganda remained out of step with combatants' sensory and bodily realities in the late war. *Krasnaia Zvezda* provided no indication of how fighting men should deal with the women in their ranks, but affirmed the masculine character of the front and combatant roles therein.

Conclusion

Red Army soldiers struggled to deal with the reality of total war that confronted them after the German invasion in June of 1941. Their sensory experiences of the duration, lethality, and scale of violence of war demanded complete commitment as a combatant, and inevitably changed who they were over the course of the war. Fighting men had to interpret their sensory experiences while struggling to survive and fight alongside comrades they often had not met before reaching the front. Attempting to guide Red Army troops throughout this process was a propaganda apparatus separated from that which the civilian population encountered. Despite the apparent specificity of frontline propaganda, the flagship publication for soldiers, *Krasnaia Zvezda*, failed to address their concerns or comprehensively shape their interpretation of the frontlines. This failure stemmed from a combination of propagandists' limited experience of combat or front life, rigid ideological priorities, and a failure to consider the embodied reality of soldiers' experiences of war. Incongruity between soldiers' views and propaganda persisted throughout the war, and produced a dynamic that was distinct among the war efforts of both allied and enemy countries.

The nature of total war diminished the distinctiveness of sensory experiences among different national armies. The sophistication of weaponry troops had to master, the high casualty rates of frontline units, and development of a masculine, small-unit, frontline culture characterized the war experience of the main belligerents. The Red Army's main adversary, the German Wehrmacht, operated differently in a few crucial aspects that contributed to the distinctiveness of the Soviet experience. Most German soldiers accepted ideological interpretations of the war effort, meaning there was no significant difference between official and soldierly understandings of the front experience.[67] Moreover, women played a minor role in even auxiliary services of the military, which provided no jarring experience of isolation and then re-introduction to the sight of women within the ranks.[68] The US Army, as the Red Army's primary allied fighting force, also fought with significant structural differences that affected US soldiers' understanding of the war. The configuration of US media differed dramatically from that of the Soviet propaganda state, and US coverage of the war proved entirely more honest about issues of soldiers' wounds, deaths, and sexual interest in women.[69] The US military also engaged in less intense and less deadly fighting for a shorter period than the Red Army, and never experienced sustained isolation from women in the European Theatre of Operations.[70] The differences of its primary adversary and primary ally highlight the Soviet struggle between official and soldierly interpretations of the sensory experiences of war and the challenge of integrating a sizeable cohort of women combatants and auxiliaries into a fighting force that began with men alone.

A study of sensory experiences in the Red Army in the Second World War highlights several key facets of a notoriously brutal conflict. The lens of embodiment reveals how the senses not only registered the extreme horror and physical danger that confronted Red Army men in battle but also the embodied practices that enabled them to survive and cope with the threat of a violent death. Likewise, scrutiny of the embodied, or more often disembodied, efforts of Red Army propaganda to mobilize or motivate troops helps explain its shortcomings. Alongside a general scarcity of sensory details, a mandate to infuse the physical demands of war with ideological content and pre-war practices yielded propaganda heroes who lacked the bodily needs, limits, or sexual desires of actual Russian troops. Instead, among the heroic figures troops were to emulate, ideological commitment served as a substitute for the power of the senses to induce physiological or emotional reactions. Ultimately, the contrast between propaganda in *Krasnaia Zvezda* and soldiers' embodied memories highlights how meaningful and disruptive sensory experience could be within a successful war effort.

Notes

1 Aleksandr V. Pyl'tsyn, *Shtrafnoi udar* (Moscow: Znanie, 2003), 112.
2 Martin Jay, "In the Realm of the Senses: An Introduction," *The American Historical Review* 116 (2) (2011): 309.
3 Mark M. Smith, "Still Coming to 'Our' Senses: An Introduction," *The Journal of American History* 95 (2) (2008): 379.
4 Mark M. Smith, *The Smell of Battle, The Taste of Siege: A Sensory History of the Civil War* (New York: Oxford University Press, 2013), 7.
5 All memoirs and oral history interviews were published after 1991 (most after 2000), and first appeared in print in Russian. The texts do not shy away from sensitive issues such as prisoner killing, rape, or looting by the Red Army, which strongly suggests that they have not been edited or censored. For an analysis of relationships, goals, and achievements, as well as more elaborate discussion about the limits and uses of different source types, see Steven G. Jug, "All Stalin's Men? Soldierly Masculinities in the Soviet War Effort, 1938–1945" (PhD diss., University of Illinois, 2013).
6 William A. Cohen, *Embodied: Victorian Literature and the Senses* (Minneapolis: University of Minnesota Press, 2008), xiii–6.
7 Jochen Hellbeck, *Revolution on My Mind: Writing a Diary Under Stalin* (Cambridge, MA: Harvard University Press, 2006); Anna Krylova, *Soviet Women in Combat: A History of Violence on the Eastern Front* (Cambridge: Cambridge University Press, 2010), 9–12.
8 Sean Guillory, "The Shattered Self of Komsomol Civil War Memoirs," *Slavic Review* 71 (3) (2012): 550.

9   Simon Creak, *Embodied Nation: Sport, Masculinity, and the Making of Modern Laos* (Honolulu: University of Hawai'i Press), 9.

10 Ana María Alonso, "The Politics of Space, Time, and Substance: State Formation, Nationalism and Ethnicity," *Annual Review of Anthropology* 23 (1994): 386.

11 For the standard treatment of the Stakhanovite movement, see Lewis H. Siegelbaum, *Stakhanovism and the Politics of Productivity in the USSR, 1935–1941* (Cambridge: Cambridge University Press, 1988). On athletics, see Susan Grant, *Physical Culture and Sport in Soviet Society: Propaganda, Acculturation, and Transformation in the 1920s and 1930s* (New York: Routledge, 2012). For the role of national exploits in Soviet culture, see Katerina Clark, *The Soviet Novel: History as Ritual*, 3rd ed. (Bloomington: Indiana University Press, 2000), Chapter 5.

12 I focus on newspapers and text-based propaganda materials over visual forms, such as films, plays, songs, and posters. While such materials remain evocative to postwar and non-Soviet audiences, studies of these aspects of wartime culture cannot explain how frequently they reached the front, and how widely soldiers saw them. For example, see Suzanne Ament, "Reflecting Individual and Collective Identities—Songs of World War II," in *Gender and National Identity in Twentieth-Century Russian Culture*, ed. Helena Goscilo et al. (DeKalb: Northern Illinois University Press, 2006), 115–30.

13 Karel Berkhoff argues in favor of the influence of propaganda, even if not true. Karel Berkhoff, *Motherland in Danger: Soviet Propaganda during World War II* (Cambridge, MA: Harvard University Press, 2012), 66–7. Catherine Merridale contends that official ideals were inspiring and popular because they had staying power in the same official culture that first invented them. Catherine Merridale, *Ivan's War: Life and Death in the Red Army, 1939–1945* (New York: Picador, 2007), 189–98. Roger Reese likewise focuses on truth in propaganda as the key issue. Roger Reese, *Why Stalin's Soldiers Fought: The Red Army's Military Effectiveness in World War II* (Lawrence: University Press of Kansas, 2011), 193–5.

14 Smith's approach rests on detecting those battles in which one sense came to predominate over all others, while I focus on recurrence of a specific type of meaning assigned to different sensory experiences. Smith, *The Smell of Battle*, 8.

15 Smith, *The Smell of Battle*, 67.

16 Ivan Yakushin, *On the Roads of War: A Soviet Cavalryman on the Eastern Front* (Barnsley: Pen and Sword, 2005), 70.

17 Recollections of Aleksandr Vasil'evich Rogachev in Artem Drabkin, ed., *Panzer Killers: Anti-Tank Warfare on the Eastern Front*, trans. Stuart Britton (Barnsley: Pen and Sword, 2013), 198.

18 Joseph Pilyushin, *Red Sniper on the Eastern Front: The Memoirs of Joseph Pilyushin*, ed. Sergey Anisimov, trans. Stuart Briton (Barnsley: Pen and Sword, 2010), 1.

19 Petr Mikhin, *Guns Against the Reich: Memoirs of an Artillery Officer on the Eastern Front*, trans. Bair Irincheev and Stuart Britton (Barnsley: Pen and Sword, 2010), 13–4.

20 Recollections of Vitaly Andreevich Ulianov in Drabkin, ed., *Panzer Killers*, 34.
21 Vasily Reshetnikov, *Bomber Pilot on the Eastern Front: 307 Missions Behind Enemy Lines*, ed. Serguey Anisimov, trans. Vladimir Kroupnik, John Armstrong, and Sarah Bryce (Barnsley: Pen and Sword, 2008), 12.
22 Recollections of Boris Vasil'evich Nazarov, in Drabkin, ed., *Panzer Killers*, 90.
23 Vasiliy Krysov, *Panzer Destroyer: Memoirs of a Red Army Tank Commander* (Barnsley: Pen and Sword, 2010), 108.
24 Nikolai I. Obryn'ba, *Red Partisan: The Memoir of a Soviet Resistance Fighter on the Eastern Front* (Washington, DC: Potomac Books, 2007), 16.
25 On the typical behavior of correspondents at the front, see Antony Beevor, ed., *A Writer at War: Vasily Grossman with the Red Army, 1941–1945*, trans. Luba Vinogradova (New York: Pantheon Books, 2005), xi–xiv. On the official sources of front reports, including Soviet leader Joseph Stalin's personal involvement, see Karel C. Berkhoff, *Motherland in Danger: Soviet Propaganda during World War II* (Cambridge, MA: Harvard University Press, 2012), 30–7.
26 Beevor, ed., *A Writer at War*, 16.
27 Ibid., 20.
28 Recollections of Nikolai Konstantinovich Shishkin, in Drabkin, ed., *Panzer Killers*, 135–6.
29 Recollections of Moisei Isaakovich Dorman, in Artem Drabkin, ed., *Ia dralsia s Pantservaffe* (Moscow: Iauza, 2007), 187.
30 Petr Mikhin, *Guns Against the Reich: Memoirs of a Soviet Artillery Officer on the Eastern Front* (Barnsley: Pen and Sword, 2010), 115.
31 Pyl'tsyn, *Shtrafnoi udar*, 29.
32 Recollections of Boris Vasil'evich Nazarov, in Drabkin, ed., *Panzer Killers*, 99.
33 Reshetnikov, *Bomber Pilot on the Eastern Front*, 13.
34 "At a Leningrad rally of snipers," *Krasnaia Zvezda*, February 26, 1942, 3.
35 "Master of Artillery Reconnaissance," *Krasnaia Zvezda*, January 8, 1944, 3.
36 Siegelbaum, *Stakhanovism*, chapter 6. See also, Toby Clark, "The 'New Man's' Body: A Motif in Early Soviet Culture," in *Art of the Soviets: Painting, Sculpture and Architecture in a One-Party State,* ed. Matthew Cullerne Bown et al. (Manchester: Manchester University Press, 1993), 43.
37 "Our troops break enemy resistance," *Krasnaia Zvezda* 31 January 1942, 1.
38 "The aimed fire of snipers," *Krasnaia Zvezda* May 15, 1942, 2.
39 Sonya O. Rose, *Which People's War? National Identity and Citizenship in Wartime Britain, 1939–1945* (New York: Oxford University Press, 2003), 153–9.
40 Christina Jarvis, *The Male Body at War: American Masculinity during World War II* (Dekalb: Northern Illinois University Press, 2004), 125–9.

41 Recollections of Boris Vasil'evich Nazarov in Drabkin, ed., *Panzer Killers*, 92.
42 Recollections of Dorman, in Drabkin, ed., *Panzer Killers*, 106–7.
43 Mansur Abdulin, *Red Road from Stalingrad: Recollections of a Soviet Infantryman* (Barnsley: Pen and Sword, 2004), 11.
44 Recollections of Ulianov, in Drabkin, ed., *Panzer Killers*, 28.
45 "An agitator in the trench," *Krasnaia Zvezda*, December 9, 1942, 3.
46 "The exploit of Komsomol Farafonov," *Krasnaia Zvezda*, December 16, 1942, 2.
47 "We will become masters of our domain," *Krasnaia Zvezda*, April 5, 1942, 2.
48 Eliot Borenstein, *Men without Women: Masculinity and Revolution in Russian Fiction, 1917–1929* (Durham, NC: Duke University Press, 2000), 24.
49 Recollections of Sergei L'vovich Ariia, in Artem Drabkin, ed., *Ia dralsia na T–34* (Moscow: Iauza, 2008), 96.
50 Nikolai Litvin, *800 Days on the Eastern Front: A Russian Soldier Remembers World War II* (Lawrence: University Press of Kansas, 2007), 111.
51 Recollections of Rostislav Ivanovich Zhidkov, in Artem Drabkin, ed., *Na voine kak na voine* (Moscow: Iauza, 2013), 592–3.
52 RGASPI, f. M-33. op. 1, d. 99, ll 1–2.
53 Dmitriy Loza, *Fighting for the Soviet Motherland: Recollections of the Eastern Front*, ed. and trans. James F. Gebhardt (Lincoln: University of Nebraska Press, 1998), 210.
54 "Courageous Medics," *Krasnaia Zvezda*, March 13, 1942, 2.
55 "The death of private Malinin," *Krasnaia Zvezda*, February 16, 1944, 2.
56 "The grave of a guards soldier," *Krasnaia Zvezda*, April 16, 1942, 3.
57 For estimates on the chronology of women's entry into military service, see Krylova, *Soviet Women*, 299. On women's varied frontline roles and their impact, see Roger D. Markwick and Euridice Charon Cardona, *Soviet Women on the Frontline in the Second World War* (London: Palgrave Macmillan, 2012).
58 On officer-soldier rivalries and resentments about women and their impact on Red Army gender dynamics, see Steven G. Jug, "Red Army Romance: Preserving Masculine Hegemony in Mixed Gender Combat Units, 1943–1944," *Journal of War and Culture Studies* 5 (3) (2012).
59 Mikhin, *Guns Against the Reich*, 195.
60 Cohen, *Embodied*, xvi.
61 R. W. Connell's revised formulation of the hierarchical relationship of genders distinguishes between "internal" and "external" masculine hegemony: the internal domination over subordinate masculinities that do not contribute to the maintenance of patriarchy, which reinforces external domination over the "emphasized femininity" defined in contradistinction. The emphasized femininity is defined around compliance with the subordination of women to men and presents women with traits and behaviors that accommodate the interests and desires of men. R. W. Connell and James W. Messerschmidt,

"Hegemonic Masculinity: Rethinking the Concept," *Gender and Society* 26 (6) (2005): 847–8.
62. Laura Mulvey, "Visual Pleasure and Narrative Cinema," *Screen* 16 (3) (1975): 6–18.
63. Abdulin, *Red Road from Stalingrad*, 150.
64. "An agitator's useful initiative," *Krasnaia Zvezda*, December 18, 1942, 3.
65. "A Red Army kitchen," *Krasnaia Zvezda*, April 11, 1943, 1.
66. "Young women—military cooks," *Krasnaia Zvezda*, December 5, 1944, 2.
67. Omer Bartov, *Hitler's Army: Soldiers, Nazis, and War in the Third Reich* (Oxford: Oxford University Press, 1991).
68. Karen Hagemann, "Mobilizing Women for War: The History, Historiography, and Memory of German Women's War Service in the Two World Wars," *Journal of Military History* 75 (4) (2011): 1055–93.
69. Jarvis, *The Male Body at War*.
70. From the D-day landings to the liberation of Paris, Allied losses and French civilian casualties briefly reached Eastern Front levels. Antony Beevor, *D-Day: The Battle for Normandy* (New York: Viking Penguin, 2009), 522. On the contrasting character of the US Pacific experience, see John A. Lynn, *Battle: A History of Combat and Culture* (New York: Basic Books, 2004), Chapter 7 "The Merciless Fight: Race and Military Culture in the Pacific War." On US soldiers' sexual opportunities in Europe, see Mary Louise Roberts, *What Soldiers Do: Sex and the American GI in World War II France* (Chicago: University of Chicago Press, 2014).

PART FOUR

Reconstructing Russia

CHAPTER ELEVEN

The sensory experience of martyrdom and Soviet collective memory

Adrienne Harris

In her 2011 article "Productive Death: The Necropedagogy of a Young Soviet Hero," cultural historian Maria Tumarkin details the role the Second World War martyrs played in Tumarkin's psyche:

> As I was growing up in the Soviet Union in the 1970s and 1980s, there was one death scene I compulsively reimagined and restaged in my mind, one that would not leave me alone. [...] Tortured by the Nazis, seventeen-year-old [sic] Zoya Kosmodemyanskaya, who quit her Moscow high school to join partisans as soon as the Great Patriotic War started in June 1941, does not give up the names of her comrades. While the German army advances toward Moscow and the Soviet army is in disarray, partisans are ordered to do all in their power to sabotage and derail the enemy's war effort. This includes setting fire to the occupied Soviet villages so as to destabilize the German troops stationed there. This is what Kosmodemyanskaya does, and this is how she gets caught. At the time when the enemy's onslaught seems unstoppable, partisans like her carry the hopes of the besieged nation. Taken to the gallows for a public execution, Kosmodemyanskaya shows no fear. Instead, she shouts to the villagers forced to watch her die, "Comrades! Why are you so gloomy? I am not afraid to die!" [...] Maybe because I can still "feel" the story of Kosmodemyanskaya's death not as cold and utterly explicable artifice but as what was once a hot, powerful, and unsettling presence, I am not content to reconstruct it backward [...] as a linear progression from the actual historical event to its reconstitution into a myth.[1]

Although her account of Zoia's *podvig* (feat or exploit) contains some factual errors,[2] Tumarkin captures the living resonance of Zoia's story decades after her death. She notes the reimagining and revisualization of Zoia's death and recalls both Zoia's words and her silence. She *feels* the hagiographic narrative of Zoia's last moments.

This article asks how the sensory details of Second World War hero Zoia Kosmodemianskaia's death contributed to her prominent role in Soviet collective memory. I argue that Zoia's image remained central in Soviet memory largely because the Soviet citizenry could imagine her *podvig* more clearly than those of other heroes. What does the example of Zoia Kosmodemianskaia tell us about the role of the senses in mythmaking and memory? To answer these questions, I draw on archival documents (unpublished poems and letters), public sculptures and art, and published memoirs and literary works. I situate my analysis within scholarship related to sensory history, collective memory, and war commemoration. For comparative purposes, I juxtapose Zoia with Liza Chaikina, another partisan martyr hero whom the *Komsomol* promoted. Propagandists cited the two women's names together throughout the 1940s and 1950s, yet Chaikina never achieved Zoia's permanence in Russian collective memory.[3]

How did Zoia become a symbol of Soviet wartime resilience and patriotism? In late November 1941, a young woman operating behind enemy lines in the Moscow region was captured in the process of burning down a stable in the village of Petrishchevo. Although gravely tortured and forced to march

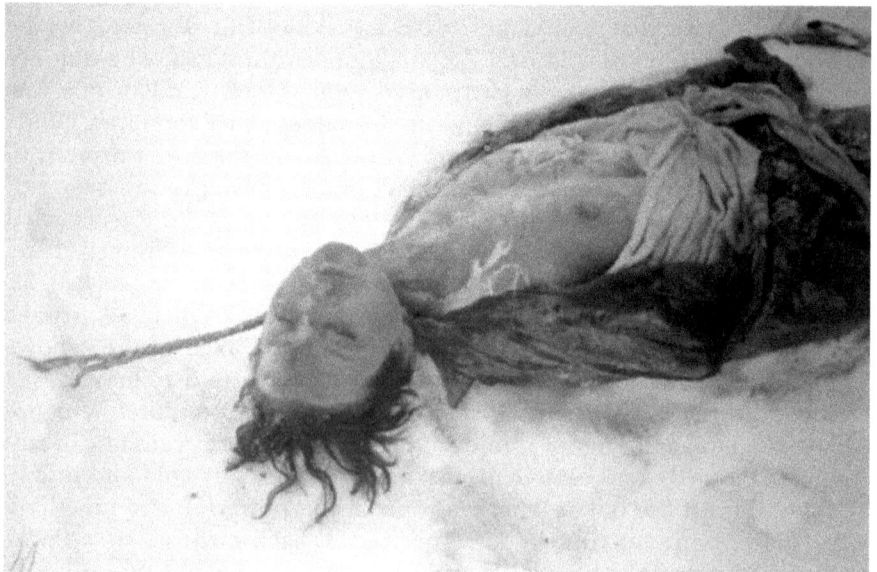

FIGURE 11.1 *Sergei Strunnikov's photograph of Zoia's exhumed body. Courtesy of the Russian State Archive of Social and Political History, Moscow (RGASPI).*

undressed and barefoot for hours in the snow, the woman who identified herself simply as "Tania" refused to divulge any information about her mission, and, instead, delivered an inspiring speech to the Russian villagers assembled to watch her be hanged on November 29. The body remained in the square a month, perhaps as a warning and on New Year's Eve, inebriated Nazis stabbed it with bayonets and cut off the left breast before finally burying it. After the area's liberation several weeks later, *Pravda* correspondent Petr Lidov visited the village and learned of "Tania's" fate. Lidov published the story in *Pravda* on January 27, 1942, and "Tania" was identified as an eighteen-year-old Moscow school girl, Zoia Kosmodemianskaia, a special forces scout serving in the 9903 partisan unit. Lidov's article contained all the hagiographic elements necessary, including Sergei Strunnikov's gruesome photograph of her exhumed body (Figure 11.1), to ensure Zoia's secular canonization as a Hero of the Soviet Union and to fix her central position in the pantheon of Soviet saints. Journalists and Komsomol officials immediately spotted the potential of Zoia's image to motivate her compatriots and they shaped its execution and her narrative accordingly.

The photograph that traumatized the nation

Early into my study of Zoia's cult, I recognized the centrality of the visual sense in her memorialization. The image of her mutilated body was imprinted on Soviet collective memory from the inception of the myth: Strunnikov's photograph has always accompanied and documented Zoia's martyrdom.[4] Strunnikov's photograph depicts the body of a young woman, her head thrown back, with a peaceful face—bruised, yet largely uncorrupted. The rope by which her Nazi executioners hanged her remains tethered to her neck. The body lies in the snow. Most horrifyingly, her open shirt reveals her breasts, one of which has been cut off from the body. When discussing Zoia Kosmodemianskaia, Russians still reference this photograph.

In her cultural analysis of pain, literary critic Elaine Scarry reminds us that we must analyze wounds within their individual cultural contexts, in relation to other cultural signs.[5] Wartime readers might not have known that the body was mutilated after death. Regardless, the image would have had a profound impact on the Russian population that, until a generation before, had believed in the sanctity of the whole body upon death, so it could enter the afterlife complete. I have posited that Zoia remains the supreme war martyr, because the Russian nation has always been able to visualize her tortured last moments and her death through media depictions of her body and detailed description of her final hours. History did not preserve images of the bodies of the other great Second World War martyrs who achieved national acclaim.

Numerous visual cultural scholars have argued that sight has occupied a central position in Western culture, in large part because of the invention of moveable type, as well as the expansion of technologies that allow one to observe.[6] While written language has little to do with the resonance of Zoia's myth in Russian culture, the Russian Orthodox heritage and the

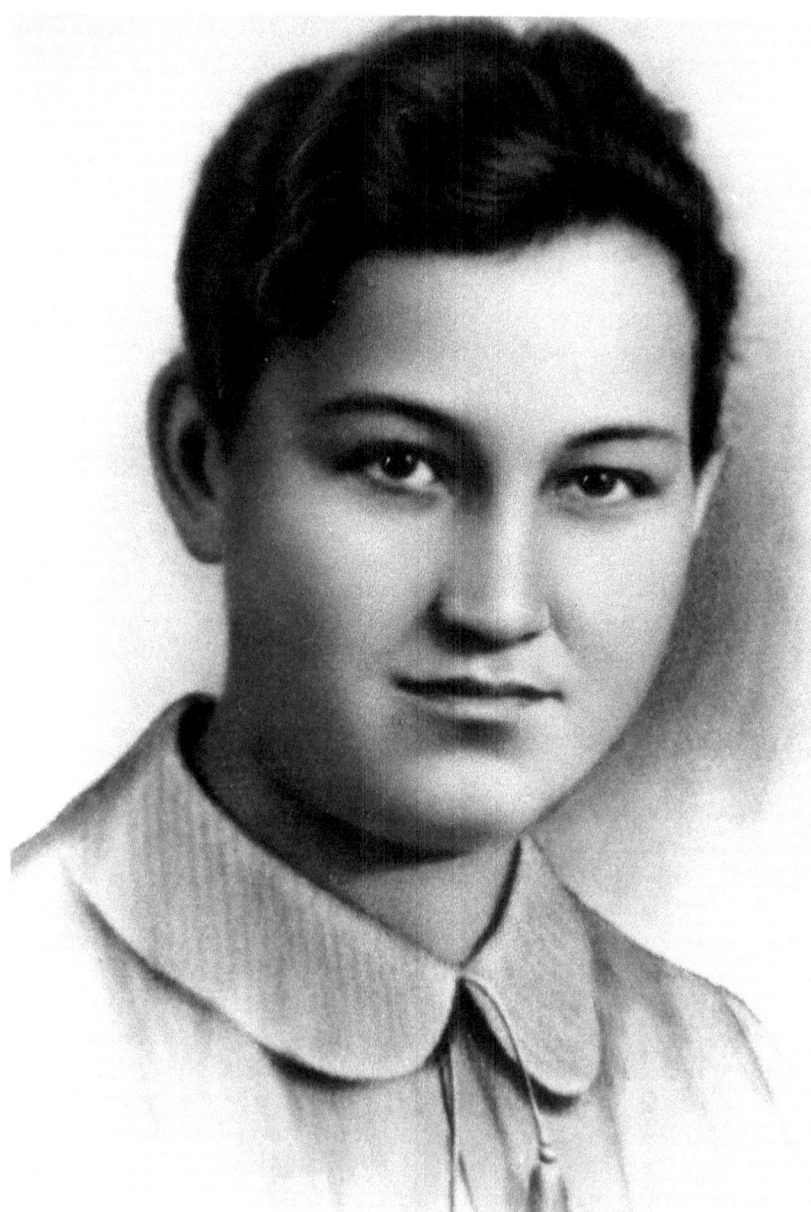

FIGURE 11.2 *Zoia's school portrait, courtesy of RGASPI.*

central role of icons played large roles in her permanence. Nina Tumarkin has shown how the makers of Soviet propaganda relied upon Orthodox models for the cult of Lenin and later Stalin, demonstrating the compatibility of Orthodox forms with communist meaning.[7] The veneration of saints, ancestors, and relics never entirely died out under Soviet rule. *Podvig*

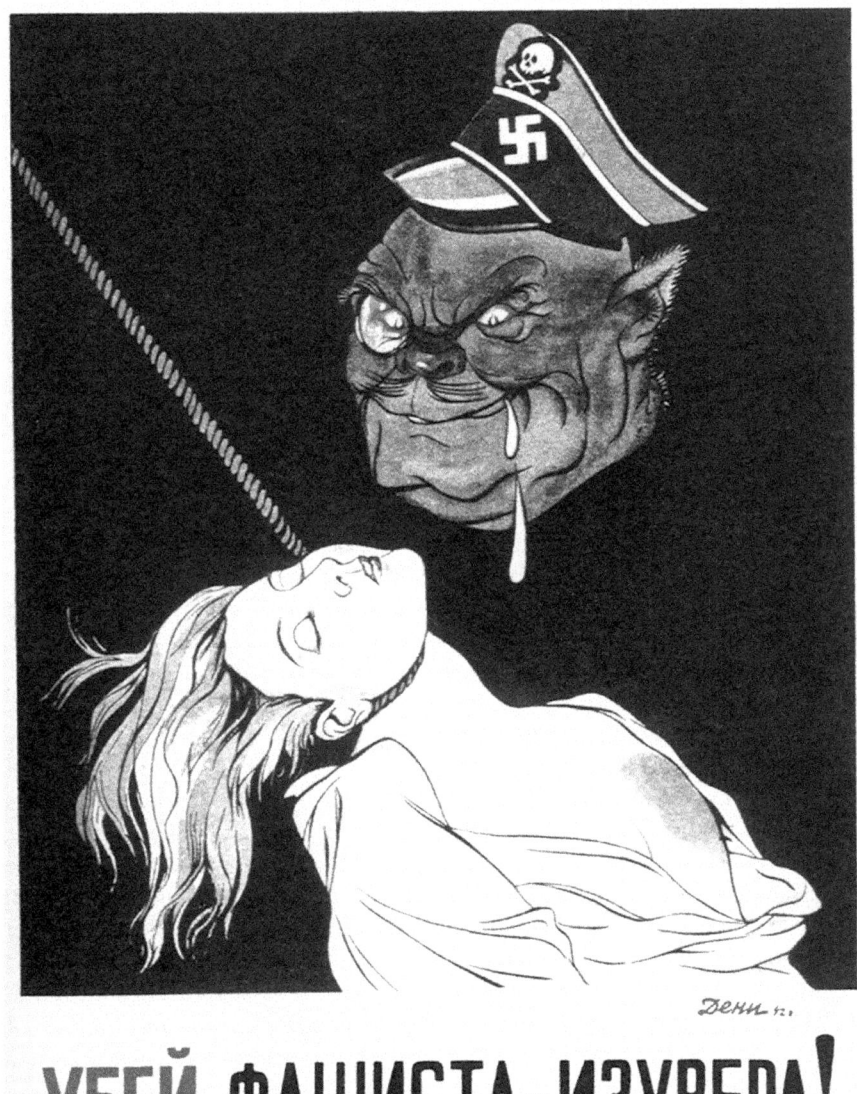

FIGURE 11.3 *Viktor Deni,* Kill the Fascist-Monster!, *1942. Courtesy of Helena Goscilo.*

itself is originally an Orthodox concept. Russian cultural historian Elina Kahla notes that "the concept of *podvig,* connoting an exploit, a feat, or the virtuousness of a person, is organically linked with the concept of vita: the vita is about the exploits of a saint."[8] Strunnikov's photograph showed a mutilated corpse with a serene, uncorrupted face, which did not go unnoticed by a people owning a long tradition of venerating uncorrupted corpses as saints and maintaining a belief that God—a belief in a higher power or Truth—enabled them to overcome their pain.[9]

Roughly two weeks after Lidov's "Tania" appeared in print, *Komsomol* authorities released the unknown partisan's identity. *Pravda* published another Lidov article, "Who was Tania?" and illustrated it with the school picture that would become iconic. The portrait (Figure 11.2) depicts an androgynous schoolgirl—a stark departure from Strunnikov's photograph. The media initially bombarded the Soviet public with these two contradictory photographs, images that contributed to a kind of schizophrenic conceptualization of Zoia. The discrepancy between these two bodies would eventually lead to the rumors that continue to this day that Zoia was not the "Tania" executed in Petrishchevo. More significantly in the early mythological process, this disconnect let her body function as an empty vessel and site for others' projections. When juxtaposed with each other, contradictory depictions of Zoia's body as both prepubescent and as curvy draw attention to her youth and her lost potential as wife and mother, a theme common to literary texts about Zoia, as this chapter will discuss below.

Immediately upon the publication of Lidov's articles, propagandists began using Zoia's image and narrative to motivate its citizenry to fight more fiercely and to work harder to avenge Zoia's death. Clearly, in public art and sculpture, artists referenced her wound from these early days. In 1942, Deni's propaganda poster referenced Strunnikov's photograph, reproducing Zoia's wound, and urged Soviet citizens to avenge Zoia (Figure 11.3). In October of that year, the renowned sculptor Matvei Manizer debuted his model of Zoia; Manizer's Zoia and almost all future sculptures would point to Zoia's breast, referencing her mutilation and reminding citizens of her horrific death (Figure 11.4). To avoid violating masculine norms, newspapers never showed disfigured male bodies, unless the men were very young or very old, however, newspapers included images of victimized women's bodies in an effort to prompt men to avenge them. The violation of women's bodies, and in particular the post-mortem mutilation of Zoia's left breast, transcended the abuse of individual bodies, or even of maidenly bodies, and can be read as an affront on the entire nation and an attack on the Soviet body's capacity to regenerate itself.

Official literary works reflect the resonance of Strunnikov's image of Zoia's body and the penetration of the media coverage of Zoia's martyrdom. Hero of the Soviet Union and Molodiaia Gvardiia commissar Oleg Koshevoi's mother describes her son's reaction to Lidov's article in her hagiographic *Story of a Son*: "Perhaps, at that moment [when he read

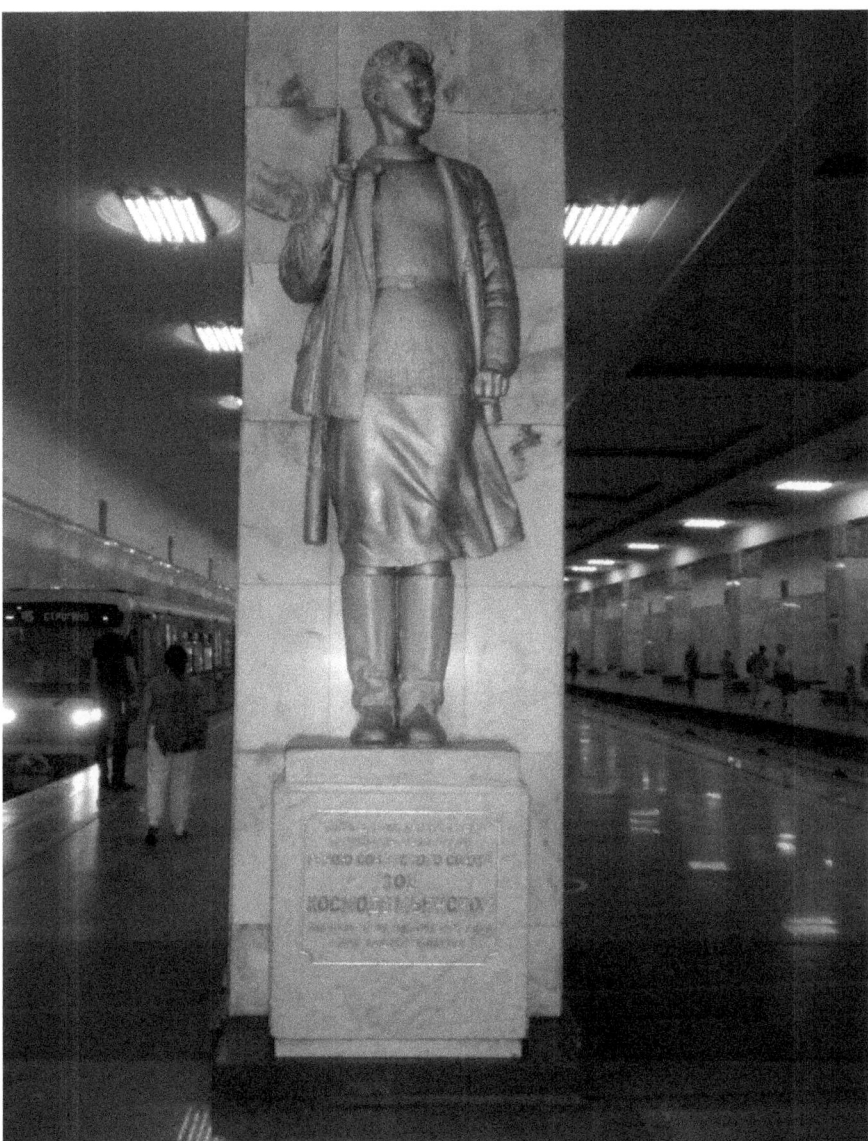

FIGURE 11.4 *Matvei Manizer's sculpture of Zoia in the Partizanskaia metro station. Photograph taken by the author.*

about the death of Kosmodemianskaia] he imagined for himself the courageous path of Zoia, and it is possible, that that was precisely when his heart became enflamed with the fire of revenge which never from that time would extinguish in his chest."[10] Elena writes that he cut her picture out of the paper, framed it, and hung it over his bed. Koshevoi was one of many who treated Zoia's image as an item of veneration—an icon.

Poet Margarita Aliger provides the strongest example of the impact Zoia's image had in elite literature. Between July and September 1942, Aliger wrote the best-known literary work about Zoia: her Stalin Prize winning "Zoia: Poema," published in 1943. The poem, rife with vivid imagery appeals to the visual sense—prompting readers to visualize Zoia as a child and an adolescent. She mentions young men noticing Zoia as she comes of age, transforming Zoia into an object of the male gaze. Toward the end of the narrative poem, she provides a poetic description of Strunnikov's photograph, but she contextualizes it within a romance. She proceeds to describe the scene in the photograph and transforms Zoia's body into a reclining woman's body, awaiting a suitor:

A maidenly body,
    Neither dead
                  Nor alive.
Zoia made of marble
    Lying quietly in the snow.
Her thin neck is broken by a merciless noose.
There's an unknown power in your face, thrown back.
As if you were awaiting your beloved,
    Growing prettier through a hidden beauty,
Illuminating from inside with a secret women's fire.
Only you didn't wait for him, snow bride.
He wears a fighter's coat
                His path lies to the West.
Maybe not far from this terrible place,
Where snowflakes lie on her rigid chest.
An inimitable unity of eternal strength and weakness.
You are entirely cold, but grief burns through me.
Maternity did not burst in to you, did not boil up in you
The hot mouth of a child did not touch your dry nipple.
You lie on the snow.
    Oh how much you gave for us,
In order to proudly recline your pure, beautiful face![11]

In this short passage, Aliger propels the Zoia pictured in Strunnikov's photograph into a dramatically different direction, out of the stillness of death and into a dynamic fantasy. She uses the visual image as inspiration to construct an entire romantic narrative, a narrative that underscores the eroticism of Zoia's position and her exposed chest. These lines address both her martyred body and the loss of the maternal experience that she would never know. I have written elsewhere that this tendency to construct fictitious romances around female war heroes conforms to a larger trend in Soviet culture in keeping with the pronatalist movement that takes shape during the war.[12] The visual sense played a key role in the feminization of these war heroes.

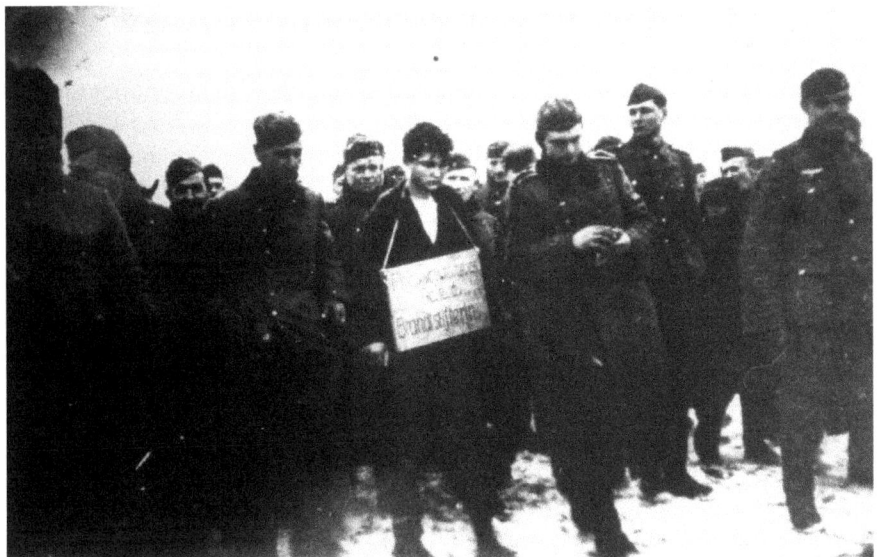

FIGURE 11.5 *One of the five photographs found in 1943 that depicted Zoia's execution. Courtesy of RGASPI.*

Aliger concludes this section with an explicit reference to Strunnikov's photograph and instructions for its treatment:

Always keep Zoia's photograph
I surely will never be able to forget it.

The visual sense shapes Aliger's memory as the image of Zoia's body has left a lasting imprint on Aliger's psyche.

Additional images surfaced in 1943 and continued to shape the memorialization of Zoia. In October 1943, Russian soldiers discovered five photographs of Zoia's execution on the body of a German officer killed near Smolensk. Newspapers reprinted these photographs, which corroborated witnesses' accounts. Viewers of the photographs are able to see Zoia's calm demeanor as she walked to her execution. They provide another side to the multifaceted image of Zoia for Soviet citizens to negotiate in their memories: the semi-erotic, mutilated body, an iconic school portrait, and the young partisan dressed for her mission in men's pants.

A call to arms and resolute silence

Perhaps because of these photographs and monuments that commemorated Zoia, particularly Komov's 1986 sculpture on Zoia's grave, I had assumed that Zoia's body had always been central in her collective memory and that the missing breast, mutilated body, bare feet, and bound hands had left the deepest impression on Zoia's contemporaries. After reading 197 pages of unpublished, archived poetry written between 1942 and 1943 and sent to *Komsomolskaia Pravda,* I discovered that her tortured body played less of a role in individuals' imaginations—at least in the early days of Zoia commemoration—than I had previously assumed. I found only one citation of a mutilated body, few mentions of torture—most quite vague, one reference to her chest, two to her lips (which she bit through as she maintained her silence under interrogation), three of her hands, and only three of her bare feet.[13] In contrast, I found twenty invocations of her words. One author even structured his lyric poem around her words. These archived documents—unofficial, unsolicited poems—prompted me to reconsider how average people processed Zoia's *podvig* and to re-examine official works created by professionals to see what role the auditory sense played; I realized that my visual bias had prevented me from understanding Zoia's impact on a deeper level.

In her chapter on wartime nursing, Laurie Stoff argues that privileging sight over other senses "has led to the unfortunate disregard of other sensory perceptions and the neglect of important elements of wartime experiences." She advocates for the addition of auditory and other senses to our analysis of wartime experience because these senses shaped memory in ways beyond the visual. A re-examination of these poems and other archived responses from 1942 give evidence that scholars should devote more attention to what Jonathan Sterne has termed "sound culture" or "sound studies." He explains this lacuna:

> Today, it is understood across the human sciences that vision and visual culture are important matters. Many contemporary writers interested in various aspects of visual culture (or, more properly, visual aspects of various cultural domains)—the arts, design, landscape, media, fashion—understand their work as contributing to a core set of theoretical, cultural, and historical questions about vision and images. While writers interested in visual media have for some time gestured toward a conceptualization of *visual culture,* no such parallel construct—*sound culture* or, simply, *sound studies*—has broadly informed work on hearing or the other senses. While sound is considered as a unified intellectual problem in some science and engineering fields, it is less developed as an integrated problem in the social and cultural disciplines.[14]

I eventually concluded that during the war, the auditory sense played a central role comparable to the visual sense and that it motivated citizens' actions to a greater degree.

During the war, Zoia's words would have held particular significance. According to the official narrative, Zoia died with a message for her compatriots. Lidov initially reported her final words as:

> Comrades! Why do you look so sad? Be braver, fight, beat the Germans, burn them, destroy them! I am not scared to die, comrades. It's happiness to die for one's nation…You will hang me now, but I'm not alone. There are 200 million of us, you cannot hang us all. They will avenge me. Soldiers! It's not too late to surrender to us. All the same, victory will be ours. They will avenge me … Goodbye, comrades! Fight, don't be afraid! Stalin's with us! Stalin will come![15]

Not surprisingly, organizations responded to Zoia's call. On February 18, 1942, immediately after the release of Zoia's identity, the Timiriazevskii regional Komsomol Committee concluded a bulletin with Zoia's call to arms: "We hear a voice: 'Be braver, fight, beat the Germans, burn them, destroy them!' We will fight, comrade Zoia! In cruel days of battles with the hated enemy, we will erect an eternal monument of glory in our hearts to you, soldier and friend."[16] Zoia grew up and lived in the Timiriazevskii region of Moscow; it was only fitting that her native Komsomol Committee, located in the metaphorical heart of the nation, responded publicly and exemplified correct behavior.

On the same day, Zoia's mother Liubov Kosmodemianskaia repeated Zoia's call on the radio. Like Strunnikov's photograph and Lidov's article, Liubov Timofeevna's address penetrated the Soviet citizenry to its core. Propagandists would reprint her address in newspapers, pamphlets, and books as "Word of a Mother" and newspapers such as *Komsomolskaia Pravda* received countless letters addressed to Liubov Timofeevna from Soviet youth swearing to answer her call to arms by avenging Zoia. Liubov Timofeevna concluded her address with an excerpt from Zoia's words: "Be braver! Fight! Beat the Germans! Death to the fascist executioners! Death to them!"[17] This conclusion, Zoia's words proclaimed by her grieving mother, helped cement Zoia's call in the consciousness of Zoia's compatriots during those dire days of early 1942. Listeners heard the convergence of voices: both the hero's and the hero's mother's.

Zoia's *podvig* prompted countless unknown compatriots to respond verbally by sending letters to Zoia's mother and by sending poems to *Komsomolskaia Pravda*. These poems and letters give us insight into how ordinary people responded to Zoia's death. Moscow children evacuated to Omsk wrote Zoia's mother: "We give our word to you, Zoia, to work like you fought against the fascist butchers. We heard your voice, Zoia! We will avenge you! And we heard you, dear Liubov Timofeevna, who raised such an extraordinary daughter."[18] These children not only heard her voice but put themselves into dialogue with her.

Soldiers and civilians alike responded to Zoia's call. Nikolai Nosov, a mechanic in the army, stationed at the front, wrote:

> Your words ring out now like copper
> They fly through all of the fatherland:
> It is not scary to die for one's people,
> It's not a waste of life to die for the happiness of all.[19]

Similarly, junior sergeant Ivan Smirnov in the army, stationed at the front, writes of Zoia's words:

> Your *podvig* inspires soldiers to battle
> Partisans take revenge on Nazis for your death.
> And to us, *komtsomoltsy*,
> Don't you fearlessly turn your dear face?
>
> Do your words not consecrate us?
> The wind carries them into cities and villages
> Native Moscow heard your call
> And *komsomolki* rose up for their turn.[20]

These poems provide clear images of Zoia's call reaching all corners of the Soviet Union. In this poem, her words carry religious significance. Mariia Ruban from Sverdlovsk in the Voroshilovgradskaia oblast wrote of the motivational nature of Zoia's voice:

> Your speech was broken off—you were unable to finish it.
> Your antemortal voice serves as an ardent alarm,
> Which called to the definitive battle
> For us, it became a flame and a cry.[21]

Interestingly, unlike Strunnikov's immobile, eternal photograph, Zoia's words have always varied although witnesses, biographers, and journalists represent each version as truth. This shifting produces fuzzy memories that individuals must negotiate for themselves. Some poets creatively played with her words fitting them into their rhyme scheme. While reworking her words, some highlighted the reference to Stalin; others cut it—just as authors would do after Stalin's death.

Although the medium of film might privilege the visual sense, Lev Arnshtam organized much of his 1944 Stalin Prize winning film *Zoia* around the development of Zoia's consciousness. Arnshtam constructs his film, which historian Richard Stites deemed a "brilliantly executed Soviet fairytale,"[22] around Zoia's pre-execution claim that "it is happiness to die for one's people." The viewer witnesses Zoia as a schoolgirl writing "What is happiness?" in her notebook. As a result of her development in the Soviet school system and the Komsomol, she eventually comes to understand that happiness is love for her country and comrades, even if this love requires one to die for his or her nation. Released after the turn of the war, Arnshtam's Zoia delivers a message of selfless devotion to one's country useful for political education in the distant postwar future.

Jonathan Sterne notes that a few scholars have begun to recognize the necessity of more attention paid to auditory studies. An understanding of the relevance of sound is particularly helpful if cultural events, in this case, the emergence of a national hero, occurred in the age of the radio. One cannot underestimate the role of radio broadcasts and moving proclamations during the Second World War. Historian Lisa Kirschenbaum has discussed the role of the radio extensively in her study of the siege of Leningrad.[23] The radio also played a central function in Liza Chaikina's narrative. Nazis allegedly captured Chaikina as she traveled from village to village relaying Stalin's November 7, 1941 speech, which she had heard on the radio. Her repetition of Stalin's words assured that peasants in her occupied territory understood that the Nazis had not captured Moscow.

Sensory history helps one understand the role of plays and performances in both Zoia commemoration and the commemoration of other heroes. Those familiar with literary works based on Zoia's life likely know that Margarita Aliger penned a narrative poem about Zoia in 1942. She also wrote two versions of a play for schoolchildren, publishing one, *Zoia: A Fairy Tale about Truth*, in 1944. Archival documents indicate that when the play was broadcast over the radio in 1951, listeners found that the play transgressed the boundaries of acceptability and complained to Komsomol authorities. In addition to complaints of an excess of "mysticism" and heartbreak over a fictional romance with a suitor, the listeners were particularly offended by the liberties Aliger took with Zoia's last words. Clearly, some Soviet citizens took these productions quite seriously in which performers, often schoolchildren, acted out a fictionalized version of Zoia's biography and final moments serving a similar spiritual role as Christ's passion. One must consider how this play and similar variants about other heroes might have shaped memories—rooted in sensory experiences—of both spectators and actors. Beyond the case of Zoia Kosmodemianskaia, an examination of commemoration through the senses informs us about Soviet mythopoesis and the roles individual heroes played in Soviet culture—specifically for Soviet youth. Sensory scholarship allows one to understand non-elite responses to heroes and myths promoted by those who crafted and shaped propaganda. One must not underestimate the role of heroes in the Soviet context: the heroes served a religious function in a secular society and the makers of propaganda controlled the official images of these heroes. Nevertheless, Soviet citizens responded both collectively and individually to these images. Accordingly, their memorialization differed from commemoration of Western war heroes who did not hold such central roles. As Western commemoration lacked the centralized nature of the Soviet situation, individuals enjoyed much greater freedom of expression and the right to dedicate monuments acting as what historian Jay Winter had termed "fictive kinship" groups, "small groups of men and women ... whose presence antedated these monuments and whose bonds frequently endured long after they were unveiled."[24]

Finally, while Zoia's words motivated her compatriots to action and the recitation of both her words and the narrative of her *podvig* over the radio certainly helped cement her central position in the pantheon of Soviet martyrs, one cannot overlook the role of the absence of sound in her *podvig*. Her silence under immense torture would remain an equally integral part of her narrative. This resolute silence served as an example of what one should endure for one's nation and played a key role in memorialization. Maria Tumarkin references "Zoia not giving up the names of her comrades" in the passage quoted in the epigraph—clearly, it had become an integral part of the narrative memorized by children. The saying "remain silent like a partisan" stems from Zoia's resolute silence. In *Comrade Pavlik: The Rise and Fall of a Soviet Boy Hero*, literary scholar Catriona Kelly defines Zoia's ability to keep silence as "emotional management" and discusses the pedagogical usefulness of her exemplary self-control in raising children during the last years of the war and the immediate postwar period.[25]

Activity and passivity, art and witnesses

Attention to the senses allows one to reconsider activity and passivity in Zoia's narrative—both Zoia's and her witnesses'. While those focused on the visuals vacillate between a focus on activity and passivity—an active patriot to emulate or a passive victim to avenge—the auditory reproduction of Zoia's words creates an active agent. Deni's wartime propaganda poster contrasts strongly with versions of a portrait finished in 1947, by the artistic collective Kukryniksy. In "Tania (The Feat of Zoia Kosmodemianskaia)," Zoia looks intensely toward those gathered around the scaffolding as she prepares to speak. She holds the sign that reads "Arsonist" with one hand and clenches her empty hand in a fist.[26] She maintains an erect posture and projects defiance, bravery, and strength. Rather than referencing her mutilated body, the artists of the Kukryniksy captured the active resistance that transcended death.

Numerous works of visual art—paintings, sculptures, and illustrations—capture Zoia's resolute silence and exist at the intersection of multiple senses: the visual, auditory, and tactile. For example, those depicting Zoia in a state of undress point to the cold she experienced and her frostbitten feet. A painting preserved in Zoia's museum in Petrishchevo includes an oil lamp in the picture next to the resolutely silent young woman, reminding the viewer that Zoia refused to give away valuable information even as her torturers burned her.[27] Monuments in Petrishchevo, Volgograd, and Kiev all remind viewers of Zoia's physical suffering and her active, unyielding resistance.

Witnesses also bridge the senses as transmitters of Zoia's narrative—again Tumarkin captures them, as did Kukryniksy. These witnesses originally recited the narrative of Zoia's execution that led to Lidov's visit to Petrishchevo and they have always played a role in the narrative, representing the Soviet nation, forced to witness Nazi atrocities. Lidov reproduced witnesses' words as they detailed hearing Zoia's moans and the slashing of belts across her skin as Nazis tortured her. In Lidov's narrative, Nazi soldiers rounded up the townspeople and forced them to watch her public execution. In the Kukryniktsy painting, we gaze upon these witnesses as they observe a martyr's death and listen to her words; they would later fulfill the role of Christ's disciples, telling listeners touring Petrishchevo what they saw and heard in Petrishchevo. These witnesses would continue to play an integral role for years to come: constructing the narrative and passing it on as evangelists. For decades following Zoia's execution, newspaper editors deemed witnesses'—or supposed witnesses'—reports worthy of publication. A self-identified witness, A. S. Shmatkov describes Zoia's speech in the December 2, 1966, Kaluzhsky *oblast'* version of *Krasnoe Znamia*: "And seeing Zoia Kosmodem'ianskaia's death before my *very* eyes was staggering."[28] He describes the effect her words had on him: "I don't remember *what* the partisan said word for word. But her last words, her immortal speech, cut into my memory, not to cry, that there were many of us, that they would not hang us, that we would be victorious."[29] Witnesses were key—as parts of not only the official narrative but also functionally.

People mediate their individual perceptions of Zoia through their senses and the reports of the sensory experience of others. During the war, she served as a catalyst for action; some visualized her body, imagined her pain, and strove to avenge her. Others heard her words and recited them for themselves and heeding her call, they fought or worked harder for the war effort. Witnesses and the creators of art and literature reproduced all aspects of her *podvig*, ensuring that it would remain relevant in the postwar period.

Intersensorality and memorialization in Petrishchevo

The confluence of senses that historian Mark Smith calls "intersensorality"—the fact that senses act in concert—helps us understand more deeply how Soviet citizens would relive her torture and death after the war. From January 1942 on, when Lidov and Strunnikov first arrived in Petrishchevo to investigate the rumors of Zoia's death, witnesses played key roles in passing on Zoia's *podvig* orally and unofficially as citizens flocked to Petrishchevo to venerate and mourn Zoia. Initially, people came individually, yet in 1944, the Komsomol began shaping Petrishchevo into a monument denoting triumph and marked her execution site, the location of her *podvig*, with a wooden obelisk. By not marking Zoia's physicality, the Komsomol directed attention away from Zoia the individual and toward Zoia the national symbol of self-sacrificial duty, especially pertinent during the war years. Unlike monuments to Zoia in other places, this wartime memorial celebrates Zoia's words. The four sides of the obelisk mark nationally significant moments in her plot of self-sacrificial torture and death and resulting decoration and eternal glory. The monument combines inscriptions that compel the visitor to conjure up visual images, to imagine physical suffering, and to hear words. The side facing the site of her torture reads "Here, on 29 November 1941, German fascists executed *komsomolka*-partisan Zoia Kosmodemyanskaya," prompting visitors to reflect upon Zoia's torment. The other three sides point to Zoia's wartime political function and denote the triumphant nature of the site. Zoia's inspiring words "I am not scared to die, comrades. It is happiness to die for one's people" are written on the side that faces the forest from which Zoia came and fulfilled her duty. A third side references her decoration as a Hero of the Soviet Union and the fourth side, bearing the words "Eternal glory to the heroes who fell in the battle for freedom and independence of our Motherland," faces the location where the Komsomol would erect a museum to serve as a depository for the "relics," that would demonstrate that Zoia had been a moral, communist young woman.

After the war, Zoia remained relevant to both the Komsomol and individuals, but her official, public purpose evolved. Zoia's political usefulness as an exemplary *komsomolka* would transform from the war period into the postwar period and her image would develop as individuals negotiated her memory for themselves within the context of Soviet propaganda. Although educators hoped that Zoia would motivate Soviet youth to continue fighting the metaphorical battle for socialism, they realized that Zoia's primary postwar use lay in her act as an ideal role model rather than a victim to avenge. As the years passed, Zoia came to function as a type of quasi-patron saint for *komsomolki* in the atheist, Soviet context. Her voice, motivating the Soviet citizenry to war, receded while the visual reminders of her sacrifice persisted.

Historian Peter Charles Hoffer argues that "by engaging in sensory history we can stimulate our powers of imagination to their fullest extent" and "histories of the senses would fulfill the highest purpose of historical scholarship: to make the past live again."[30] By studying how people perceived Zoia, one understands the complexity of their commemoration. Early on, Komsomol authorities planned to dedicate a museum in Petrishchevo and as stated previously, Soviet citizens visited the site and talked to witnesses unofficially. Many of the initial plans came to fruition slowly, if ever. Calls for a museum came as early as 1942. In the 1950s at the suggestion of Komsomol secretary Nikolai Mikhailov, a museum opened and the facilities saw improvements in preparation for the 1957 international youth festival. In 1961, School 201 in Moscow opened a Zoia and Aleksandr Kosmodemianskii museum under the guidance of pedagogue Nikolai Borisov.

While curators intended both museums for patriotic, educational purposes, each acted as reliquaries. The Petrishchevo museum, in particular, served an almost sacred purpose as the site of Zoia's *podvig,* the reliquary that held items on which Zoia had shed blood. In her discussion of interactive seventeenth-century museums, Classen finds that "the museum, along with other exhibition sites, is treated as a kind of gymnasium for the senses,"[31] but that curators restricted museums to the visual as museums began to open publicly to members of lower classes. While visitors to Petrishchevo could not touch exhibits, they could approach and examine relics laden with meaning that would bring Zoia's narrative to life and embody her story in their memories: the table on which she was tortured, the bench on which she spent her final night. Cultural anthropologist C. Nadia Seremetakis has described memory as "a culturally mediated material practice that is activated by embodied acts and semantically dense objects. This material approach to memory places the senses in time and speaks to memory as both meta-sensory capacity and as a sense organ in-it-self."[32] Petrishchevo became a sacred space, and appeals to the senses helped visitors—namely children born after the war—negotiate meaning for themselves.

Schools in the Moscow area and pioneer groups made regular trips to Petrisichevo to visit the Zoia Kosmodemianskaia museum, but as part of the construction of the Moscow museum in School 201, Borisov had his pupils march through the snow where Zoia marched. They recorded witnesses' accounts and sketched her execution spot. This experience of "living history" became a martyr's pilgrimage, and surely helped the children experience Zoia's *podvig* on a deeper level: not only could they visualize the Petrishchevo about which they had read, they could feel the piercing cold and smell the peasant huts in which she spent her last hours.

In the introduction to her *The Deepest Sense: A Cultural History of Touch,* cultural historian Constance Classen details the benefits of the history of the senses and notes that "When we allow historical figures to be of flesh and blood we make it possible to relate to them as fellow beings and, therefore, to make meaningful comparisons between their lives and situations and our own."[33] Museums in Petrishchevo and Moscow, along with a focus on Zoia's corporality, certainly helped make her relatable to Soviet children. As they sat in her desk in Moscow or stared at the table on which she was tortured in Petrishchevo, they almost certainly could imagine themselves in her place. The children fortunate enough to visit these museums likely experienced Zoia on a deeper level than those who were only able to read about her.

Sculpture and the enduring role of the senses

As discussed earlier, commencing with Manizer, sculptors almost always referenced Zoia's left breast in some way. Later sculptures also captured key themes from Lidov's narrative: a nightshirt or dress referencing the undershirt or slip, the only item of clothing left after Nazis stripped her,[34] and the bare feet, on which she marched through the snow fulfilling Nazi orders. To this day, the image of the nearly-naked, beaten, bleeding partisan, walking barefoot through the snow touches people as they imagine the unbearable cold, as evidenced in the most recent monument to date on Russian soil: Viktor Fetisov's sculpture in Volgograd. Like Strunnikov's photograph of Zoia's reclining body, Zoia's march through the snow combined unimaginable strength with victimhood and contains erotic undertones.

The Volgograd sculpture, dedicated in 2008 on a square adjacent to School 130, holds particular significance as it replaces an earlier sculpture and takes commemoration in a more sensory direction. Near that location, two years ago, vandals had destroyed statues of both Kosmodemianskaia and another young Soviet hero, Pavlik Morozov. School children had collected funds to erect the original plaster statue in 1963 and in keeping with monuments to Zoia erected during the 1960s, it was a simple bust— it neither referenced her *podvig* or the treatment of her body; rather, it replicated her iconic school portrait. Ardent protests from veterans' organizations and groups with communist leanings resulted in Fetisov's "Return of Zoia Kosmodemianskaia."[35] In the years following the vandalism, the media had personified the sculpture, equating the statue with Zoia's body, and the act of vandalism with her torture and execution: "A Monument Suffered" and "The Execution of Zoia in Volgograd."[36] Fetisov incorporated this bodily focus and the monument references the wounds that characterize her narrative. The figure's arms are bound. The fabric of her shift is wrinkled and her jacket pulled back and bunched up in a manner that places emphasis on her left breast, the breast missing in Strunnikov's photograph. Like previous depictions, the folds of fabric clothe a strong body; her bound hands are clenched in fists. Like statues in Petrishchevo, the figure's bare feet recall the hours she spent marching barefoot in the snow on her last night. Fetisov constructed his three-meter statue out of white marble, a much more permanent substance than the plaster of the original. The white stone also alludes to the figure's innocence, in spite of its scantily clad state. The statue stands rooted to the ground on eye level and invites passersby, including children who attend School 130, to remember the agony Zoia experienced. The lack of an elevated podium eliminates the distance between the viewer and the statue, removes her from mythology, and brings her into the present. The inscription which reads "to young unconquerable patriots," synedochially represents Zoia's generation with her image and reminds today's children how the young patriots of the past suffered for their nation.

Why Zoia?

An examination of Zoia's function in collective memory though the lens of sensory experience has revealed much more precisely how she inspired her compatriots both during the war and during the postwar period. Sensory scholarship helps us understand how she penetrated memory for the long-term, unlike similar heroes such as Liza Chaikina. According to the official narratives, Liza Chaikina served as the Komsomol secretary of the Peno region of the Kalinin (now Tver) *oblast'*. During Nazi occupation, she organized underground activities and fought as a partisan. After being tortured, she was executed by shooting on November 22, 1941 at the age of twenty-three. The Soviet people learned about her *podvig* on March 7, 1942 in *Pravda*. Like Zoia, she was named a Hero of the Soviet Union. During the war, the Komsomol invested significant resources into the cultivation of her memory, even sending a correspondent to Ryno to interview her mother. Only months after Chaikina was named a Hero of the Soviet Union, Komsomol secretary Mikhailov himself published a biography of the young woman, and *Komsomolskaia Pravda* featured poet Mikhail Svetlov's narrative poem about her *podvig* in its pages. During the war and immediate postwar period, she and Zoia often appeared side-by-side in periodicals: the collective farm worker and the urban schoolgirl—both martyrs for their fatherland, both martyrs for a symbolic father, Stalin. Regardless of Komsomol efforts, both during the war and at the height of the 1960s cult of the Second World War, to cite Nina Tumarkin, Chaikina never achieved a lasting permanence in Soviet collective memory. The Soviet citizenry could neither visualize her tortured body nor could they hear her words, which no one seems to remember precisely. Although the Nazis surely treated her cruelly, explicit witnesses' accounts of her treatment—blow by blow—do not exist.

Zoia likely retains her cultural prominence because of the flexibility of her body. Marina Warner writes of Joan of Arc, who has long fulfilled a similar role in French culture as multifaceted national symbol, "in the transformation of her body, and in the different emphases of different times, we have a diviner's cup."[37] Warner could be writing about Zoia and, in fact, cultural scholar Daniela Rathe has compared the role of Zoia in

Russian culture to the role that Joan of Arc plays in French culture.[38] The disconnect between Strunnikov's photograph, Zoia's school portrait, and the five photographs found in 1943 that depict her execution left room for individual projections and a range of portrayals, unlike, for instance, Liza Chaikina's body, which was unmistakably womanly.

Conclusion

The case of Zoia Kosmodemianskaia demonstrates clearly how sensory studies might enrich our understanding of memory, memorialization, and mythopoesis, especially within an authoritarian state in which individuals must mediate official messages for themselves. C. Nadia Seremetakis writes that "There is no such thing as one moment of perception and then another of memory, representation or objectification. Mnemonic processes are intertwined with the sensory order in such a manner as to render each perception a re-perception. Re-perception is the creation of meaning through the interplay, witnessing, and cross-metaphorization of co-implicated sensory spheres."[39] The striking visual image of Zoia's mutilated body shocked her compatriots in early 1942 and continues to disturb people today, serving as a testimony of Nazi cruelty and the suffering borne by Soviet citizens. A close reading of archival documents shows the importance of sound, frequently overlooked, in her mythopoesis. The auditory and visual senses allow us to understand more deeply the dual active/passive nature of both Zoia and the witnesses that would recreate her narrative for visitors to Petrishchevo.

Intersensorality and the tactile sense increase in importance in the memorialization of Zoia during the postwar years. Regarding touch, Classen argues that "the intention is rather to explore how the corporeal practices of any particular period relate to the cultural context of the time, and how this relationship changes under the influence of new factions."[40] As Zoia became a memory and a historical figure, the intersensual experience of the museum replaced the wartime significance of her voice, calling her compatriots to battle. Museums enlivened her for postwar generations of Soviet children who were able to witness for themselves relics and the place of her death and relive her words as they read them to themselves. They could imagine what it would feel like to sleep on the bench on which she spent her last night, walk barefoot through the snow, and withstand bodily abuse on the table preserved in Petrishchevo. They could smell the wooden huts and the fresh air of the Podmoskovian countryside. To this day, sculptures, primarily visual representations, reference significant, torturous moments in Zoia's narrative, as well as the final abuse her corpse suffered. When millions of Soviet citizens perished in the Second World War, many of them heroically, some just as Zoia died, one must ask why Zoia's death so shocked her compatriots during the war and through which means did she retain her place in the Soviet pantheon of martyrs. A reading of her narrative through the lens of the senses helps one understand more deeply the processes of collective and individual remembering.

Notes

1   Maria Tumarkin, "Productive Death: The Necropedagogy of a Young Soviet Hero," *The South Atlantic Quarterly* 110 (4) (2011): 886.
2   "Quitting school to become a partisan" simplifies Zoia's path to service. The war broke out just as her ninth grade year was finishing. According to biographies, she tried to enlist in the army but was turned away because of her gender. She participated in a work brigade on a *kolkhoz* and helped dig trenches. Eventually, she was accepted as a special-forces scout in the 9903 unit and underwent training in November 1941. Although she was seventeen when the war began, she achieved her *podvig* in Petrishchevo at age eighteen.
3   For more on Zoia Kosmodemianskaia, see Daniela Rathe, "Soja— eine 'Sowjetische Jeanne d'Arc'? Zur Typologie einer Kriegsheldin," in *Sozialistische Helden: Eine Kulturgeschichte von Propagandafiguren in Osteuropa und der DDR*, ed. Silke Satjukow and Rainer Gries (Berlin: Ch. Links Verlag, 2002), 45–59; Ann Livschiz, "Children's Lives after Zoia's Death: Order, Emotions and Heroism in Children's Lives and Literature in the Postwar Soviet Union," in *Late Stalinist Russia: Society between Reconstruction and Reinvention,* ed. Juliane Fürst (London: Routledge, 2006), 192–208; Adrienne M. Harris, "The Myth of the Woman Warrior and World War II in Soviet Culture" (PhD diss., University of Kansas, 2008), 69–121; Adrienne M. Harris, "The Lives and Deaths of a Soviet Saint in the Post-Soviet Period: The Case of Zoia Kosmodem'ianskaia," *Canadian Slavonic Papers* 53 (2–4) (2011): 292–5; Adrienne M. Harris, "Memorializations of a Martyr and her Mutilated Bodies: Public Monuments to Soviet War Hero Zoya Kosmodemyanskaya (1942–the present)," *The Journal of War and Culture Studies* 5 (1) (2012): 73–90; Jonathan B. Platt, "Zoia Kosmodem'ianskaia mezhdu istrebleniem i zhertvoprinosheniem," *Novoe literaturnoe obozrenie* 124 (2013): 54–78; Andrei Shcherbenok, "Psikhika bez psikhologii: 'Zoia,' ideologiia i Stalinskoe kinoprostranstvo," *Novoe literaturnoe obozrenie* 124 (2013): 79–92; Adrienne Harris, "Stalinskaia liniia i vydumannye zhenikhi: Rol' liubovnoi linii v povestvovaniiakh o geroiakh vtoroi mirovoi voiny," *Novoe literaturnoe obozrenie* 124 (2013): 93–110; Adrienne M. Harris, "Evolution of the Immortal: Dynamic Images of World War II Heroes," in *Post-Communist Transition and Women's Agency in Eastern Europe*, ed. Cynthia Simmons (Dordrecht: The Republic of Letters, 2013), 15–26; Anja Tippner, "Girls in Combat: Zoia Kosmodem'ianskaia and the Image of Young Soviet Wartime Heroines," *Russian Review* 73 (2014): 371–88. For more on Chaikina, see Harris, "Stalinskaia linia" and "Evolution of the Immortal."

4   Rosalinde Sartorti compares Strunnikov's photograph to hagiographic depictions in her article "On the Making of Heroes, Heroines, and Saints," in *Culture and Entertainment in Wartime Russia*, ed. Richard Stites (Bloomington: Indiana University Press, 1995), 185.
5   *The Body in Pain: The Making and Unmaking of the World*, as cited in Christina S. Jarvis, *The Male Body at War: American Masculinity During World War II* (Dekalb: Northern Illinois University Press, 2003), 87–8.
6   Mark M. Smith, *Sensing the Past: Seeing, Hearing, Smelling, Tasting, and Touching in History* (Berkeley: University of California Press, 2007), 9, 19.
7   Nina Tumarkin, *Lenin Lives! The Lenin Cult in Soviet Russia* (Cambridge, MA: Harvard University Press, 1993).
8   Elina Kahla, *Life as Exploit: Representations of Twentieth-Century Saintly Women in Russia* (Helsinki: Kikimora Publications, 2007), 46.
9   In her analysis of partisan Liudmila Dediukhina's inclusion of a recent anthology "Realost' sviatosti," Kahla finds that "the representation of one major virtue, such as fighting Nazism, is the most important common denominator in Russian politically oriented neo-hagiography." Ibid., 50.
10 Elena Koshevaia, *Povest' o syne* (Donetsk: Donbas, 1985), 56.
11 Margarita Aliger, "Zoia" (Leningrad: Lenizdat, 1948), 79. The Russian text reads:
        Eto devich'e telo,
                Ne mertvoe
                        I ne zhivoe
        Eto Zoia iz mramora
                Tikho lezhit na snegu.
        Besposhchadnoi petlei pererezana tonkaia sheia.
        Neznakomaia vlast' v zaprokinutom like tvoem.
        Tak liubimogo zhdut,
                Sokrovennoi krasoi khorosheia,
        Iznutri ozariaias' tainstvennym zhenskim ognem.
        Tol'ko ty ne dozhdalas' ego, snegovaia nevesta.
        On—v boitsovskoi shineli,
                Na zapad lezhit ego put'.
        Mozhet byt', nedaleko ot etogo strashnogo mesta,
        Gde lozhilis' shezhniki na stroguiu devich'iu grud'.
        Vechnoi sily i slabosti nepovtorimo edinstvo.
        Ty sovsem kholodna, a venia prozhigaet toska.
        Ne vorvalos' v tebia, ne vskipelo v tebe
                Materinstvo,
        Teplyi rotik rebenka ne tronul sykhogo soska.
        Ty lezhish' na snegu.
                O, kaka mnogo za nas otdala ty,
        Shtoby gordo otkinut'sia chistym, prekrasnym litsom!
12 See Harris, "Stalinskaia liniia."
13 One author claims to always see her image in front of him and visualizes her childlike eyes and the farewell wave of her hand. Rossiiskii gosudarstvennyi

arkhiv sotsial'no-politicheskoi istorii (RGASPI), f. M-7, op. 2, d. 649/13, ll. 34–5.

14 Jonathan Sterne, *The Audible Past: Cultural Origins of Sound Reproduction* (Durham, NC: Duke University Press, 2003), 3.

15 P. Lidov, "Tania," *Pravda*, January 27, 1942, 3. These words would evolve from their initial appearance in Lidov's communiqués through the duration of the Soviet period.

16 RGASPI, f. M-7, op. 2, d. 649/5, l. 30.

17 *Narodnaia geroinia* (Moscow: Molodaia Gvardiia, 1943), 38.

18 RGASPI, f. M-7, op. 2, d. 649/8, l. 118. These particular children claimed to have known her personally having been Octobrists in a troop she led.

19 RGASPI, f. M-7, op. 2, d. 649/13, l. 2.

20 RGASPI, f. M-7, op. 2, d. 649/13, l. 30.

21 RGASPI, f. M-7, op. 2, d. 649/13, l. 60.

22 Richard Stites, *Russian Popular Culture* (New York: Cambridge University Press, 1994), 114.

23 Lisa Kirschenbaum, *The Legacy of the Siege of Leningrad, 1941–1995: Myth, Memories, and Monuments* (Cambridge: Cambridge University Press, 2006).

24 Jay Winter, *Remembering War: The Great War Between Memory and History in the Twentieth Century* (New Haven, CT: Yale University Press, 2006), 145.

25 Catriona Kelly, *Comrade Pavlik: The Rise and Fall of a Soviet Boy Hero* (London: Granta Books, 2005), 185–6.

26 One can access the Kukryniksy collective's "Tania" here: "Megabook: Megaentsiklopediia Kirilla i Mefodiia," http://megabook.ru/stream/mediaprev iew?Key=%D0%9A%D1%83%D0%BA%D1%80%D1%8B%D0%BD%D0 %B8%D0%BA%D1%81%D1%8B%20(%D0%A2%D0%B0%D0%BD%D 1%8F)&Width=10000&Height=10000 (accessed July 26, 2015).

27 T. Zhispar, "Tania."

28 Aleksandr Iur'evich Krivitskii, "Svidetel' gibeli Zoi," *Krasnoe znamiia (Kaluzhskaia oblast')*, RGALI, f. 3126, op. 1, ed. khr. 566.

29 Ibid.

30 Peter Charles Hoffer, *In Sensory Worlds of Early America* (Baltimore, MD: Johns Hopkins University Press, 2004), 8–10.

31 Constance Classen, *The Deepest Sense* (Champaign: University of Illinois Press, 2012), 169.

32 C. Nadia Seremetakis, ed., *The Senses Still: Perception and Memory as Material Culture in Modernity* (Boulder, CO: Westview Press, 1994), 9.

33 Classen, *The Deepest Sense*, xii.

34 The *sorochka* actually sanitizes the narrative. The emphasis on the undressed young woman in the *sorochka* simultaneously adds an erotic element to the narrative.

35 *Argumenty i fakty—Nizhnee Povolzh'e*, September 9, 2008, http://www.aif.ru/culture/news/25507

36 "Postradal pamiatnik," *Argumenty i fakty Kuzbass*, September 1, 2010, http://www.kuzbass.aif.ru/archive/1786414 (accessed February 26, 2016), print; and A. Donskoi, "Kazn' Zoi v Volgograde," *Voennyi vestnik luga Rossii*, August 14, 2006: 8.

37 Marina Warner, *Joan of Arc: The Image of Female Heroism* (New York: Alfred A. Knopf, 1981), 7.

38 Daniela Rathe, "Soja—eine "sowjetische Jeanne d'Arc"? Zur Typologie einer Kriegsheldin," in *Sozialistische Helden. Eine Kulturgeschichte von Propagandafiguren in Osteuropa und der DDR*, ed. Silke Satjukow and Rainer Gries (Berlin: Links, 2002), 45–9.

39 Seremetakis, *The Senses Still*, 9.

40 Classen, *The Deepest Sense*, xiv.

CHAPTER TWELVE

Stalinism's sights and smells in the films of Aleksei German, Sr.

Tim Harte

Smell, as Vladimir Nabokov emphasized in his first novel *Mary* (1926), can serve as a powerful form of inspiration: "She used a cheap, sweet perfume called 'Tagore.' Ganin now tried to recapture that scent again, mixed with the fresh smells of the autumnal park, but, as we know, memory can restore to life everything except smells, although nothing revives the past so completely as a smell that was once associated with it."[1] For Nabokov (and his protagonist Ganin), smell remains a sense firmly embedded in the present yet also capable of reviving, in an instant, the past. Our memories, unable to invoke a specific scent without some prompting, are indeed at the beck and call of smell, easily overwhelmed by a fragrant whiff of a familiar odor that transports us back to a very particular time and place. It is this lopsided and somewhat paradoxical relationship between smell and memory that has proven particularly germane to the work of the recently departed Soviet-Russian filmmaker Aleksei German, Sr. (1938–2013), who in many respects tried to overcome the inaccessibility of the redolent past by resurrecting bygone smells cinematically. While German could not, of course, recapture on screen the scents of former times, he visually evoked odor as he sought out powerful, visceral means for resurrecting Soviet history in his films.

A filmmaker inordinately preoccupied with Russia's dark Stalinist period, German strove to conjure up a distinct historical atmosphere before his viewers' eyes, appealing to the senses—not only sight and hearing, as one would naturally expect in cinema, but also smell—to probe the essence of Stalinism and collective memories of these dark Stalinist years. For German, smell signified a convenient, albeit somewhat illusive avenue to the past. In *My Friend Ivan Lapshin* (1984) and *Khrustalev, My Car!* (1998), two of the mere six films German made over the course of his long directorial career, this visionary filmmaker increasingly evoked and amplified smell as he dug deeper and deeper into the complex—and very fragrant—tyrannical underpinnings of Soviet society. As I will argue in what follows, smell constitutes a fundamental component of German's films, serving as a conspicuous focus of his cinematic work while also providing a helpful prism through which to experience and comprehend his frequently confounding, yet undeniably vivid, filmic evocations of the Soviet past. Although the multifarious smells evoked by German may at times repulse viewers, it is a repugnant odor that ultimately unites the past with the present, as German uses the sense of smell to transport audiences back to his country's past and the heavy, redolent air of Stalinism.

Film, of course, hardly seems an ideal vehicle for conjuring up scents. Yet in comparison to other artistic media, save literature perhaps or, one might imagine, installation art with a provocative, aromatic twist, cinema offers a very effective means for showing people sniffing, reacting to certain smells, and even emitting odors. Moviegoers may not be able to directly appreciate a fragrance (other than that of popcorn), but they can indirectly gain access to a whole array of olfactory sensations triggered by a given image or scene. According to film scholar Laura Marks, who has written extensively on touch, scent, and the other senses in the arts, smell is the sense "most likely to operate mimetically" and can be conveyed on screen in three distinct ways.[2] First, the filmmaker might show in a straightforward mimetic fashion a character smelling or sniffing. Second, a director can rely on a synaesthetic appeal to other senses that subsequently evoke an olfactory effect, such as a sound closely connected to this smell (the snorting of a pig, for example) or an image of something distinctly fragrant (such as a loaf of bread straight out of the oven). And third, filmmakers can place particular emphasis on the haptic appreciation of close-up images that in their proximity to the viewer and through their detailed visual texture evoke or at least hint at certain smells. By haptic, Marks implies anything related to touch, and it is indeed an olfactory tangibility that cinema is capable in certain instances of invoking, particularly when a given film shot undermines conventional ways of viewing or hearing. As Marks explains, "By resisting control of vision, for example being blurry, haptic images encourage the 'viewer' to get close to the image and explore it through all of the senses, including touch, smell and taste."[3] In instances when sight and sound do not allow viewers to grasp the meaning of a film scene due to blurriness or, to cite several of German's signature methods, due to muffled voices and dizzying imagery produced by a rapid traveling shot, audiences can be compelled to rely upon other senses to process what transpires on screen and thus perceive a given sequence not simply diagetically or conceptually but also sensorially. Therefore a conspicuous shift away from traditional forms of cinematic representation potentially triggers within viewers a collective, visceral form of memory, whereby smell can bolster the intricate rendering of the past that, as Soviet and Russian audiences have been well aware of, materializes in virtually every Aleksei German film.

In German's complex cinematic work, smell—or, as the case may be, visual, haptic references to smell—are indeed at the heart of the viewing experience for audiences, whom German challenges through his films' disorienting images and scenes. By recreating the past and evoking collective memories of the Soviet Union's troubled history, German accordingly relies on all three of Marks's well-defined methods for cinematically triggering film viewers' senses and olfactory recollections. From a brief, tender sequence of a woman carefully cutting a loaf of Russian black bread in *The Seventh Companion* (1968), German's first film, to shots of boiling pots on the stove of a crowded communal apartment in *Twenty Years without War* (1977), to close-ups of a naked behind in a decrepit outhouse shown during the opening credits of *Hard to be God* (2013), the director's final film, imagery associated with smells—some familiar to all audiences but many familiar only to Russian and Soviet viewers—have always occupied a prominent place in German's work.[4]

The most Russian of filmmakers, German created images and very specific sensorial impressions of the Soviet past that have often proven visually challenging to Western audiences. All shot in black and white (save several sequences with faded colors from *My Friend Ivan Lapshin*) along the principle that our memories are colorless, German's films vividly evoke bygone scents.[5] This emphasis on smell is especially pronounced in *My Friend Ivan Lapshin* and *Khrustalev, My Car!* Throughout both films characters not only find themselves in very odorous situations but also actively sniff and snort, as if to ground themselves in the disorienting, threatening environment of Stalinism. In the latter of these two films, moreover, the focus repeatedly falls on noses, be they sniffing, sniffling, or, thanks to the secret police (the NKVD), bashed and bloodied. Indeed, German's Stalin-era personae smell, taste, and feel their way through cold, murky landscapes and cramped spaces that so often appear to be emitting a bewildering mix of both pleasant and noxious odors, well in accordance with Marks's notion of cinema synaesthetically appealing to the other senses to evoke olfactory sensations.

As if reinforcing Marks's contention that haptic images can indirectly conjure up smell, German frequently hones in on everyday objects and body parts in ways that indirectly allude to familiar odors, many of them unpleasant ones from the repressive Stalinist era, while he also stimulates viewers' senses by means of his characters' inaudible speech, disquieting actions, and angry outbursts. Insinuation of smell likewise arises out of German's penchant for claustrophobic spaces through which his camera gymnastically maneuvers, presenting the past in a visually unorthodox, unsettling fashion. By relying on these untraditional means of haptic representation to transport his viewers back to the Stalinist past, German repeatedly privileges smell in both *My Friend Ivan Lapshin* and *Khrustalev, My Car!*

My Friend Ivan Lapshin, German's most celebrated and broadly appreciated film, has been resoundingly praised for its innovative form of nostalgia. As literary scholar Anthony Anemone writes, "Rooted in the historical revisionism of the Khrushchev period, the film may be unique in all of post-Stalinist Russian culture for its historical accuracy, subtlety and the depth of its critique of Stalinist utopianism."[6] In *Lapshin*, German recreates in painstaking detail the unique atmosphere of a provincial town in 1930s Soviet Russia, replicating the language and mannerisms of the time, along with the textures and smells of the early Stalin years. German, writes Russian film critic Anton Dolin, "is the sole practitioner of a genre of his own invention: 'film recollection'."[7] A hybrid form of cinema that is hyper-realistic (and inspired by old photographs of the era) yet at the same time dreamlike in nature, German's cinematic recollections go well beyond conventional cinema's typical, commercially popular "period piece" in that he establishes a vivid, highly-personal portrait of the past that simultaneously underscores a collective vision of Soviet history. *Lapshin*, the plot of which is loosely based on fiction by the filmmaker's father (the well-known Soviet writer Yuri German), begins with an adult reminiscing in the present day (the 1980s) about his childhood in the mid-1930s, when Soviet society stood on the threshold of the Stalinist purges and era of Great Terror that resulted in the disappearance and death of so many Communist officials and others in the Soviet hierarchy.

Right from the outset of *My Friend Ivan Lapshin*, odors of a bygone era waft through the film and its vision of the past, fondly recalled by German's narrator as he reminisces about his pre-Purge childhood. In the film's brief present-day prelude, this narrator remarks that in moments of idleness the distinct fragrance of Lapshin's cigarettes suddenly come to him as he returns to the past.[8] German, however, will quickly dispense with, or at least de-emphasize, the first-person narrative, as he works to establish a collective, rather than individual vision of the Soviet Union's redolent, yet very anxious past. The plot of German's film subsequently involves a series of events from the mid-1930s in Unchansk, a fictional Soviet town, where the eponymous police chief pursues a vicious band of criminals headed by a shadowy figure named Solov'ev. Lapshin, clumsy and quite awkward when it comes to women, falls for an actress performing at the town's theater in a semi-successful staging of a socialist realist play (Lapshin has better luck capturing criminals than he does capturing the heart of this actress). Although Stalinism lurks only in the background of the film, with mere whiffs of the upcoming purges in the air, the small-town atmosphere and tense interrelationships of the characters suggest that Stalinist authoritarianism has slowly been working its way into people's lives. A semi-sweet nostalgia for the sounds and scents of the early Soviet era permeates the film, but these sounds and scents ultimately prove somewhat ominous, even oppressive, as if the essence of the Stalinist era can be found in its minor, everyday details and plethora of smells.

Mention of cat odors, a fragrant prostitute, and the stench from a man who has had his fill of vodka after a night of revelry provide a background of relatively harmless, albeit unpleasant odors in the film, as does the cheerful atmosphere—so carefully recreated by German—of a fortieth birthday party for Lapshin that occurs early on in the film. In this early scene, a host of characters, mostly police officers, sit at a cluttered table in a crowded, smoke-filled room, as German, using one relatively lengthy, slow panning shot, moves through the party, capturing bits and pieces of various conversations (one of which, incidentally, involves cat smells) before slowly zooming in on Lapshin (Figure 12.1). Nostalgia floats through the air, as the polyphonic mix of voices, songs, whistling, and joyful clinking of glasses produces a tangible, albeit somewhat confusing tapestry of life in 1930s Soviet Russia. As in so many other scenes from the film, smell comes not only from direct mention of various stenches and such, but also from the evocative black-and-white images and diverse, discordant sounds of day-to-day life under Stalin.

The everyday odors of provincial Stalinist Russia and its somewhat repressive atmosphere, however, give way to more malodorous smells, particularly when Lapshin discovers an underground vault containing two dead bodies. These two corpses, the grisly result of Solov'ev's criminal activity, provide a fitting, albeit gruesome embodiment of German's ambiguous nostalgia and retrospective attitude toward the Stalinist era. Police carry the bodies out of the vault and into the open air, as if conveying metaphorically—embodying, one might say—the filmmaker's urge to expose the rot and stench of Stalinism (Figure 12.2). Since the scene transpires in the heart of winter, the odors of these rotting corpses are masked by the frost, but German's camera hones in on the bodies as

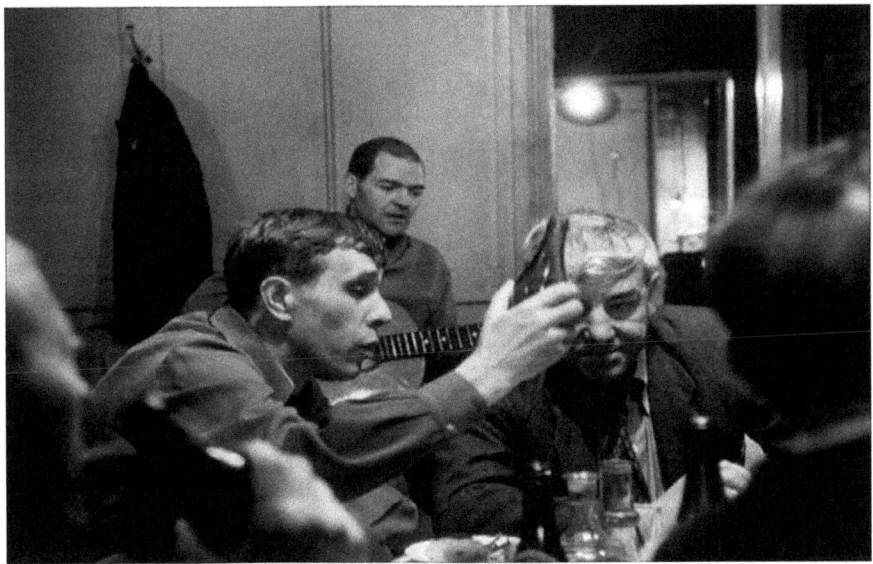

FIGURE 12.1 *Scene from* My Friend Ivan Lapshin. *Courtesy of Lenfilm.*

the police place them in the back of a truck, thus providing viewers with a stark, sensorial reminder of the era's brutality. A crowd of bystanders lingers, their frosty breath and the exhaust from the truck beautifully captured in the scene amidst harsh cries coming from a distraught women, thus creating considerable dissonance in the sequence. And quite tellingly, it is immediately following this scene with the corpses that Lapshin, racing on a motorcycle through Unchansk's barren, wintery landscape, blurts out a Stalinist-inspired slogan: "No matter, we'll clean this place out, we'll plant a garden, and we'll live to stroll in this garden." This slogan only accentuates the emerging discrepancy between utopian propaganda and reality in the country's emerging dystopia. After the rotting corpses and harsh shouting, Lapshin's words notionally reek of irony, for it is death, not a flower, which blossoms in this spoiled garden of Stalinism.

The foul air of crime and authoritarianism gradually pervades German's film, as evidenced by the scene in which Lapshin leads his men to the ramshackle lodgings of Solov'ev's gang. Having surrounded the building, Lapshin and his fellow officers approach and surround the criminals' hideout, whereby the police themselves emerge as a gang ready to do what is necessary to get their man. The camera, lingering at the threshold of these dilapidated lodgings, reveals the comings and goings of the police and various suspicious characters before accompanying Lapshin as he enters the building (German uses a lengthy handheld traveling shot to increase the scene's dizzying sense of confusion). Pitch-black shots prevail for several seconds before the camera proceeds quickly down a faintly lit corridor. In line with Marks's notion that an audience's sense of smell can be triggered

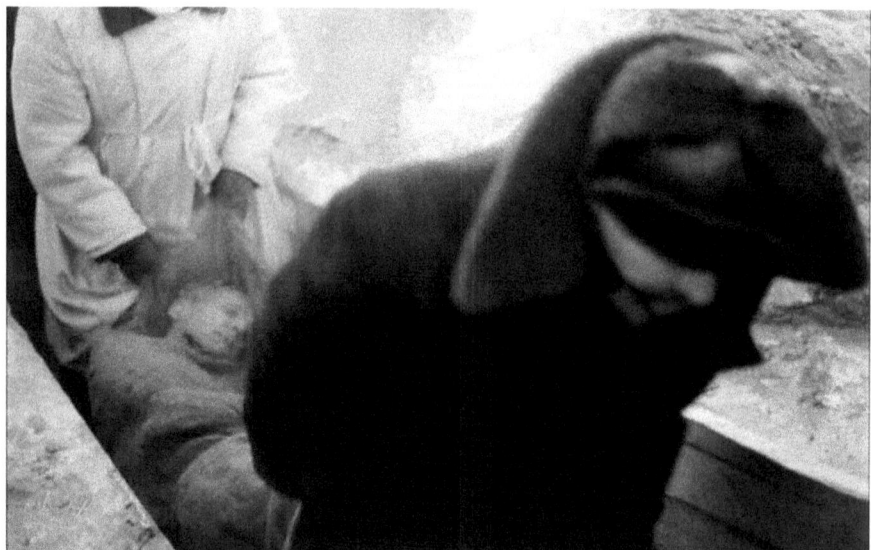

FIGURE 12.2 *Scene from* My Friend Ivan Lapshin. *Courtesy of Lenfilm.*

through disorienting, haptic imagery, the traveling camera shots create a bewildering scene of chaos in which the odors of the criminal environment again prove disturbingly tangible. In the semi-darkness, Lapshin and his fellow officers aggressively bang down the doors of various rooms, yet Solov'ev manages to escape (and then stab Lapshin's good friend Khanin) before eventually being gunned down by Lapshin himself. This thwarting of Solov'ev, however, will be only a pyrrhic victory, for a similar fate surely awaits Lapshin; it is implied that he will perish in the upcoming purges, as the violent practices of the police come back to haunt Lapshin and others amidst an intensification of the era's repressive atmosphere.[9]

Whereas in *My Friend Ivan Lapshin* German makes sporadic, subtle use of smell through haptic images of dark, musty crime scenes, crowded rooms, and cramped communal apartments, in 1998's *Khrustalev, My Car!* the smells have become all the more pungent, unavoidable, and unsettling. Developing on the sensorial complexities of *Lapshin*, German goes much further with these olfactory sensations in his later *Khrustalev*, whereby he links history and smell in a comprehensive, conspicuous, and unmistakably redolent fashion. Indeed, intense smells waft through the entire film, as scene after scene places a heavy emphasis on the penetrating odors of corruption in the late Stalinist era. At the same time, all the smelling and overwhelming attention paid to scent in *Khrustalev* establishes a direct link between the film's grotesque cast of characters and contemporary viewers, who must implicitly breathe in the same air and react to the same smells as German's semi-historical figures. The smells being sniffed in both a diagetical and extra-diagetic fashion ultimately emanate from the rotting body of the state, a stench that for German has wafted well into the present day. In interviews, in fact, German has admitted that *Khrustalev* has great relevance to the present-day situation in Russia.[10] And by leading his viewers, via his murky plot, straight to the stench of the dying Stalin, he will provide both his fictional characters and his audience with a strong, often overwhelming whiff of Soviet tyranny.

The odors in *Khrustalev* may be explicit, but the narrative threads of this beguiling film, which took German over a decade to make, prove anything but straightforward. Replete with muffled whispers, sharp yells, and threatening innuendo, *Khrustalev* remains baffling to many viewers (especially those who did not grow up in the Soviet Union).[11] The semi-autobiographical, semi-historical action, loosely based on German's own memories of childhood in Moscow as the son of a prominent Soviet writer, defies easy comprehension. In various respects, a good understanding of the film requires multiple viewings, as well as a very solid grasp of Soviet history. Discussion of *Khrustalev*, therefore, must begin with a brief synopsis of the film's narrative (the screenplay for which German co-wrote with his wife Svetlana Karmalita), particularly given the obscure, confusing nature of so many of the film's scenes. The events of *Khrustalev*, told as a series of dreamlike reminiscences belonging to the protagonist's son (a stand-in for the young German), take place in late February and early March of 1953, when an ill Stalin lay on his deathbed and the Stalinist, anti-Semitic "Doctor's Plot" targeted various physicians, among them the film's fictional protagonist General Yuri Klensky, a prominent Moscow brain surgeon (although not a Jew) and Red Army general. Amidst a swirl of subplots, whispers, and snow, Klensky finds himself under suspicion, as the NKVD monitors his whereabouts and eventually arrests him (after his son has implicitly informed on him following a visit from a Swedish journalist).

In the second half of *Khrustalev*, the authorities transport Klensky through a labyrinth of checkpoints, vehicles, and snowy roads before pushing him into the back of a Soviet Champagne truck, where a gang of prisoners brutally rapes and sodomizes him. Soon after this grotesque, violent rape scene, however, Klensky is ostensibly freed and delivered to a heavily guarded complex near Kuntsevo, the town outside of Moscow where an ailing Stalin, having suffered a stroke, lies dying in bed at his dacha. Instructed by Lavrentii Beria, Stalin's main henchman, to minister to the ailing leader in a cramped, cluttered room, Klensky attempts to aid his soiled and comatose patient, who breathes his last breaths—officially, at least, on March 5, 1953, but most likely several days earlier—before the anxious, agitated Klensky and the fat, morose Beria. The title of the film, appropriately obscure, comes from these climactic scenes at the Kuntsevo dacha, where Beria shouts to Stalin's real-life, eponymous bodyguard, "Khrustalev, my car!"; German does not even show Khrustalev, who remains off screen during this momentous point in the film. Klensky subsequently returns as a free man to his family in Moscow, but he then vanishes, and it is in the final scenes of the movie that Klensky is shown, some time later, on a creaky train traveling through the stark Soviet landscape, now rather desperate and depraved, but still a charismatic figure who drinks with fellow revelers on an open-air train car. While performing a drunken stunt with a shot glass balanced on his head, Klensky asks a traveling companion to wipe his nose, with which he seemingly hopes to breathe in the fresh, post-apocalyptic air of the post-Stalinist era (Figure 12.3).

From the first shot to the last, *Khrustalev* is a very idiosyncratic cinematic work, as it merges autobiography and Soviet history. Profoundly modern in its use of space and its evocation of the past, the film exudes a visual power that largely emanates from the claustrophobic atmosphere created early on in the opening scenes of Moscow's dark, snowy streets. As in his earlier work, particularly *Lapshin*, sweeping long takes and constricted settings full of ominous figures and shadows enable German to generate a distinct spatial component that visually challenges audiences. Confining the gaze of viewers through his frequent dispensing with standard lighting and through shots of crowded apartments, Moscow's ornate baths, and a truck's dark cargo bay, among other tight places, German establishes a highly elaborate, often oppressive *mise-en-scène* in *Khrustalev*. Startling, unconventional pirouettes by German's camera prove especially disconcerting, as the

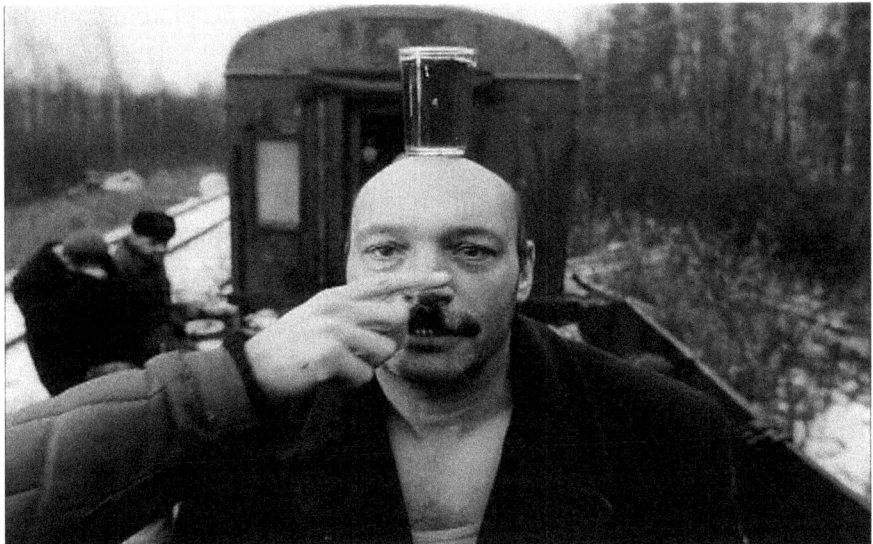

FIGURE 12.3 *Scene from* Khrustalev, My Car! *Courtesy of Lenfilm.*

filmmaker provides his audience with highly visceral impressions of life under Stalin. Throughout the film, black-and-white imagery, the headlong flow of the camera through narrow spaces, and erratic behavior from virtually every character enable German to convey so much of the horror and repressiveness of late Stalinism. Fellini-esque in nature, given the way the camera navigates the hellish, decadent world of late Stalinist Moscow à la *La Dolce Vita* (or, as Phillip Lopate has nicely put it, "like a hellish version of *Amarcord*"), *Khrustalev* presents a disorienting, carnivalesque portrait of life under Stalin.[12] And as witnesses to all the claustrophobic scenes and grotesque imagery, German's viewers find themselves trapped in the Stalinist era, their senses engulfed in the era's violence, threatening sounds, and repellant odors.

In comparison to *Lapshin*, the emphasis on smell throughout *Khrustalev* has increased noticeably. In the first half of the film, for instance, aromas and smelling abound, particularly in a series of overcrowded Moscow apartments and buildings, which offer a disorienting maze of smell-filled dining rooms, baths, toilets, and offices through which German's acrobatic camera guides the viewer. Consider, for instance, one crucial scene in the hospital where Klensky works as the chief of medicine. Parading through the hospital with his underlings in tow, the General somewhat inexplicably breaks down the door into another ward in an adjacent part of the hospital, where within the "enema room" he discovers his double, a man who looks remarkably similar to him (prominent figures under suspicion often had doubles who would appear on their behalf at show trials to ensure the delivery of proper testimony). Against a portentous backdrop of seemingly noxious steam that rises throughout the hospital and amidst various references to the smell of death, odors implicitly permeate this highly chaotic scene that is made all the more disorienting and unnerving to the senses by the rapid, flowing movement of German's traveling camera. Over the course of this bewildering hospital sequence background figures jump unexpectedly out of the shadows. "Death, is that you?" Klensky asks a worker ("Death" is evidently this individual's moniker) before he encounters another attendant holding (and then dropping) two cats by the scruff of their necks, whereby the head surgeon barges into the room where his double stands. Klensky sits down with his double and offers him a cigar, but the imposter passes on the cigar to someone else, remarking that it smells awful ("It smells like shit") (Figure 12.4). Other smelling ensues here as well, for instance when Klensky's subordinates attempt to get a whiff of his "tea" to discern whether it contains some cognac. But the most significant odor sensed here by Klensky and his subordinates is a threatening, metaphorical one: they now know with great certainty that he is under suspicion and in serious danger of being arrested.

Upon discovering his double, Klensky instinctually senses—as do German's viewers—that he is a marked man. The most immediate method of self-preservation in the unsettling, suspicious atmosphere of Stalinist Russia indeed appears to be an olfactory one, as a variety of the film's characters attempt to smell and snort their way to safety. In analysis of *Khrustalev*, French film scholar Georges Nivat has remarked, "Everyone sniffs at things; if noses are more active than intellects it is because an animalistic resistance to annihilation exists, as life triumphs, irrespective

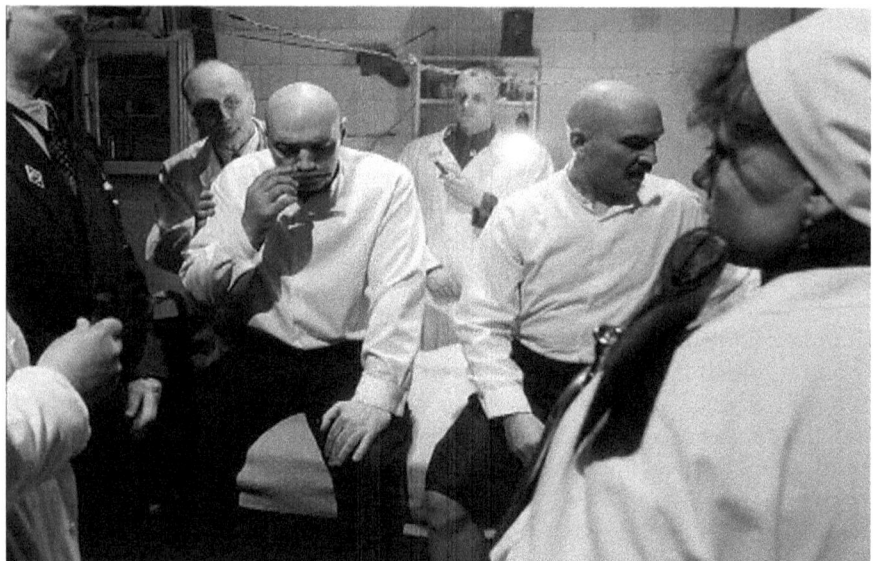

FIGURE 12.4 *Scene from* Khrustalev, My Car! *Courtesy of Lenfilm.*

of anything and above all."[13] All the overt sniffing in *Khrustalev*, Nivat suggests, conveys the reflexive, animalistic response of Soviet citizens to the repressive order established under Stalin, as German accentuates the dehumanizing, degrading effects of Stalinism on the Soviet people. The underlying suspicion and brutality of the Soviet state have transformed its populace into wild animals who must smell and scrape for their survival.

General Klensky senses danger all around him, as rumors, threats, and the realization that he is under suspicion propel him forward through the labyrinth of constricted spaces comprising German's conception of Stalinist Moscow. In one crucial scene toward the end of Part One of this approximately two-and-a-half hour film, Klensky attends a party in the ornate, yet crowded Moscow apartment of an aging, well-to-do woman, the academic Shishmareva, who is, as it turns out, a specialist in extending the lives of human beings.[14] Klensky and Shishmareva, along with her Great Dane, quietly retreat to a cluttered little room where the doctor offers Shishmareva's dog some cognac in a bowl and then lets the big animal lick his face for a treat. As if to emulate this dog, the intoxicated Klensky sniffs at Shishmareva's fist (Figure 12.5). Odors, both actual and metaphorical, permeate this sequence, given the tight space (accentuated by a model of a miniature theater into which Klensky places a shoe) and the fact that Klensky, in discussion with Shishmareva about extending the life of a human and about his recently discovered double, mumbles that "death reeks." And together with these smells and morbid thoughts comes a veiled conversation between Klensky and Shishmareva regarding Stalin's fragile health, impending death, and the immediate threat lurking in the air for doctors like Klensky ("When Nero dies," Klensky whispers, "there are executions, executions. Who needs these insignificant little doctors here?"). Speaking to Klensky somewhat inexplicably through a large plate of glass, Shishmareva scolds her interlocutor for cynically speaking of Stalin's death, and as a coughing Klensky looks to exit this small, redolent space, Shishmareva repeatedly tells the doctor that he is sick.

Following Klensky's cryptic scene with Shishmareva, the phantasmagorical, carnivalesque tone of the film dissipates somewhat, as decadent scenes of feasting (seemingly in the time of the plague) give way to more nightmarish musings but also something less personal for German, as the film takes on a more implicitly collective theme. Night turns to day, but in place of the ominous, threatening shadows of Part One, it is now unadulterated brutality and death that materializes. Odors accordingly grow in intensity throughout Part Two of *Khrustalev*, for instance when Klensky finds himself in the hands of the NKVD. Having been viciously sodomized in the back of the Soviet Champagne truck (I will refrain from delving into the smells evoked throughout this dark, disturbing rape scene, given that the sensorial emphasis is far more physical than olfactory), Klensky is dragged away from the other prisoners and revived by several officers so that he can medically attend to Stalin. An officer pours cologne into one of Klensky's

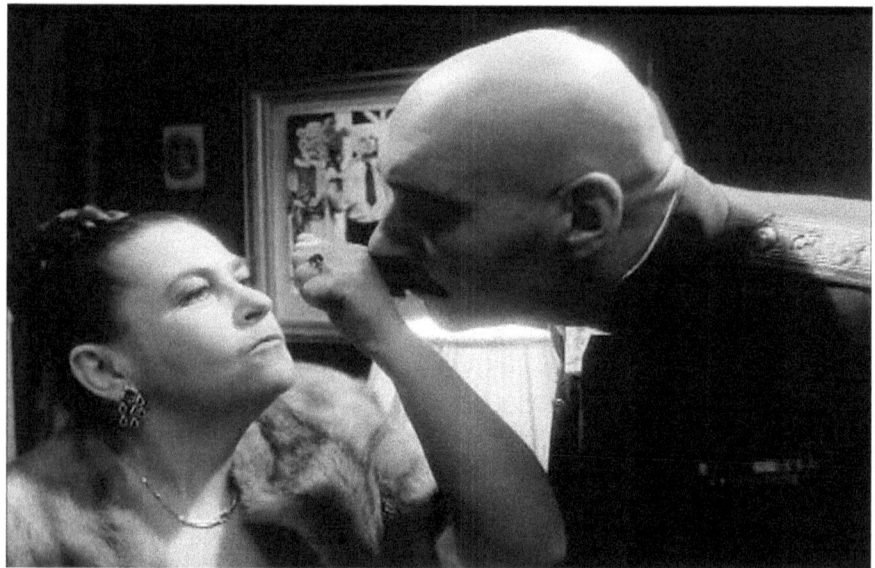

FIGURE 12.5 *Scene from* Khrustalev, My Car! *Courtesy of Lenfilm.*

boots to help make them fit, for these boots actually belong to Klensky's double encountered earlier in the hospital. The cologne surely hides the reek arising from Klensky's violated body and ruptured anus, while it also masks much more widespread smells. And it is this cologne that catches the attention of a guard on the long road leading toward Stalin's dacha. Accompanying Klensky from one automobile to another at a guardhouse along the beautiful, snow-packed approach to Stalin's abode, the guard asks Klensky why he stinks of perfume. Klensky can only shrug and mutter, "It happens," as he sits in the car and gazes pitifully at this guard, whose hand twitches as he momentarily dozes off before Klensky. Only the fragrance of the cologne, which will be mentioned several more times in the film, can overpower, albeit temporarily, the vile smells of the brutal Stalinist system, so disturbingly embodied by the earlier rape sequence in the truck and the scene to come by the side of Stalin's deathbed.

At Stalin's dacha, a Dante-esque ninth circle of hell, Klensky at last discovers the fundamental source of all the vile smells pervading the Soviet landscape. In this climactic scene with the comatose Stalin, in fact, German focuses inordinately on each of the five human senses, as sight, sound, touch, smell, and even taste all play a role in the protracted scene of Stalin's last moments, thus enabling German to create a sensorial smorgasbord of death. Hence the sight of the Soviet leader is a remarkable one for Klensky, who at first does not even know that he is in fact in the presence of Stalin (he asks Beria if the patient is his father, whereupon Beria replies, "Father? ... You said that very well"). It is only when a gust of cold air blows open a wardrobe door in the room to reveal the leader's uniforms that Klensky realizes that it is indeed Stalin lying before him (and that he has also been dealing with Beria). Several times Klensky rubs his eyes, as if doubting the veracity of what he sees. Sounds likewise predominate, as Stalin's moaning, gurgling belly, and passing of noxious gas resonate loudly throughout the room, as do Beria's frantic screams and yelling. German similarly amplifies touch in this climactic scene, as Beria pours disinfectant over the hands of Klensky, who proceeds to thrust a finger into Stalin's mouth, rub the dying man's bloated belly, and then press down on the belly in an attempt to save his patient's life (Beria beseeches Klensky to extend Stalin's life, but the frantic doctor refuses and says it is impossible) (Figure 12.6). Once Klensky realizes that it is indeed Stalin who lies before him, he quickly gives himself an injection before placing multiple kisses on the General Secretary of the Communist Party's decaying body. And taste, meanwhile, also seems to figure in the action, as bubbles come oozing out of Stalin's mouth and then, once Stalin has died, when Klensky eats a quick, interrupted meal with the distraught Beria.

Above all, however, it is a sense of smell that most significantly underlies the tumultuous, early March 1953 events in *Khrustalev*. As he does in so many instances throughout this film and his other work, German offers a *mise-en-scène* of a small, cramped space within the Kuntsevo dacha, undoubtedly to make the pervasive odors seem all the more intense and suggestive. A vile, unpleasant stench conspicuously wafts through the enclosed space of the room, and Beria on several occasions over the course of this approximately five-minute scene complains about the awful odor. Desperately recoiling from the stench, he has an attendant nurse pour

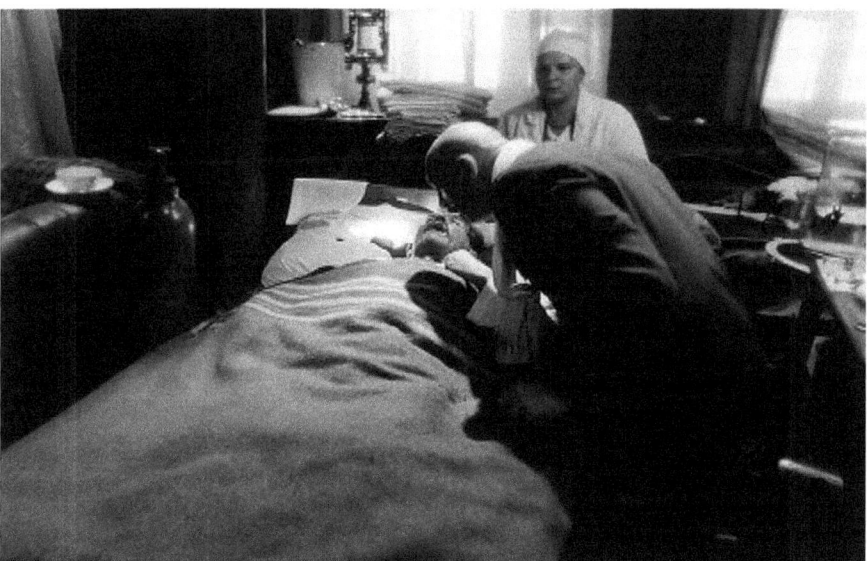

FIGURE 12.6 *Scene from* Khrustalev, My Car! *Courtesy of Lenfilm.*

disinfectant on his hands, which he then splashes over his face. Klensky too is well aware of the smell. Asked to administer to the dying man, he immediately begins to sniff the Soviet leader up and down. Upon thrusting his finger into Stalin's mouth, Klensky uses his nose to inspect this finger carefully, while he also pulls back the sheets on Stalin's bed, only to find the General Secretary lying in his own excrement. The attendant nurse tries to explain to Beria that she had recently changed the now-soiled Stalin ("He was clean! He was clean!"), whereby she receives a whack on the head (and probably worse) from Beria for her troubles. To alleviate the stench, Beria opens the window, as a burst of fresh air wafts through the room (and forces open Stalin's wardrobe); this is one of the film's rare moments of tranquility, as German's camera focuses for several seconds on the window curtains while they billow in the wind. A sublime moment amidst all the horror, death, and depravity of the time, these images of the billowing curtains hint at the fresh air needed throughout the entire country (and in the film itself, one might contend).

Over the course of this climactic scene of death, German's camera remains relatively immobile, sporadically blocked by various figures and seemingly a startled bystander to this momentous event in Soviet history. In the end, there is no need for German to insinuate smell through disorienting camera work and indirect haptic images, for smell occupies a foremost position in the scene. As it becomes clear at the Kuntsevo dacha, we have at last come to the primary source of the smell that the film continually privileges, for the stench from Stalin's excrement, rotten farts, decaying body, and, in a metaphorical sense, his moral turpitude implicitly fill the room and beyond. Beria, like Klensky, cannot escape the stench, and in certain respects, neither can German's viewers, who have been thrust—via the film's overt olfactory references to Soviet history and via haptic insinuation of scent—into the Stalinist past. For many viewers, this stench may be unbearable (and thus the profound difficulty audiences have had with this film), but German, like Klensky, has traveled to the heart of Stalinism in such a vivid, cinematically compelling fashion.

The collective memories of Stalinism that German uncovers and probes so vividly in *Khrustalev, My Car!*, as well as *My Friend Ivan Lapshin*, hinge greatly upon viewers' visceral reactions to the noxious odors of repression. In certain respects, the emphasis on smell in these two films, particularly *Khrustalev*, offers audiences an active way to reassess the Soviet past. "Smell," film scholar Paul Elliott maintains, "is inextricably linked to memory and, through this, to our sense of space, place, and identity; but it is also constantly in flux, existing in a continual becoming that avoids being tied to specific meaning and thus to semiological processes."[15] A smell-induced flux and shifting sense of the Soviet Union's historical "space, place, and identity" indeed lie at the heart of *Lapshin* and *Khrustalev*. In both films, semiological processes fluctuate in accordance with Elliott's supposition that olfactory memories resist any fixed, rigid meaning. Thus smell provides German—and those viewers willing to engage in a sensorial fashion with his films—the opportunity to defy, conceptually and viscerally, the authoritarian essence of Stalinism. The smells may be overwhelming at times, as are the sights and sounds of these two films, but through active memory and through a willingness to grapple with a filmic vision of the past that is in constant flux, viewers can ultimately escape the stench, much like General Klensky does in the concluding scene of *Khrustalev*.

Notes

1 Vladimir Nabokov, *Mary*, trans. Michael Glenny (New York: Vintage Press, 1989), 60.
2 Laura U. Marks, *Touch: Sensuous Theory and Multisensory Media* (Minneapolis: University of Minnesota Press, 2002), 115.
3 Ibid., 118.
4 Discussing the then in-progress *Hard to be God*, German remarked, "From the very beginning I said, let's try and shoot a film with smell." Anton Dolin, *German: Interv'iu. Esse. Tsenarii* (Moscow: Novoe literaturnoe obozrenie, 2011), 274. As German's final film, *Hard to be God* is the only work by the filmmaker that does not harken back to a former time but rather, ostensibly in sci-fi fashion, recounts events on a distant planet that eerily resembles the Middle Ages on Earth. As for earlier work by the filmmaker, the events of *The Seventh Companion*, which German co-directed with the well-established, albeit conventional, Soviet filmmaker Grigori Aronov, take place during the Civil War soon after the 1917 Revolution. *Twenty Years without War*, a more mature work by German, recounts the making of a propagandistic film during the Second World War and a fleeting love affair, both of which transpire in the eastern Soviet city of Tashkent (now part of Uzbekistan). Meanwhile, German's second film, *Trial on the Road* (*Proverka na dorogakh*, 1971/86), transpires during the Second World War, but it places far less emphasis on a sensorial recreation of the past in comparison to German's other films.
5 In a 1999 interview, German remarks, "Close your eyes. Imagine [your deceased relatives] in color. You won't have any luck with this. Recollections don't have color. One can try and film them in color. Sometimes it seems pretty, but after 300 meters [of film] you realize that you are ruining the film. It's strange, but color kills reality." See Maria Bozhovich, "Aleksei German: 'Izgoniaushchii d'iavola'," *Iskusstvo kino* 6 (June 1999).
6 Anthony Anemone, "*Moi drug Ivan Lapshin*/*My Friend Ivan Lapshin*," in *The Cinema of Russia and the Former Soviet Union*, ed. Birgit Beumers (London: Wallflower Press, 2007), 203.
7 Anton Dolin, "The Strange Case of Aleksei German," trans. Oleg Dubson, *Film Comment* 48 (2) (March/April 2012): 31. Dolin's article on German initially appeared in the Russian newspaper *Moskovskie novosti*.

8   German's narrator states: "Only infrequently, when I write or read, or when, like today, there's no work, suddenly for no reason at all I recall the sound of my childhood steps in the long corridor of our apartment, the smell of those 'Bliuming' cigarettes, which Lapshin smoked." This perhaps contradicts Nabokov's point on smell from *Mary*, but it surely points to the prominence of smell in German's film.

9   Discussing his decision to have the relatively unknown actor Andrei Boltnev play the role of the central, eponymous protagonist in *Lapshin*, German remarked, "He had to have the face of a man from the Red List, a man who would soon be killed." Quoted in Dolin, "The Strange Case," 30.

10 See, for instance, J. Hoberman's discussion of German's film, which draws upon an interview Hoberman conducted with German. Hoberman writes, "I asked German if *Khrustalyov* was about present-day Russia. 'Of course,' he replied, adding that 'maybe things are simpler now—they just shoot you.'" See J. Hoberman, "Exorcism: Aleksei German Among the Long Shadows," *Film Comment* 1 (January/February 1999).

11 In fact, it is not unusual to see *Khrustalev, My Car!* and have only a minimal sense of what is transpiring in the film. Reaction to *Khrustalev*, given the confusing nature of the film, was initially quite negative, although appreciation for it has grown steadily, now that people have gotten a second look. The film, in fact, received loud, derogatory boos during its premiere at the Cannes Film Festival in 1998, and many in the audience walked out midway through its screening; Harlan Kennedy, discussing the 1998 Cannes Film Festival that year in the journal *Film Comment*, writes, "Even the rubbish this year at Cannes was lively ... Alexei Guerman's *Khoustaliov, My Car!* [*sic*], a political satire from Russia, was like escaped early Dick Lester. (Some of the audience escaped early, too)." See Harlan Kennedy, "Idiot's Delight," *Film Comment* 34 (4) (July/August 1998): 7. (Dick Lester is an American filmmaker.) But French film critics subsequently apologized for their harsh initial reaction to *Khrustalev*. For more on the negative reaction to *Khrustalev* at Cannes and the subsequent about-face of French film critics, see Irina Rubanova, "Davai uletim!" *Iskusstvo kino* 3 (March 2000): 55–62.

12 Phillip Lopate, "New York," *Film Comment* 34 (6) (November/December 1998): 52.

13 George Nivat, "Popugai v kommunal'noi pustote," trans. from French by V. Bozhovich, *Iskusstvo kino* 2 (February 2000): 56.

14 For more on the scientific and artistic preoccupation with immortality in early Soviet culture that presaged the Stalinist-era experiments in longevity alludes, see Nikolai Krementsov, *Revolutionary Experiments: The Quest for Immortality in Bolshevik Science and Fiction* (New York: Oxford University Press, 2014).

15 Paul Elliott, *Hitchcock and the Cinema of Sensations: Embodied Film Theory and Cinematic Reception* (New York: I.B. Tauris, 2011), 125.

SELECTED BIBLIOGRAPHY

Ackerman, Diane. *A Natural History of the Senses*. New York: Random House, 1990.
Attali, Jacques. *Noise: The Political Economy of Music*. Minneapolis: University of Minnesota Press, 1985.
Bacci, Francesca and David Melcher, eds. *Art and the Senses*. New York: Oxford University Press, 2011.
Baldwin, Peter C. "How Night Air Became Good Air, 1776–1930." *Environmental History* 8 (3) (2003): 412–29.
Barnes, David S. *The Great Stink of Paris and the Nineteenth-Century Struggle against Filth and Germs*. Baltimore, MD: Johns Hopkins Press, 2006.
Bello, Patrizia di and Gabriel Koureas, eds. *Art, History, and the Senses: 1830 to the Present*. Burlington, VT: Ashgate, 2011.
Bentley, Amy. *Eating for Victory: Food Rationing and the Politics of Domesticity*. Champaign: University of Illinois Press, 1998.
Biesold, Horst. *Crying Hands: Eugenics and Deaf People in Nazi Germany*. Trans. William Sayers. Washington, DC: Gallaudet University Press, 1999.
Biltekoff, Charlotte. *Eating Right in America: The Cultural Politics of Food and Health*. Durham, NC: Duke University Press, 2013.
Borrero, Mauricio. *Hungry Moscow: Scarcity and Urban Society in the Russian Civil War, 1917–1921*. New York: Peter Lang, 2003.
Bourdieu, Pierre. *Distinction: A Social Critique of the Judgement of Taste*. Trans. Richard Nice. Cambridge, MA: Harvard University Press, 1984.
Brant, Clare. "Fume and Perfume: Some Eighteenth-Century Uses of Smell." *Journal of British Studies* 43 (4) (2004): 444–63.
Burch, Susan. "Transcending Revolutions: The Tsars, the Soviets and Deaf Culture." *Journal of Social History* 34 (2) (2000): 393–9.
Bynum, W. F. and Roy Porter. eds. *Medicine and the Five Senses*. Cambridge: Cambridge University Press, 1993.
Campen, Cretien van. *The Proust Effect: The Senses as Doorways to Lost Memories*. Trans. Julian Ross. Oxford: Oxford University Press, 2014.
Camporesi, Piero. *Exotic Brew: The Art of Living in the Age of Enlightenment*. Trans. Christopher Woodall. Cambridge: Polity Press, 1994.
Carlisle, Janice. *Common Scents: Comparative Encounters in High-Victorian Fiction*. New York: Oxford University Press, 2004.
Chaplin, Joyce E. "Natural Philosophy and an Early Racial Idiom in North America: Comparing English and Indian Bodies." *The William and Mary Quarterly* Third Series 54 (1997): 229–52.

Chiang, Connie Y. "The Nose Knows: The Sense of Smell in American History." *The Journal of American History* 95 (2008): 405–16.

Christian, David. "Prohibition in Russia, 1914–1925." *Australian Slavonic and East European Studies* 9 (2) (1995): 89–118.

Classen, Constance. *The Deepest Sense: A Cultural History of Touch*. Urbana: University of Illinois Press, 2012.

Classen, Constance, David Howes, and Anthony Synnott. *Aroma: The Cultural History of Smell*. London: Routledge, 1994.

Cockayne, Emily. *Hubbub: Filth, Noise and Stench in England, 1600–1770*. New Haven, CT: Yale University Press, 2007.

Cohen, Esther. "Towards a History of European Physical Sensibility: Pain in the Later Middle Ages." *Science in Context* 8 (1995): 47–74.

Cohen, William A. *Embodied: Victorian Literature and the Senses*. Minneapolis: University of Minnesota, 2008.

Cook, James W. "Seeing the Visual in U.S. History." *The Journal of American History* 95 (2008): 432–41.

Corbin, Alain. *The Foul and the Fragrant: Odor and the French Social Imagination*. Trans. Miriam Kochan. Cambridge, MA: Harvard University Press, 1986.

Corbin, Alain. *Village Bells: Sound and Meaning in the Nineteenth-Century French Countryside*. Trans. Martin Thom. New York: Columbia University Press, 1998.

Coveney, John. *Food, Morals and Meaning: The Pleasure and Anxiety of Eating*. New York: Routledge, 2000.

Cowan, Alexander and Jill Steward. eds. *The City and the Senses: Urban Culture since 1500*. Aldershot: Ashgate, 2007.

Dainotto, Roberto M. *Europe (In Theory)*. Durham, NC: Duke University Press, 2007.

Das, Santanu "'The Impotence of Sympathy': Touch and Trauma in the Memoirs of the First World War Nurses." *Textual Practice* 19 (2) (2005): 239–62.

Dillon, Emma. *The Sense of Sound: Musical Meaning in France, 1260–1330*. New York: Oxford University Press, 2012.

Douglas, Mary. "A Distinctive Anthropological Perspective." In *Constructive Drinking: Perspectives on Drink from Anthropology*. ed. Mary Douglas, 3–15. New York: Cambridge University Press, 1987.

Douglas, Mary. *Purity and Danger: An Analysis of Concepts of Pollution and Taboo*. London: Routledge, 2002.

Duden, Barbara. "Medicine and the History of the Body." In *The Social Construction of Illness: Illness and Medical Knowledge in Past and Present*, ed. Jens Lachmund and Gunnar Stollberg, 39–51. Stuttgart: Franz Steiner Verlag, 1991.

Dugan, Holly. *The Ephemeral History of Perfume: Scent and Sense in Early Modern England*. Baltimore, MD: The Johns Hopkins University Press, 2011.

Earle, Rebecca. *The Body of the Conquistador: Food, Race and the Colonial Experience in Spanish America, 1492–1700*. Cambridge: Cambridge University Press, 2012.

Elias, Norbert. *The Civilizing Process: Sociogenetic and Psychogenetic Investigations*. Trans. Edmund Jephcott. Oxford: Blackwell Publishers, 2000.

Elliott, Paul. *Hitchcock and the Cinema of Sensations: Embodied Film Theory and Cinematic Reception.* New York: I.B. Tauris, 2011.
Ely, Christopher. *This Meager Nature: Landscape and National Identity in Imperial Russia.* DeKalb: Northern Illinois University Press, 2002.
Falkenhausen, Lothar von. *Suspended Music: Chime Bells in the Culture of Bronze Age China.* Berkeley: University of California Press, 1993.
Ferguson, Priscilla Parkhurst. "The Senses of Taste." *The American History Review* 116 (2) (2011): 371–84.
Fitzgerald, Gerard J. and Gabriella M. Petrick. "In Good Taste: Rethinking American History with Our Palates." *The Journal of American History* 95 (2008): 392–404.
Foucault, Michel. *Madness and Civilization: A History of Insanity in the Age of Reason.* Trans. Richard Howard. New York: Vintage Books, 1988.
Freedman, Paul, ed. *Food: The History of Taste.* Berkeley: University of California Press, 2007.
Frierson, Cathy. *Peasant Icons: Representations of Rural Russia in Late Nineteenth Century Russia.* New York: Oxford University Press, 1993.
Garrioch, David. "Sounds of the City: The Soundscape of Early Modern European Towns." *Urban History* 30 (1) (2003): 5–25.
Glantz, Musya and Joyce Toomre, eds. *Food in Russian History and Culture.* Bloomington: Indiana University Press, 1997.
Goldstein, Darra. "Gastronomic Reforms under Peter the Great. Toward a Cultural History of Russian Food," *Jahrbücher für Geschichte Osteuropas* 48 (4) (2000): 481–510.
Gorham, Michael. *Speaking in Soviet Tongues: Language Culture and the Politics of Voice in Revolutionary Russia.* Dekalb: Northern Illinois University Press, 2003.
Goubert, Jean-Pierre. *The Conquest of Water: The Advent of Health in the Industrial Age.* Trans. Andrew Wilson. Princeton, NJ: Princeton University Press, 1989.
Gronow, Jukka. *Caviar with Champagne: Common Luxury and the Ideals of the Good Life in Stalin's Russia.* Oxford: Berg, 2003.
Hamlin, Christopher. *Public Health and Social Justice in the Age of Chadwick: Britain, 1800–1854.* Cambridge: Cambridge University Press, 1998.
Harrison, Mark. *Climates and Constitutions: Health, Race, Environment and British Imperialism in India, 1600–1850.* New York: Oxford University Press, 1999.
Harvey, Elizabeth D. "The Portal of Touch." *The American History Review* 116 (2) (2011): 385–400.
Harvey, Elizabeth D., ed. *Sensible Flesh: On Touch in Early Modern Culture.* Philadelphia: University of Pennsylvania Press, 2003.
Harvey, Susan Ashbrook. *Scenting Salvation: Ancient Christianity and the Olfactory Imagination.* Berkeley: University of California Press, 2006.
Herlihy, Patricia. *Alcoholic Empire: Vodka and Politics in Late Imperial Russia.* New York: Oxford University Press, 2002.
Hernandez, Richard L. "Sacred Sound and Sacred Substance: Church Bells and Auditory Culture of Russian Villages during the Bolshevik *Velikii Perelom*." *The American Historical Review* (2004): 1475–504.
Higgins, Paul C. *Outsiders in a Hearing World: A Sociology of Deafness.* Beverly Hills, CA: Sage, 1980.

Higonnet, Margeret. "Authenticity and Art in Trauma Narratives of World War I." *Modernism/Modernity* 9 (1) (2002): 91–107.
Hilton, Marjorie L. *Selling to the Masses: Retailing in Russia, 1880–1930.* Pittsburgh, PA: University of Pittsburgh Press, 2012.
Hoffer, Peter Charles. *Sensory Worlds in Early America.* Baltimore, MD: Johns Hopkins University Press, 2003.
Hosler, Dorothy. *The Sounds and Colors of Power: The Sacred Metallurgical Technology of Ancient West Mexico.* Cambridge, MA: MIT Press, 1994.
Houston, Stephen and Karl Taube. "An Archaeology of the Senses: Perception and Cultural Expression in Ancient Mesoamerica." *Cambridge Archaeological Journal* 10 (2) (2000): 261–94.
Howes, David. "Can These Dry Bones Live? An Anthropological Approach to the History of the Senses." *The Journal of American History* 95 (2008): 442–50.
Howes, David. *The Varieties of Sensory Experience: A Sourcebook in the Anthropology of the Senses.* Toronto: University of Toronto Press, 1991.
Howes, David, ed. *Empire of the Senses: The Sensual Culture Reader.* London: Bloomsbury, 2014.
Hynes, Samuel. *The Soldiers' Tale: Bearing Witness in Modern War.* New York: Penguin, 1998.
Jarvis, Christina S. *The Male Body at War: American Masculinity during World War II.* DeKalb: Northern Illinois University Press, 2003.
Jay, Martin. "In the Realm of the Senses: An Introduction," *American Historical Review* 116 (2) (2011): 307–15.
Jenner, Mark S. "Civilization and Deodorization? Smell in Early Modern English Culture." In *Civil Histories: Essays Presented to Sir Keith Thomas*, ed. Peter Burke, Brian Harrison, and Paul Slack, 127–44. New York: Oxford, 2000.
Jenner, Mark S. "Follow Your Nose? Smell, Smelling, and Their Histories." *The American History Review* 116 (2) (2011): 335–51.
Johnson, James H. *Listening in Paris: A Cultural History.* Berkeley: University of California Press, 1995.
Jütte, Robert. *A History of the Senses: From Antiquity to Cyberspace.* Trans. James Lynn. Cambridge: Polity 2005.
Kaganovsky, Lilya and Masha Salazkina, eds. *Sound, Speech, Music in Soviet and Post-Soviet Cinema.* Bloomington: Indiana University Press, 2014.
Kahla, Elina. *Life as Exploit: Representations of Twentieth-Century Saintly Women in Russia.* Helsinki: Kikimora Publications, 2007.
Kayiatos, Anastasia. "Sooner Speaking than Silent, Sooner Silent than Mute: Soviet Deaf Theatre and Pantomime after Stalin." *Theatre Survey* 51 (1) (2010): 5–31.
Korsmeyer, Carolyn. *Making Sense of Taste: Food and Philosophy.* Ithaca, NY: Cornell University Press, 1999.
Krementsov, Nikolai. *Revolutionary Experiments: The Quest for Immortality in Bolshevik Science and Fiction.* New York: Oxford University Press, 2014.
Krentz, Christopher. *Writing Deafness: The Hearing Line in Nineteenth-Century American Literature.* Berkeley: University of California Press, 2007.
Kupperman, Karen Ordahl. "Fear of Hot Climates in the Anglo-American Colonial Experience." *The William and Mary Quarterly* Third Series 41 (2) (1984): 213–40.
Ladd, Paddy. *Understanding Deaf Culture: In Search of Deafhood.* Clevedon: Multilingual Matters, 2003.

Lane, Harlan. *When the Mind Hears: A History of the Deaf*. New York: Random House, 1984.
Le Guerer, Annick. *Scent: The Mysterious and Essential Powers of Smell*. New York: Turtle Bay Books, 1992.
LeBlanc, Ronald D. *Slavic Sins of the Flesh: Food, Sex, and Carnal Appetite in Nineteenth-Century Russian Fiction*. Lebanon: University of New Hampshire Press, 2009.
Levenstein, Harvey A. *Paradox of Plenty: A Social History of Eating in Modern America*. Berkeley: University of California Press, 2003.
Levenstein, Harvey A. *Revolution at the Table: The Transformation of the American Diet*. Berkeley: University of California Press, 2003.
Lévi-Strauss, Claude. "The Culinary Triangle." Trans. Peter Brooks. In *Food and Culture: A Reader*, ed. Carole Counihan and Penny van Esterik. New York: Routledge, 1997.
Lotman, Yuri and Jelena Pogosjan. *High Society Dinners: Dining in Tsarist Russia*. Trans. Marian Schwartz, ed. Darra Goldstein. Totnes: Prospect Books, 2014.
Lovell, Stephen. "Broadcasting Bolshevik: The Radio Voice of Soviet Culture." *Journal of Contemporary History* 38 (1) (2013): 78–97.
Lovell, Stephen. "How Russia Learned to Listen: Radio and the Making of Soviet Culture." *Kritika: Explorations in Russian and Eurasian History* 12 (3) (2011), 591–615.
MacKay, John. *True Songs of Freedom: Uncle Tom's Cabin in Russian Culture and Society*. Madison: University of Wisconsin Press, 2013.
Maiorova, Olga. *From the Shadow of Empire: Defining the Russian Nation through Cultural Mythology, 1855–1870*. Madison: University of Wisconsin Press, 2010.
Marks, Laura U. *Touch: Sensuous Theory and Multisensory Media*. Minneapolis: University of Minnesota Press, 2002.
Martin, Alexander M. *Enlightened Metropolis: Constructing Imperial Moscow, 1762–1855*. Oxford: Oxford University Press, 2013.
Martin, Alexander M. "Sewage and the City: Filth, Smell, and Representations of Urban Life in Moscow, 1770–1880." *The Russian Review* 67 (2008): 243–74.
Mazow, Leo G. "Sensing America." *American Art* (Fall 2010): 1–11.
McCagg, William O. and Lewis Siegelbaum, eds. *The Disabled in the Soviet Union: Past and Present, Theory and Practice*. Pittsburgh, PA: University of Pittsburgh Press, 1989.
Merridale, Catherine. "The Collective Mind: Trauma and Shell-Shock in Twentieth-Century Russia." *Journal of Contemporary History* 35 (1) (2000): 39–55.
Milner, Matthew. *The Senses and the English Reformation*. Burlington, VT: Ashgate, 2011.
Monaghan, Leila et al., eds. *Many Ways to Be Deaf: International Variation in Deaf Communities*. Washington, DC: Gallaudet University Press, 2003.
Nakamura, Karen. *Deaf in Japan: Signing and the Politics of Identity*. Ithaca, NY: Cornell University Press, 2006.
Nordenfalk, Carl. "The Five Senses in Late Medieval and Renaissance Art." *Journal of the Warburg and Courtauld Institutes* 48 (1985): 1–22.

Padden, Carol and Tom Humphries. *Deaf in America: Stories from a Culture.* Cambridge, MA: Harvard University Press, 1988.

Parr, Joy. "Smells Like? Sources of Uncertainty in the History of the Great Lakes Environment." *Environmental History* 11 (2) (2006): 269–99.

Pentcheva, Bissera. *The Sensual Icon: Space, Ritual, and the Senses in Byzantium.* University Park: Pennsylvania State University Press, 2011.

Rabinbach, Anson. *The Human Motor: Energy, Fatigue, and the Origins of Modernity.* Berkeley: University of California Press, 1992.

Rath, Richard Cullen. "Hearing American History." *The Journal of American History* 95 (2008): 417–31.

Rath, Richard Cullen. *How Early America Sounded.* Ithaca, NY: Cornell University Press, 2003.

Rindisbacher, Hans J. *The Smell of Books: A Cultural-Historical Study of Olfactory Perception in Literature.* Ann Arbor: University of Michigan Press, 1992.

Riskin, Jessica. "The Divine Optician." *The American History Review* 116 (2) (2011): 352–70.

Romaniello, Matthew P. "Customs and Consumption: Russian Tobacco Habits in the Seventeenth and Eighteenth Century." In *The Global Lives of Things: Materiality, Material Culture and Commodities in the First Global Age*, ed. Anne Gerritsen and Giorgio Riello. London: Routledge, 2015.

Romaniello, Matthew P. and Tricia Starks, eds. *Tobacco in Russian History and Culture: From the Seventeenth Century to the Present.* New York: Routledge, 2009.

Rosenfeld, Sophia. "On Being Heard: A Case for Paying Attention to the Historical Ear." *The American History Review* 116 (2) (2011): 316–34.

Sandomirskaja, Irina. "Skin to Skin: Language in the Soviet Education of Deaf–Blind Children, the 1920s and 1930s." *Studies in East European Thought* 60 (4) (2008): 321–37.

Sanger, Alice E. and Siv Tove Kulbrandstad Walker, eds. *Sense and the Senses in Early Modern Art and Cultural Practice.* Burlington, VT: Ashgate, 2012.

Schafer, R. Murray. *The Tuning of the World: Toward a Theory of Soundscape Design.* New York: Knopf, 1977.

Schiebinger, Londa. *Nature's Body: Gender in the Making of Modern Science.* New Brunswick, NJ: Rutgers University Press, 1993.

Schmidt, Leigh Eric. *Hearing Things: Religion, Illusion, and the American Enlightenment.* Urbana: University of Illinois Press, 1992.

Scott, James. *Seeing Like a State: How Certain Schemes to Improve the Human Condition Have Failed.* New Haven, CT: Yale University Press, 1999.

Segal, Boris M. *Russian Drinking: Use and Abuse of Alcohol in Pre-Revolutionary Russia.* New Brunswick, NJ: Rutgers Center of Alcohol Studies, 1987.

Seremetakis, C. Nadia. *The Senses Still: Perception and Memory as Material Culture in Modernity.* Boulder, CO: Westview Press, 1994.

Shaw, Claire. "'Speaking in the Language of Art': Soviet Deaf Theatre and the Politics of Identity during Khrushchev's Thaw." *Slavonic and East European Review* 91 (4) (2013): 759–86.

Shaw, Claire. "'We Have No Need to Lock Ourselves Away': Space, Marginality, and the Negotiation of Deaf Identity in Late Soviet Moscow." *Slavic Review* 74 (1) (2015): 57–78.

Silverman, Lisa. *Tortured Subjects: Pain, Truth and the Body in Early Modern France*. Chicago: University of Chicago Press, 2001.
Smith, Alison K. "Public Works in an Autocratic State: Water Supplies in an Imperial Russian Town." *Environment and History* 11 (2005): 319–42.
Smith, Alison K. *Recipes for Russia: Food and Nationhood under the Tsars*. DeKalb: Northern Illinois University Press, 2008.
Smith, Mark M. "Getting in Touch with Slavery and Freedom." *The Journal of American History* 95 (2008): 381–91.
Smith, Mark M. *How Race is Made: Slavery, Segregation, and the Senses*. Chapel Hill, NC: University of North Carolina, 2006.
Smith, Mark M. "Making Sense of Social History." *Journal of Social History* 37 (1) (2003): 165–86.
Smith, Mark M. "Producing Sense, Consuming Sense, Making Sense: Perils and Prospects for Sensory History." *Journal of Social History* 40 (4) (2007): 841–58.
Smith, Mark M. *Sensing the Past: Seeing, Hearing, Smelling, Tasting, and Touching in History*. Berkeley: University of California Press, 2007.
Smith, Mark M. *The Smell of Battle, The Taste of Siege: A Sensory History of the Civil War*. New York: Oxford University Press, 2015.
Snyder, Sharon L. and David T. Mitchell. *Cultural Locations of Disability*. Chicago: University of Chicago Press, 2006.
Starks, Tricia. *The Body Soviet: Propaganda, Hygiene, and the Revolutionary State*. Madison: University of Wisconsin Press, 2008.
Sterne, Jonathan. *The Audible Past: Cultural Origins of Sound Reproduction*. Durham, NC: Duke University Press, 2003.
Stites, Richard. *Serfdom, Society, and the Arts: The Pleasure and the Power*. New Haven, CT: Yale University Press, 2005.
Stoler, Ann Laura. *Carnal Knowledge and Imperial Power: Race and the Intimate in Colonial Rule*. Berkeley: University of California Press, 2002.
Stoff, Laurie S. *They Fought for the Motherland: Russia's Women Soldiers in World War I and the Revolution*. Lawrence: University Press of Kansas, 2006.
Stone, Helena. "The Soviet Government and Moonshine, 1917–1929." *Cahiers du Monde russe et soviétique* 27 (3–4) (1986): 359–79.
Transchel, Kate. *Under the Influence: Working-Class Drinking, Temperance, and Cultural Revolution in Russia, 1895–1932*. Pittsburgh, PA: Pittsburgh University Press, 2006.
Tumarkin, Maria. "Productive Death: The Necropedagogy of a Young Soviet Hero." *The South Atlantic Quarterly* 110 (4) (2011): 885–900.
Vroon, Piet. *Smell: The Secret Seducer*. New York: Farrar, Straus and Giroux, 1994.
Ward, Megan. "Feeling Middle Class: Sensory Perception in Victorian Literature and Culture." PhD Diss., Rutgers University, 2008.
West, Sally. *I Shop in Moscow: Advertising and the Creation of Consumer Culture in Late Tsarist Russia*. Dekalb: Northern Illinois University Press, 2011.
Williams, Howard G. "Founders of Deaf Education in Russia." In *Deaf History Unveiled: Interpretations from the New Scholarship*, ed. John Vickrey Van Cleve, 224–36. Washington, DC: Gallaudet University Press, 1993.
Woolgar, Chris. *The Senses in Late Medieval England*. New Haven, CT: Yale University Press, 2006.

INDEX

The letter *f* following an entry denotes a figure

Abdulin, Mansur 229, 233
activity 256–7
advertising 4
   tobacco and 106–10, 107*f*, 109*f*
aesthetics 100
alcohol 178 *see also kumyshka*
   Gorbachev, Mikhail and 179
   prohibition 149–54
   Soviet control and 154
Aleksinskaia, Tatiana 134
Aliger, Margarita 250, 255
   Zoia: A Fairy Tale about Truth 255
   "Zoia: Poema" 250–1
All Russian Society of the Deaf
   (*Vserossiiskoe obshchestvo glukhikh*, VOG) 194, 197, 202
Alonso, Ana María 220–1
Amarcord (Fellini, Frederico) 275
America
   army and 235
   cinema and 10
   food and 7–8, 170, 174
   nutrition and 169, 170, 173–4
   sites of memory and 6
   war propaganda and 227, 235
Anemone, Anthony 270
Appert, Nicolas 45
Arnshtam, Lev: *Zoia* 254–5
art 7
Atwater, Wilbur O. 168
autobiography 220, 274
Avdeeva, Katerina 56

backwardness 11, 144, 148, 196
   cold and 25–6
   deafness and 200
   sign language and 204

   smell and 99
   speech and 207
   taste and 58
   Udmurts and 146–8, 150, 152, 153, 157, 158
bania 34–6
Barabintzes 28
Bashutskii, Aleksandr Pavlovich 72, 74–5
bathhouses 34–6
bathrooms 11
BELIP (Proteinic Product of the Nutritional Institute of the Academy of Medical Sciences of the USSR) 180
Bell, John 30
Benjamin, Walter 4, 10, 70
Bentham, Samuel 36
Berestev, Andrei 155
black market 11
body *see also* embodiment
   cold and 23–34, 37–8 *see also* bania
   war and 118–19, 120, 125
Bocharskaia, Sofia 122, 123, 124, 126–7, 128, 132–3, 134
Bogin, Mikhail: *Two, The* 204
Bolton, Ivan 58
Bondarev, G. I. 183
Book of Tasty and Healthy Food 174, 175
Borenstein, Eliot 230
Borisov, Nikolai 259
Borisov, T. K. 153
Bourdieu, Pierre 70, 105, 141
bread 178
Bremner, Robert 53

brewing 145, 146f, 147, 151 *see also* fermentation
bricolage 98
Brillat-Savarin, Jean Anthelme: *Physiology of Taste* 49–50
Britain
  class and 106
  diplomats of 30, 31–4
  tobacco and 106
  war propaganda and 227
Britnieva, Mary 125
Bruce, Peter Henry 34–5
Bukharans 28
Bulgarin, Faddei 58
Buriats, the 29

cabbage
  drying 57
  sour 51–2, 55–7
canning 45
capitalism 4
Carmichael, John 32–3
Chaikina, Liza 244, 255, 261–2
Chantreau, Pierre Nicolas 36
Chappe d'Auteroche, Jean-Baptiste 35
Charukovskii, Akim 50, 52–3
cheese 50
Chelakova, N. 117–20, 122, 126, 133
children, speech and 207
cigarettes 100–1, 102–3, 105, 110–11
cinema *see also* German, Aleksei, Sr.
  America and 10
  color and 269
  haptic images and 268–9, 272–3
  Kosmodemianskaia, Zoia and 254–5
  memory and 267–70, 280
  propaganda and 272
  smell and 267–9, 270–3, 275–81
  taste and 279
city 10
  Moscow 99
  Paris 68
  St. Petersburg 67–70
  social mobility and 69–70
  sound and 122
  tobacco and 102
civic nationalism 5

civilization 14
Civilizing Process, The (Elias, Norbert) 4
Clarke, Edward 58
class 4
  consumption and 106
  food and 8, 132–3
  kumyshka and 154–5
  smell and 102
  taste and 141
  tobacco and 102, 105, 106
  wartime nursing and 120–1, 132–3
Classen, Constance 259
  Deepest Sense: A Cultural History of Touch, The 259
climate 23–5
  health and 23–34, 37 *see also* bania
clothing 11, 12
Cohen, William 220, 233
cold 23–5 *see also* bania; winter
  backwardness and 25–6
  body, and the 23–34, 37–8
  food and 169
  health and 23–34, 37–8
  human nature and 25–6
  Kosmodemianskaia, Zoia and 256, 260
  West Europeans and 30–8
collective memory 6, 14, 244, 245, 255–6, 261–2, 280 *see also* Kosmodemianskaia, Zoia
collectivization 170
Collins, Samuel 25
colonialism 141, 148
commemoration 255–6, 258–9
Committee on Food Habits 173
commodity fetishism 4
communism 2
Comrade Pavlik: The Rose and Fall of a Soviet Boy Hero (Kelly, Catriona) 256
comradeship 230–2
Congress of Small Peoples of the Volga Region 153
Connell, R. W. 239 n.61
consumerism 10–11
  St. Petersburg and 69–70, 71–2, 78, 84–7
  women and 78, 84–7

consumption 69–70, 76, 105–6 *see also* consumerism; luxury
context and 98
Corbin, Alain 1–2, 102
corn 177, 178
Coveney, John 168
Coxe, William 52
Creak, Simon 220
cultural modernity 11
culture, taste and 58–9
Culture of Consumption, The (Khodosh, Iulia) 181
cultured sign language 203–5
cultured speech 203

Dal, Vladimir I. 143, 147
Das, Santanu 127, 128
Davidson, Alan 46
Davydov, P. 57
deafness 12–13, 193, 199, 207
   achievements and 202
   backwardness and 200
   creativity and 201–2
   education and 198
   eugenics and 200
   "golden age" 201
   hearing aids and 205–6
   identity and 193–7, 201, 206, 211
   labor and 197–8, 199f, 202
   rights and 197
   services and 202
   sign language 194, 196, 197–9, 199f, 200–5, 206–7, 209, 210–11
   society and 196, 199–200, 209
   sovietness and 195, 197, 201, 202, 211
   spying and 200
   technology and 205–10, 211
   theatre and 201–2, 204, 205, 209–10
death 118–19, 124, 231–2, 245, 278
Deepest Sense: A Cultural History of Touch, The (Classen, Constance) 259
democratic social engineering 173–4
Deni, Viktor 247f, 248
Denmark 170
Dimsdale, Elizabeth 23

diplomats, health and 30–4
Dmitriev, Valentin Grigor'evich 203–4
Dolce Vita, La (Fellini, Frederico) 275
Dolin, Anton 270
Dorman, Moisei 228
Dostoyevsky, Fyodor 168
Douglas, Mary 46, 142
drink 9 *see also* food
   brewing 145, 146f, 147, 151 *see also* fermentation
   kumys 143
   kumyshka see kumyshka
   kvas 51–2, 53–5, 57, 58, 157
   lim kumyshka 143
   nebyt kumyshka 143
   portrayal of 157–8
drunkenness 153
"Dulce et Decorum Est" (Owen, Wilfred) 125
Dumas, Alexandre, *fils*: *Dame Aux Camélias, La* 79

eating habits 11–12
Eating With an Appetite 182, 183
Elias, Norbert 4
   Civilizing Process, The 4
Elliot, Paul 280
embodiment 233, 236, 252 *see also* body
emotions 1 *see also* feelings
Enchanted Island (play) 209
enemy 227–8
England, taste and 100
Estonians 28
ethnography 145–7
eugenics 200

famine 170 *see also* poverty
Farmborough, Florence 123, 125–6, 127, 129, 130, 131, 133
feelings 243–4 *see also* emotions
Fellini, Frederico
   Amarcord 275
   Dolce Vita, La 275
Ferguson, Priscilla Parkhurst 99, 102, 132
fermentation 45–7, 51–7, 59 *see also* brewing; game

Fetisov, Viktor: "Return of Zoia Kosmodemianskaia" 260–1
feuilletons 77–9, 81
film recollection 270
Finch, Edward 31–2
First World War 3, 13, 128–9, 130–1 *see also* wartime nursing
  alcohol and 149–50
  nutrition and 170
Fitzpatrick, Sheila 175
Five-Year Plan (1928–32) 170, 173
food 11–12, 179 *see also* drink; nutrition; taste
  bread 178
  cheese 50
  class and 169
  cookbooks 172, 174–5, 182
  corn 177, 178
  culture and 47
  drying 57
  embargos 179, 183
  fermentation 45–7, 51–7, 59
  game 47, 49–51
  Germany and 173
  grain 179
  Italy and 173
  kvas 51–2, 53–5, 57, 58
  luxury and 174, 175–6
  meat economy 179–80
  national identity and 7–8, 11, 47–8, 58–9, 167–8
  potatoes 58
  poverty and 168–71
  preservation 45–6
  psychology and 173–4
  putrefaction 45–9, 56, 59
  rabbit 172–3
  rye bread 51–3, 57, 58
  sausages 175–6, 175f, 177–8, 180, 182
  science and 171–2
  seafood 180
  Second World War and 174–5
  shchi 58
  shortages 154–5, 167, 169–72, 174–5, 178, 182–3
  sour cabbage 51–2, 55–7
  soy 171–2
  state control and 167–9, 179–80
  sukharki 131, 133
  unfamiliar 167, 169, 170, 171–3, 174–5, 177–8, 180, 182–3
  vegetarianism 182
  war and 130–3, 234
  writings and 48, 50, 52
  yeast 172
Food Program of the USSR for the Period up to 1990 179, 181
Foucault, Michel 5
France
  food and 8, 49
  panoramic literature and 68
  taste and 100
freedom 151–3
French Revolution 2

game 47, 49–51
gastronomy 48, 49–51
gaze *see* male gaze
Geil'man, Iosif Florianovich 193–4, 202–3, 206
Geling, Karl 54, 56
gender 10–11, 12 *see also* men; women
  brewing and 151
  disfigurement and 248
  German army and 235
  Red Army and 232–4
  St. Petersburg and 78–82, 84
  wartime nursing and 128
Georgi, Johann Gottlieb 37
  Russia: Or A Compleat Historical Account of All of the Nations which Compose that Empire 26–9
Geraci, Robert 147
Gerd, Kuzebai 157
  "It's Better to Die" 157
German, Aleksei, Sr. 14, 267
  haptic images and 268–9, 272–3
  Hard to be God 269
  Khrustalev, My Car! 267, 269, 273–81, 275f, 276f, 278f, 279f
  memory and 267–70, 280
  My Friend Ivan Lapshin 267, 269–73, 271f, 272f, 280
  Seventh Companion, The 269
  smell and 267–9, 270–3, 275–81

taste and 279
Trial on the Road 281 n.4
Twenty Years without War 269
German, Mikhail 175–6
German, Yuri 270
Germany
   army and 235
   food and 173
   taste and 100
   women and 235
Gmelin, Johann Georg 26
Gogol, Nikolai 86
Goldstein, Darra 100
Goodfellow, Charles 30
Goodman, Steve 123
Gorbachev, Mikhail 179
Gordon, Alexander 35
Graebner, William 173–4
grain 179
Grakhova, Marta 204
Grossman, Vasily 223–4
Guillory, Sean 220
Gushev, S. 205
Guthrie, Maria 37
Guthrie, Matthew 23, 24, 29, 37, 57

Hahn, Barbara 101
Halbwachs, Maurice 6
hallucinations 120, 133–5
Hanbury Williams, Charles 33
haptic images 268–9, 272–3
hapticity 24, 81
Hard to be God (German, Aleksei, Sr.) 269
Harley-Davidson 4
Harris, Adrienne 233
Harris, James 33
Harris, Katherine Gertrude 33, 36–7, 38
Harris, Steven 177
Harrison, Mark 25
health 25 *see also* bania; water
   cabbage and 55–6
   categorizing 26–8
   cold and 23–34, 37–8
   fermentation and 57
   kumyshka and 147–8, 149–50, 153
   kvas and 54
   tobacco and 100, 110

   vegetables and 55
   water and 48
   West Europeans and 30–8
hearing 196, 210 *see also* deafness; sound
hearing aids 205–6
Helstosky, Carol 173
Henningsen, Charles 52
heroes 255–6, 261 *see also* martyrdom; national sacrifice
Herzen, Alexander 146
Higonnet, Margaret 129
Hilton, Matthew 106
Hindhede, Mikkel 170
historical fiction 1
Hoffer, Peter Charles 258
Howes, David 70, 106, 119
human nature 25–6
humoral theory 23–4, 25, 28–30, 34, 37–8
Hynes, Samuel 118

icons 247, 249
identity *see also* national identity
   sound/hearing and 193–7, 201, 206, 211
   war and 225–6, 233
Ides, Eberhard Isbrand 26
In Search of Lost Time (Proust, Marcel) 6
individualism 106
industrialization 11
intersensoriality 119, 257–8, 262
Italy 173
"It's Better to Die" (Gerd, Kuzebai) 157

Jay, Martin 98, 119, 220
Jenner, Mark S. R. 99
Jerrman, Edward 54, 74
Joan of Arc 261–2
Jourdier, A. 54
Jug, Steven 130
Jünger, Ernst 118, 124
Jungle Book, The (Kipling, Rudyard) 207–9, 208f
Jutte, Robert 100

Kahla, Elina 248

Kalmyks 28, 29
Kant, Immanuel 100
Karmalita, Svetlana 273
Kaufman, Konstantin Petrovich von 147
Kayiatos, Anastasia 209
Keith, Robert 33
Kelly, Catriona 203
  Comrade Pavlik: The Rose and Fall of a Soviet Boy Hero 256
Khodosh, Iulia 181
  Culture of Consumption, The 181
Khrustalev, My Car! (German, Aleksei, Sr.) 267, 269, 273–80, 275*f*, 276*f*, 278*f*, 279*f*
Kipling, Rudyard: *Jungle Book, The* 207–9, 208*f*
Kirghiz 29
Kirschenbaum, Lisa 255
Klioutchkine, Constantine 110
Knight, Nathaniel 146
Kohl, Johann Georg 52, 54, 74
Kol'tsov, Mikhail 171
Komarova, Anna 210
Komov, Oleg 252
Komsomol 258, 261
Korolenko, Vladimir 147
Korsmeyer, Carolyn 100, 108
Koshevaia, Elena: *Story of a Son* 248–9
Koshevoi, Oleg 248–9
Kosmodemianskaia, Liubov 253–4
Kosmodemianskaia, Zoia 14, 233, 243–5
  activity and 256–7
  cinema and 254–5
  commemoration of 258–9, 262
  images of 244*f*, 245, 246*f*, 247*f*, 248, 251, 251*f*, 256–8, 262
  literature and 248–52, 253–4, 255, 256
  museums and 259–60, 262
  passivity and 256–7
  propaganda and 247*f*, 248, 253–5, 258
  sculpture and 248, 249*f*, 260–1, 262
  sound and 256, 262
  witnesses and 257–8
  words of 253–4, 256, 258
Krainin, Viktor 210
Krasnaia Zvezda (Red Star) 223–4, 227, 235, 236
Krushchev, Nikita 177–8
Kuchebei, Viktor P. 145
Kukryniksy: "Tania (The Feat of Zoia Kosmodemianskaia)" 256, 257
kumys 143
kumyshka 9, 141–2, 146*f*
  brewing 145, 146*f*, 147, 151
  drunkenness and 153
  ethnography and 145–6
  gender and 151
  grain shortages and 154–5
  health and 147–8, 149–50, 153
  media portrayal of 151–3
  national identity and 143, 145–6, 148–9, 153, 157
  popularity of 150–1
  recipes 143
  Soviet state and 154–7
  spiritual practices and 141, 142, 143–4, 145, 147, 149, 154
  state control and 145, 149–56
  Udmurts and 141–9, 150–4, 155–7
kvas 51–2, 53–5, 57, 58, 157

LaBlanc, Ronald 168
labor 197–8, 199*f*, 202
language hierarchy 194
LeClerc 58
Leningrad Rehabilitational Center (LVYs) 193, 206
Lévi-Strauss, Claude 47, 98
Lewin, Kurt 173–4
Lidov, Petr 245, 257
  "Who was Tania?" 248
Liebig, Justus von 168
Life of the Deaf 203
life writing 220
lim kumyshka 143
literature 10 *see also* poetry
  Kosmodemianskaia, Zoia and 248–52, 253–4, 255, 256
  memoirs 220
  romantic narratives and 250
Liubimov, Valerii 204

logocentrism 210–11
Lopate, Phillip 275
Lovell, Stephen 195
Lunacharskii, Anatolii 199
luxury 68, 71–2, 74–5, 84, 85
  food and 174, 175–6
  tobacco and 105
Lyall, Robert 58

Mackenzie, George 30
male gaze 233, 250
Manizer, Matvei 248, 249f
Marbault 35
Marceau, Marcel 201
markets 67–8, 69, 72–4, 76
Marks, Laura 268–9, 272
marriage 78–80
Martin, Alexander M, 38, 69, 99, 110–11
martyrdom *see* Chaikina, Liza; Kosmodemianskaia, Zoia
Marx, Karl 4, 196
Mary (Nabokov, Vladimir) 267
Masterovoy, Anton 11, 58, 100, 141, 195, 234
Meade, Margaret 173
meat economy 179–80
medicine 24–5, 36 *see also* health
Mekke, A. V. 209, 210
memoirs 220
memorialization *see* commemoration
memory 1, 6, 259, 262
  cinema and 267–70, 280
  color and 269
  smell and 267–9, 280
men 78, 81, 84 *see also* gender; male gaze
  war and 128–9, 133, 134, 232–3, 248
Merridale, Catherine 134
Mikhailov, Nicolai 259, 261
Mikhailov, Vladimir 182–3
Mikhin, Petr 222, 233
Mikoyan, Anastas 174, 175
mime 201–2, 209
mineral waters 48
minority groups 12–13
modernity 11, 12, 144, 154
Morozov, Pavlik 260

Moscow, smell and 99
Mowgli (play) 208f, 209
Multan Case 147, 162 n.53
Mulvey, Laura 233
museums 259–60, 262
music 7, 11, 12
Muzafarov, Mudaris Zagirovich 208f, 209
My Friend Ivan Lapshin (German, Aleksei, Sr.) 267, 269–73, 271f, 272f, 280

Nabokov, Vladimir: *Mary* 267
"Natasha in Petersburg" 80, 84–5
national identity 5
  food and 7–8, 11, 47–8, 58–9, 100
  kumyshka and 143, 145–6, 148–9, 153, 157–8
  Russia and 2, 6–7, 47–8
  Soviet identity 195, 197, 201, 211
  Soviet state and 157
  taste and 141–2, 167
  tobacco and 104, 106
national movements 153
national sacrifice 220–1 *see also* Kosmodemianskaia, Zoia
national symbols *see* Joan of Arc; Kosmodemianskaia, Zoia
nationalism 5
  Russia and 9
nature 14–15
Nazarov, Boris 226
nebyt kumyshka 143
Neuburger, Mary 101
New Economic Policy 170
New Soviet Person 195
Nivat, Georges 276–7
Nora, Pierre 6
Nordman, Natalia 169
Nosov, Nikolai 254
nostalgia 270–1
nutrition 168–9, 179–80 *see also* food
  America and 169, 170, 173–4
  famine and 171–2
  Germany and 173
  Italy and 173
  World War I and 169

odor *see* smell
On the Cultivation and Fabrication of Tobacco 102–4
oralism 194
Ostiaks 26, 28
other 102, 108–10, 109f, 158
  deafness and 200, 209, 210
Owen, Wildred: "Dulce et Decorum Est" 125

pain 245
Pallas, Peter Simon 29
panoramic literature 68–9, 71–3
Paris 68
Parkinson, John 36
Passazh (Stenbock-Fermor, Iakov I. Essen-) 10–11, 67, 70, 75–7, 79–84, 85–6
passivity 256–7
Pasteur, Louis 45
Paul, R. B. 53
perfume 1–2
personal memory 6
Petrishchevo 258–9
Pevzner, Emmanuel 168
photography 118, 244f, 245, 248, 251
Physiology of Taste (Brillat-Savarin, Jean-Anthelme) 49–50
Piliushin, Joseph 221
place, tobacco and 101–2, 103–5, 106–8, 110–11
Plamper, Jan 129
podvig 247–8
poetry 250–2, 254, 261
police 82
potatoes 58
poverty 168–71
power 5
Prakhov, G. 155
Preobrazhenskii, S. A. 135
primitivism *see* backwardness
"Productive Death: The Necropedagogy of a Young Soviet Hero" (Tumarkin, Maria) 243–4
prohibition 149–54
pronatalism 250
propaganda 220–1 *see also* Soviet propaganda

Proust, Marcel: *In Search of Lost Time* 6
"Proust effect" 6
purity 45–6, 48
Pursglove, Michael 210
Pushkarev, Ivan Il'ich 71–2, 73–4
Putiatina, Olga 123
putrefaction 45–7, 56, 59 *see also* game
  taste and 48–9
Pyl'tsyn, Aleksandr V. 219

quass 58 *see also* kvas

rabbit 172–3
radio 11, 253–4, 255
Rathe, Daniel 261
Red Army 219–21, 235–6
  comradeship 230–2
  death and 231
  effect of danger and 229
  medics and 232
  national sacrifice and 220–1, 227
  pen pal program 234
  propaganda and 220–1, 226–7, 229–30, 232, 234, 235–6
  sight and 222, 225, 228–9, 231, 232–4
  smell and 222
  soldiers' experiences 223–4
  Stakhanovism and 227
  taste and 231, 234
  touch and 229, 230, 231–2
  training and 228–30, 234
  violence and 224–8
  women and 232–4
Red Cross 121, 130
Red Star (Krasnaia Zvezda) 223–4, 227, 235, 236
religion 246–8, 254
  taste and 168
  Udmurts and 141, 142, 143–4, 145, 147, 149
Reshetnikov, Vasily 226
Retish, Aaron 100
"Return of Zoia Kosmodemianskaia" (Fetisov, Viktor) 260–1
Richard, John 36
Richards, Ellen 169

Richardson, William 29
ritual 141, 142, 143–4, 154, 231–2
Roberts, Mary Louise 87
Romaniello, Matthew 51, 103, 104, 145
romantic nationalism 5
Romeo and Juliet (Shakespeare, William) 204
Rondeau, Claudius 31
Rosenfeld, Sophia 123
Rousseau, Jean-Jacques 14
Ruane, Christine 105–6
Ruban, Mariia 254
Rubner, Max 168
Rudy, Jarrett 106
Russia, encounters with 2
Russia: Or A Compleat Historical Account of All of the Nations which Compose that Empire (Georgi, Johann Gottlieb) 26–9
Russian Academy of Sciences 26
Russian Orthodoxy 246–8 *see also* religion
Russian Society of the Red Cross 121
Russolo, Luigi 122, 124
rye bread 51–3, 57, 58

St. Petersburg 10, 30, 71*f*
  artifice and 71–5, 86
  city center 68–9
  cosmopolitanism and 68, 71–2
  gender and 78–82, 84
  Gorokhovaia Street 72
  Gostinyi Dvor 73–6, 77
  Haymarket Square 71*f*, 72–3
  lighting and 75–6, 86
  markets 67–8, 69, 71*f*, 72–4, 76
  marriage and 78–80
  Nevsky Prospekt 67, 68, 70, 71–2, 74–5, 80–4, 86
  newspapers and 76, 77–81, 83–5
  panoramic literature and 68–9, 71–3
  Passazh 10–11, 67, 70, 75–7, 79–84, 85–6
  police and 82–3
  sex trade 70, 78–87
  shopping and 10–11, 67, 70, 71–5
  society and 68, 69–72, 74–8

Samoyeds 26
sausages 175–6, 175*f*, 177–8, 180, 182
Scarry, Elaine 245
School 21 259
Schrader, Abby 10–11
science 5
  deafness and 205
  food and 171–2
scientific-technological revolution 205
scurvy 23, 26
seafood 180
Second World War 13–14, 221 *see also* Red Army
  comradeship 230–2
  death and 231–2
  effect of danger and 229
  feelings and 243–4
  food and 174–5
  gender and 232–4, 243–4, 250 *see also* Kosmodemianskaia, Zoia
  identity and 225–6, 233
  literature and 250–2
  martyrs *see* martyrdom
  medics and 232
  memoirs and 220
  national sacrifice and 220–1, 227 *see also* martyrdom
  newspaper correspondents and 223–4
  pen pal program and 234
  propaganda and 220–1, 226–7, 229–30, 232, 234, 235–6, 253–5
  radio and 255
  smell and 221–2
  soldiers' experiences 223–4
  sound and 225, 228, 252–3, 255
  taste and 231, 234
  touch and 229, 230, 231–2
  violence and 224–8, 248
  vision and 222, 225, 228–9, 231, 232–4
Semina, Khristina 125, 131
sensory theory 99
Seremetakis, C. Nadia 259, 262
Seventh Companion, The (German, Aleksei, Sr.) 269
sex trade 70, 78–87

Shaternikov, Mikhail 168
Shaw, Claire 124, 157
shchi 58
Shishkin, Nikolai 124
Shmatkov, A. S. 257
shopping 87 *see also* consumerism; markets
   malls 10–11, 67, 70, 74
   Passazh 10–11, 67, 70, 75–7, 79–84, 85–6
   St. Petersburg and 10–11, 67, 70, 71–5
sight *see* visual perception
sign language 194, 196, 197–8, 199f, 200–5, 206–7, 209, 210–11
silence 195, 201–2, 256
simple sign language 203–5
sirens 1
sites of memory 6, 14
slavery 108
smell 1–2, 11, 99, 267
   cinema and 267–9, 270–3, 275–81
   confinement and 14–15
   historiography 99, 100
   kumyshka and 143, 147
   memory and 267–9, 280
   putrefaction and 47, 49
   tobacco and 99, 102, 104–5
   trenches and 1
   war and 126–7, 221–2
   winter and 15
Smirnov, Ivan 254
Smith, Alison 38, 100, 104, 141, 143, 145, 167, 168
Smith, Mark M. 98, 99, 119, 193, 220, 221, 257
social engineering 9–13
   democratic social engineering 173–4
   taste and 167–71, 173–5, 177–9, 181–3
social history 119
society 77
   deafness and 196, 196, 199–200, 209
   speech and 196
   urban life and 68, 69–72, 74–8
Sokolovskii, A. 52
sound *see also* deafness; hearing

identity and 193
   Kosmodemianskaia, Zoia and 256, 262
   war and 122–6, 225, 228, 252
sound studies 252, 255
sour cabbage 51–2, 55–7
Soviet identity 195, 197, 201, 211
Soviet ideology 126–7
Soviet People's Commissariat of Nationalities 156
Soviet propaganda 247
   cinema and 272
   Kosmodemianskaia, Zoia and 247f, 248, 253–5, 258
   war and 220–1, 226–7, 229–30, 232, 234, 235–6
Soviet regime 11–14
   kumyshka and 154–6
Soviet Union 196
   cinema and *see* German, Aleksei, Sr.
soy 171–2
speech 193–8, 200, 203–4, 206–7, 210
   acquisition of 207
   theatre and 209
Spiridonov, Petr 201
Sprenzhin, Kornilii 147–8
Stakhanovism 220, 227
Stalin, Joseph 170, 175, 200, 255, 274
   death of 277, 278–80
Stalinism, cinema and *see* German, Aleksei, Sr.
Starks, Tricia 168
state control 144–5
   food and 167–9, 179–80
   kumyshka and 145, 149–56
   taste and 167–71, 173–5, 177–9, 181–3
   Udmurts and 145, 149–54, 155–6
   war and 220–1
statist nationalism 5
Stellar, Georg Wilhelm 26
Stenbock-Fermor, Iakov I. Essen- 67, 75–6
Stepanova, Vanda 133
Sterne, Jonathan 252, 255
Stevens, Scott Manning 24
Stites, Richard 254–5
Stoff, Laurie 222, 252
Stolpianskii, Peter Nikolaevich 73

Stone, Helena 155
Story of a Son (Koshevaia, Elena) 248–9
Strunnikov, Sergei 244f, 245, 248, 250, 251
sukharki 131
Sungarin, V. 201
Svetlov, Mikhail 261
Sweet Dishes without Sugar 175

"Tania (The Feat of Zoia Kosmodemianskaia)" (Kukryniksy) 256, 257
taste 45, 97 *see also* food; tobacco
   backwardness and 58
   bad tastes 48–9, 59
   cheese and 50
   cinema and 279
   class and 141
   culture and 58–9
   engineering 167–71, 173–5, 177–9, 181–3
   fermentation and 46–7, 51–7
   game and 47, 49–51
   historiography 99–100
   kumyshka and 142–3, 157
   morality and 168–9
   national identity and 141–2, 167–8
   rotten food and 48–9
   sour 51–9, 142
   soy and 172
   state control and 167–71, 173–5, 177–9, 181–3
   technology and 171
   tobacco and 97–104
   war and 130–3, 231, 234
   water and 45, 48
   yeast 172
technology 5, 13 *see also* radio
theatre 201–2, 204, 205, 209–10
   radio and 255
Theatre of Sign and Gesture (TMZh) 201, 204, 209–10
Thurstan, Violetta 132, 135–6
Timofeevna, Liubov 253–4
tobacco 8–9, 97–8
   advertising and 106–10, 107f, 109f
   blends 97, 101–4, 111

Britain and 106
cigarettes 100–1, 102–3, 105, 110–11
class and 102, 105, 106
health and 100, 110
historiography and 99–100
manufacturing and 102–3, 110
other, and the 108–10, 109f
place and 101–2, 103–5, 106–8, 110–11
sauces and 103–5
smell and 99, 102, 104–5
varieties of 101
Tolstaia, Aleksandra 126, 128
Tolstoy, Leo 168
Tooke, William 37–8
totalitarianism 2
touch 24, 262 *see also* haptic images
   advertising and 108
   museums and 259
   sex trade and 81–2
   war and 127–30, 229, 230, 231–2
Trial on the Road (German, Aleksei, Sr.) 281 n.4
Tumarkin, Maria 247, 256
   "Productive Death: The Necropedagogy of a Young Soviet Hero" 243–4
Tungus 28–9
Twenty Years without War (German, Aleksei, Sr.) 269
Two, The (Bogin, Mikhail) 204
Tyrawley, Lord 32

Udmurts 141–3
   backwardness and 146–8, 150, 152, 153, 157, 158
   ethonography and 146–7
   kumyshka and 141–9, 150–4, 155–7
   media portrayal of 151–3
   Multan Case, the 147
   Soviet state and 155–7
   spiritual practices and 141, 142, 143–4, 145, 147, 149, 154
   state control and 145, 149–54, 155–6
   women 151, 155–6
umami 46–7

urban environment 102 *see also* city
USA *see* America
Usachev, Sergei 202

vegetarianism 182
Vereshchagin, G. E. 143
violence 224–6
Virgin Lands campaign 177
visual culture 118, 252
visual perception 209, 210–11, 246
    see also literature; photography
  haptic images 268
  Kosmodemianskaia, Zoia and 244*f*, 245, 246*f*, 247*f*, 248, 249*f*, 250, 256–7
  museums and 259
  war and 118, 222, 225, 228–9, 231, 232–4
VOG (*Vserossiiskoe obshchestvo glukhikh*, All Russian Society of the Deaf) 194, 197, 202
VOG Studio of Fine and Applied Arts 201
Voit, Carl 168
Volgograd 260
Vygotskii, Lev Semenovich 196–7

war 13–15, 119–20, 128–9, 220 *see also* First World War; Second World War; wartime nursing
  enemy, and the 227–8
  gender and 128–9, 133, 232–4, 250 *see also* Kosmodemianskaia, Zoia
  hallucinations and 120, 133–5
  images of 244*f*, 245, 246*f*, 247*f*, 248
  skills and 228–30
  smell and 126–7, 221–2
  sound and 122–6, 225, 228, 252–3
  taste and 130–3, 231, 234
  touch and 127–30, 229, 230, 231–2
  vision and 118, 222, 225, 228–9, 231, 232–4
Warner, Marina 261

wartime nursing 117–18, 120–2, 135–6, 233
  hallucinations and 134–5
  propaganda and 232
  sight and 233
  smell and 126–7
  sound and 122–6
  taste and 131–3
  touch and 127–30
water 45
  health and 48
  mineral waters 48
  purity and 45
West, Sally 70, 106, 110
Western goods 11
Whitworth, Charles 30
"Who was Tania?" (Lidov, Petr) 248
Wiche, Cyril 43
Widdis, Emma 195
"Wild Boy of Aveyron" 207
Wiley, Harvey 168, 170
winter 15–15 *see also* cold
Winter, Jay 256
women 70, 78–85 *see also* Kosmodemianskaia, Zoia
  advertising and 107*f*, 108
  German army and 235
  kumyshka and 151, 155–6
  pronatalism 250
  Red Army and 232–4
  wartime nursing and 120–2, 128–30, 133

yeast 172
Yurchak, Aleksei 209

Zakharova, Lidiia 118–19, 120, 124, 127–8, 134
Zheliazevich, R. A.: *Passazh* 76
Zhuromskii, Evgenii 197
Zoia (Arnshtam, Lev) 254–5
Zoia: A Fairy Tale about Truth (Aliger, Margarita) 255
"Zoia: Poema" (Aliger, Margarita) 250